Radiology Without Tears

Radiology Without Tears

Mastering Radiology OSCEs

Satyendra Raghuwanshi, MD, DNB, MNAMS
Associate Professor
Department of Radiodiagnosis
AFMC Pune
Maharashtra, India

Sandeep Singh Awal, MBBS, MD (Gold Medalist), DNB, EDiR, DICR, FRCR
Consultant Radiologist
Bedford Hospital, Bedfordshire NHS Foundation Trust
United Kingdom

ELSEVIER

ELSEVIER

RELX India Private Limited
Registered Office: 818, Indraprakash Building, 8th Floor, 21, Barakhamba Road, New Delhi-110001
Corporate Office: 14th Floor, Building No. 10B, DLF Cyber City, Phase II, Gurgaon-122 002, Haryana, India

Radiology Without Tears: Mastering Radiology OSCEs, Satyendra Raghuwanshi and Sandeep Singh Awal

Publisher's note: Elsevier takes a neutral position with respect to territorial disputes or jurisdictional claims in its published content, including in maps and institutional affiliations.

ISBN: 978-81-312-6939-8
e-Book ISBN: 978-81-312-6940-4

Notice

Practitioners and researchers must always rely on their own experience and knowledge in evaluating and using any information, methods, compounds or experiments described herein. Because of rapid advances in the medical sciences, in particular, independent verification of diagnoses and drug dosages should be made. To the fullest extent of the law, no responsibility is assumed by Elsevier, authors, editors or contributors in relation to the adaptation or for any injury and/or damage to persons or property as a matter of products liability, negligence or otherwise, or from any use or operation of any methods, products, instructions, or ideas contained in the material herein.

Content Strategist: Mrinalini Bakshi
Content Project Manager: Tapajyoti Chaudhuri
Sr Cover Designer: Gopalakrishnan Venkatraman
Sr Production Executive: Dhan Singh

Printed in India by Rajkamal Electric Press, Kundli, Haryana.

Do or do not. There is no try.

—Yoda (*Star Wars—The Empire Strikes Back*)

CONTENTS

FOREWORD

It is with great pleasure and a deep sense of professional pride that I introduce this indispensable radiology examination 'help book' on radiology OSCE. In the dynamic and ever-evolving field of medical imaging, mastery of the nuances of radiology is not only a requisite for success in the examinations but also a cornerstone of providing exceptional patient care.

This meticulously crafted textbook is a testament to the dedication and expertise of its authors, who have distilled their vast knowledge and practical insights into a comprehensive resource tailored specifically for those preparing for radiology examinations. The challenges inherent in mastering the intricacies of this discipline are manifold, and this book serves as a beacon, guiding learners through the complexities of radiology OSCEs with precision and clarity.

The structure of the content is thoughtfully designed to provide a systematic and in-depth exploration of radiological principles. From foundational concepts to advanced imaging modalities, each chapter unfolds with a focus on clarity and relevance. The integration of previously asked questions enhances the practical applicability of the knowledge, bridging the gap between theory and the demands of applicability in examinations and clinical practice.

To the authors, I extend my sincere appreciation for their dedication to the educational advancement of our field. Aspiring radiologists as well as seasoned practitioners alike will find this book to be an invaluable companion in their pursuit of excellence. Its relevance extends beyond examination preparation, serving as a lifelong reference for continuous professional growth.

In conclusion, I commend the authors for their commitment to elevating the standards of radiological education. May this exam-oriented help book empower and inspire radiology residents to not only succeed in their DMRD/MD/DNB/EDiR/FRCR examinations but also excel in their noble mission of contributing to the well-being of those under their care. I am sure that this book will act as a platform for radiology residents to enhance their knowledge and perform well in the examinations.

Dr Bhupinder Kaur Anand
Vice Chancellor
Al-Falah University
Faridabad (Haryana), India

PREFACE

OSCE and spotters are an indispensable part of every radiology examination worldwide. Although the spectrum of diseases in any examination can be vast and challenging, the commonly asked pathologies are limited and follow a fairly predictable pattern. Despite this fact, students often perform poorly in this segment of the radiology practical examination. The basic reason is the lack of lucid, authentic and credible study material which can offer a one-stop solution to this facet of final radiology examinations. The authors have been witness to innumerable DNB and MD examinations and have observed hundreds of students getting nervous and performing poorly. There was an imperative need to develop comprehensive yet lucid study material for radiology residents so that they could pass out with flying colours in the examinations without having to shed their precious tears. This help book is designed in the most simplistic manner. The questions asked are targeted and therefore a crisp and accurate answer is expected from the candidate within the constraints of time.

Although it has taken more than 2 years to complete this book with the aim of making it credible and flawless; however, there is always scope for improvement in any work and we would be greatly obliged to suggestions and comments from learned teachers and students.

We wish you all the best in examinations and life!

Dr Satyendra Raghuwanshi
Dr Sandeep Singh Awal

ACKNOWLEDGEMENTS

The completion of this book represents the culmination of extensive effort and collaboration; it would be undeniable to express our gratitude to our parents and the infinite existence which makes us what we are.

We are sincerely appreciative of all the listed contributors for their significant contributions towards the completion of this book. Their meticulous attention to detail and profound understanding of the subject have greatly enriched the narrative. Our seniors Dr A. K. Singh, Dr P. Dhagat, Dr Ravinder Sahdev, Dr S. A. Raheem, Dr Bharat Hosur and Dr Amit Bajpai for their teachings and our colleagues Dr Ashok Narayan, Dr Nipun Rajgarhia, Dr Reshma J., Dr Akshay Kurumilla and Dr Saurabh Mishra for their steadfast support.

Special acknowledgement is reserved for Sudeep Singh Awal for providing technical expertise and enriching the book with beautiful illustrations.

To my family, whose enduring support has been a constant source of strength, I offer my deepest thanks. Your unwavering belief in my pursuits has been a motivating force, and I am truly appreciative of your encouragement.

Lastly, to the discerning readers who will engage with this work, I sincerely hope it proves to be a valuable and insightful resource. Your pursuit of knowledge fuels the scholarly endeavours of authors, and I am honoured to contribute to this intellectual discourse.

A pictorial list of contributors has been attached as a mark of our gratitude for their commitment towards enhancing radiology education. Thank you all for your meaningful contributions to this endeavour.

For images, we are thankful to:

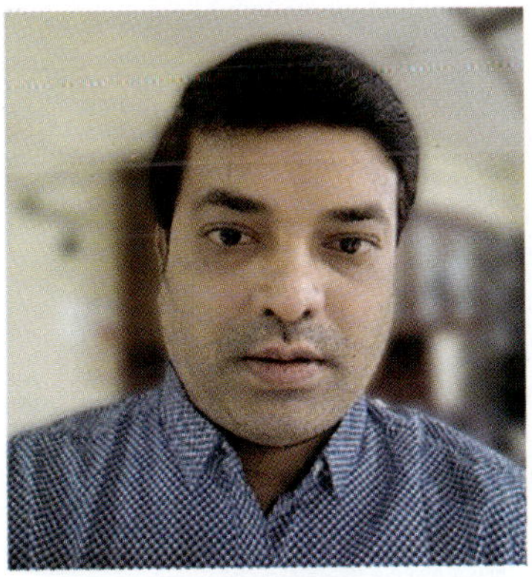

Dr Siripuram Naveen Kumar, MBBS, MD (Professor and HOD of Radiodiagnosis, CAIMS, Karimnagar and IRIA General Secretary, Karimnagar, Telangana, India)

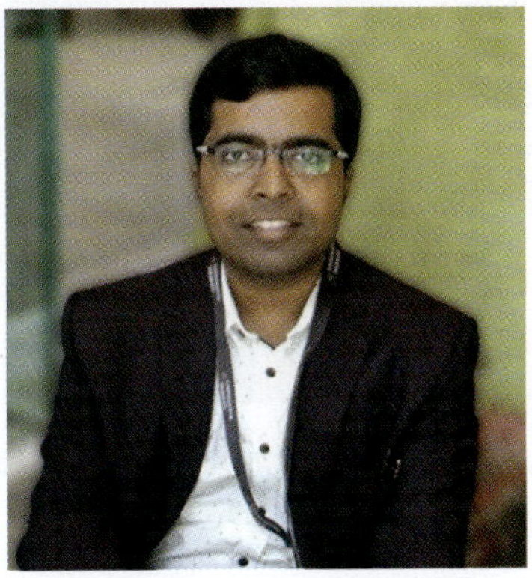

Dr Sanjay P. Yadav, MBBS, MDRD (Associate Professor, Mysore Medical College & Research Institute, Karnataka, India)

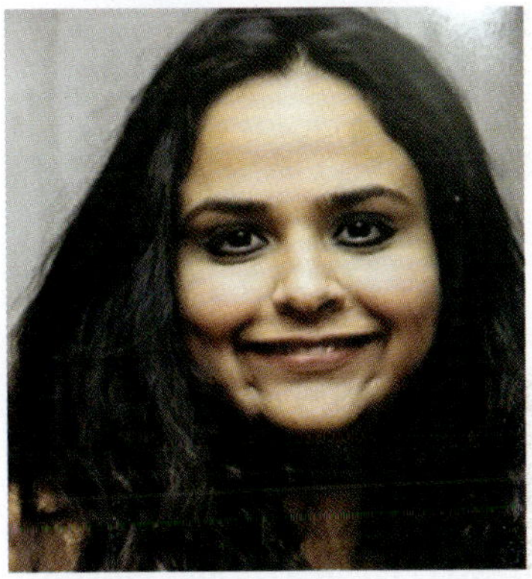

Dr Smita Nitin Borale, MBBS, MD, DMRE, FRCR, Fellowship in Body Imaging (Senior Consultant Teleradiologist)

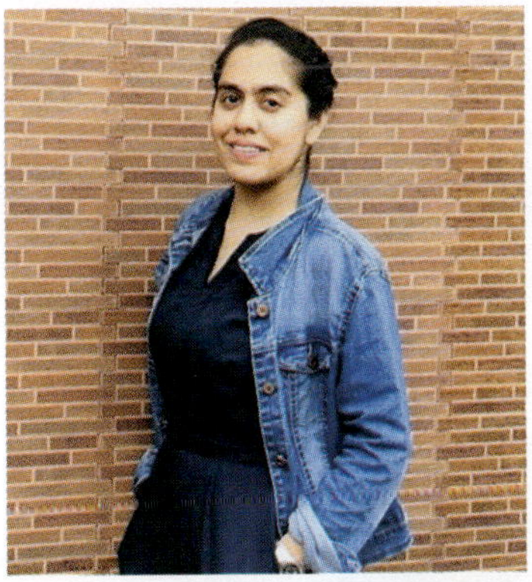

Dr Jamanjit Kaur Sidhu, MBBS, MD, FRCR (Fortis Escorts Hospital, Amritsar, India)

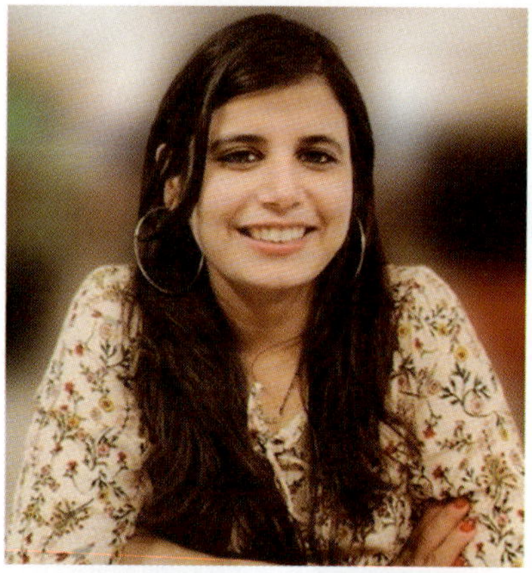

Dr Sajal Agarwal, MBBS, DMRD (Secondary DNB Resident, Fortis Hospital Noida, India)

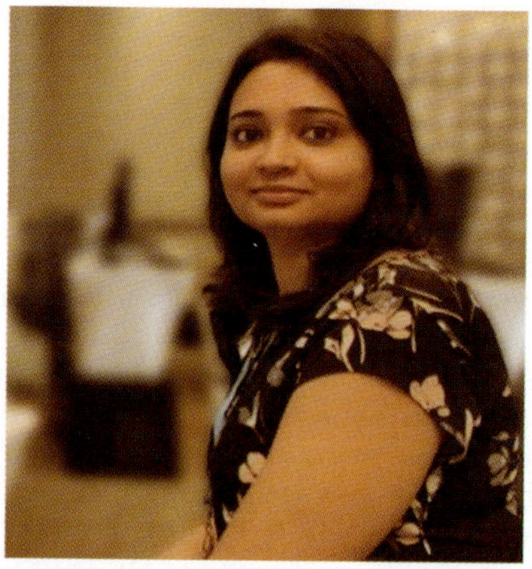

Dr Niharika Prasad, MBBS, MD, FRCR (Senior Consultant Teleradiologist)

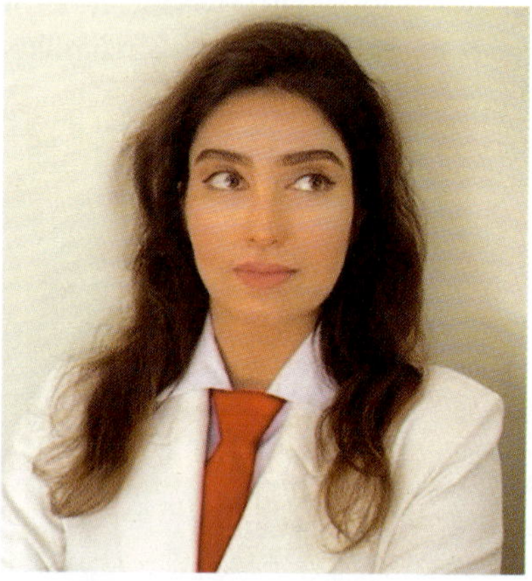

Dr Ramesh Giti, MD (Javad Al-Amee Hospital and Radiology and Sonography Clinic of Dr Giti, Kharameh, Fars, Iran)

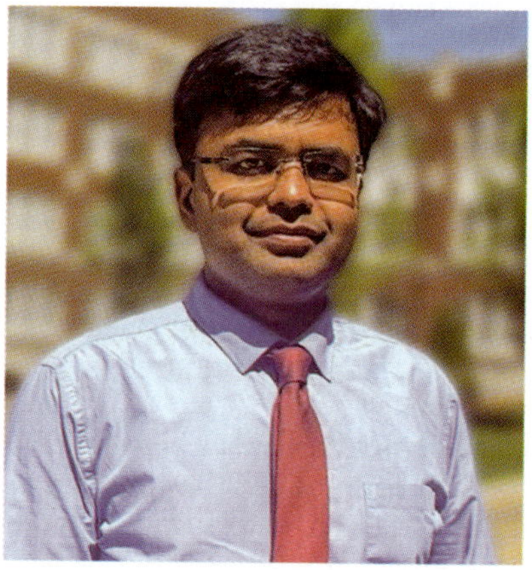

Dr Som Biswas, MBBS, MS, MD, DNB, DMRD, FPM, DCR, MBA, Fellowship in Pediatric Radiology (The University of Tennessee Health Science Centre [UTHSC])

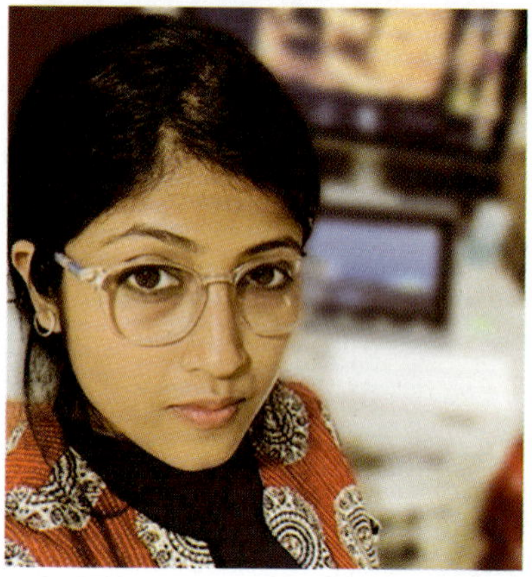

Dr Shramana Bagchi, MBBS, DNB, Fellowship in Pediatric Radiology, Fellowship in Fetal Medicine

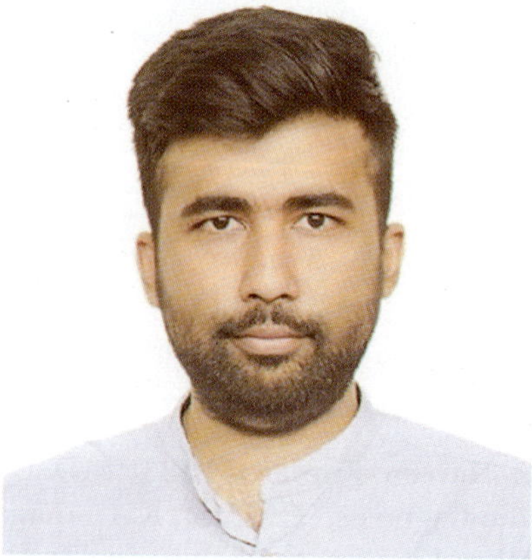

Dr Suhas C. M., MBBS, MD (Shivamogga Institute of Medical Sciences, Shivamogga, Karnataka, India)

OSCE

1

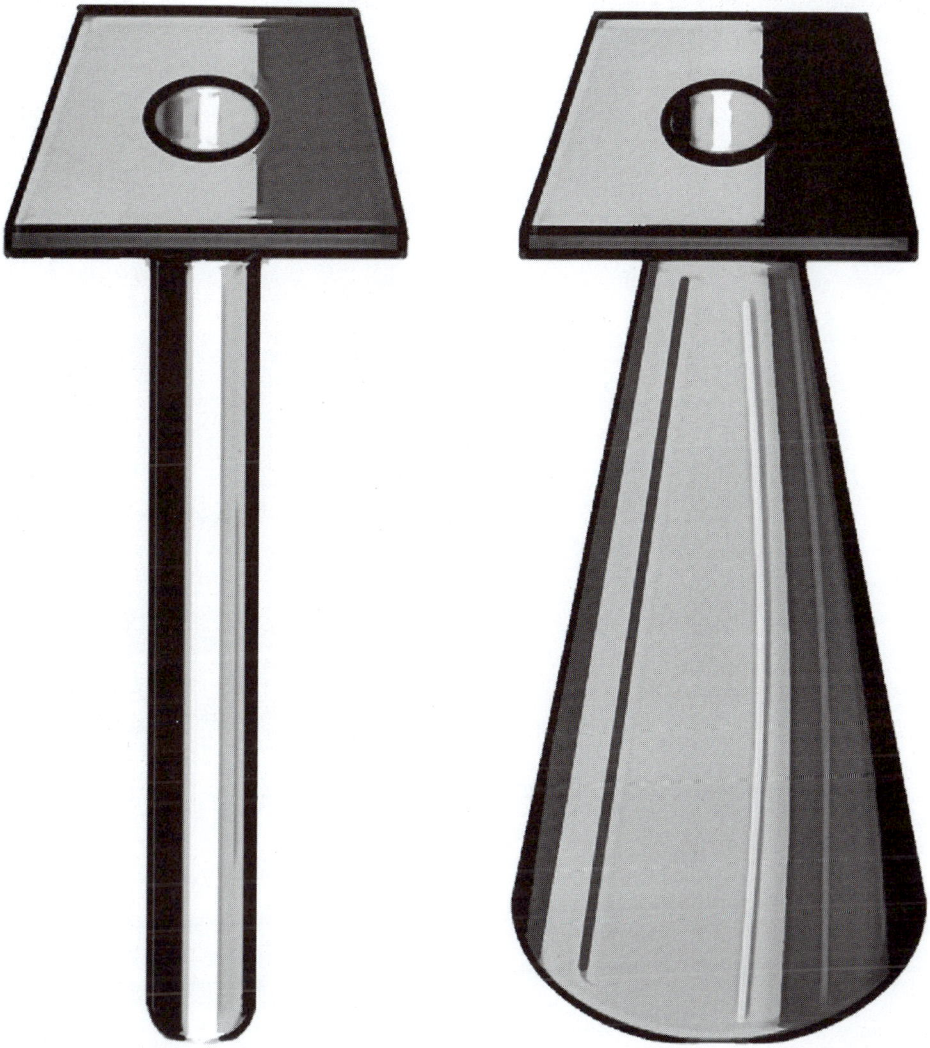

1. Identify the devices.
2. Into what broad category are these devices grouped.
3. Explain one use of each in radiology.
4. Name two other devices within the same group.

PART

A

Radiography and Physics

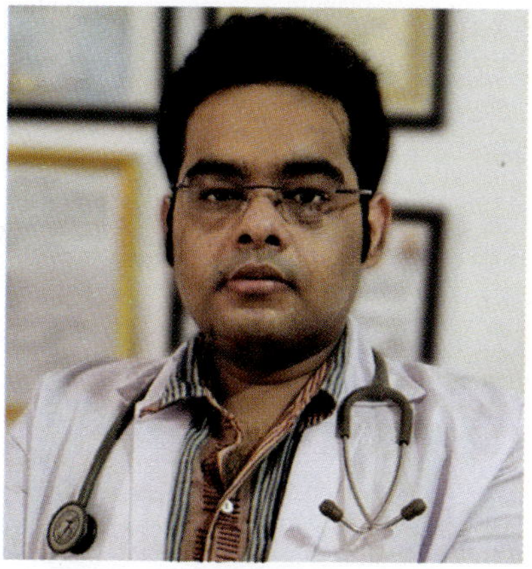

Dr Anish Choudhary, MBBS, MD, Fellow BISI (Delhi), Assistant Professor and HOD (Central Institute of Psychiatry, Ranchi)

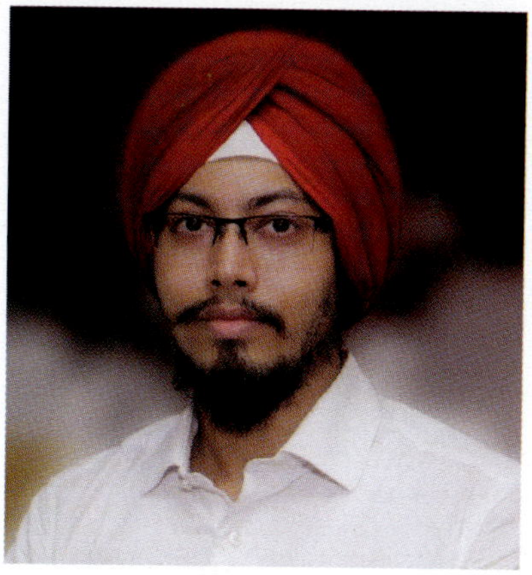

Sudeep Singh Awal – Illustrations (Mass Communication and Video Production, Karim City College, Jamshedpur, India)

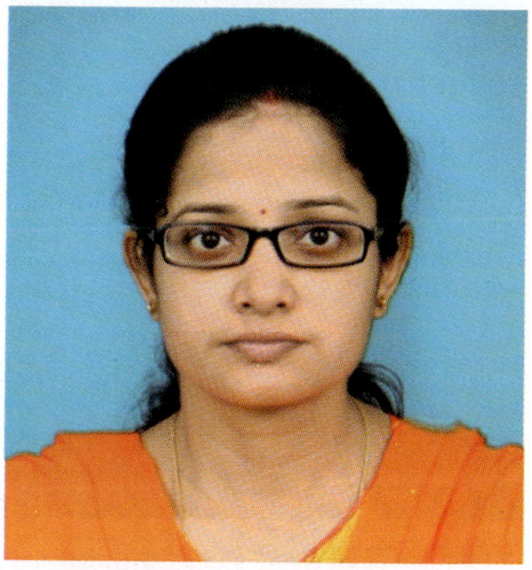

Dr Manisha Roy, MBBS, MS (MGM Medical College and Hospital, Jamshedpur, India)

Dr Satyendra Raghuwanshi

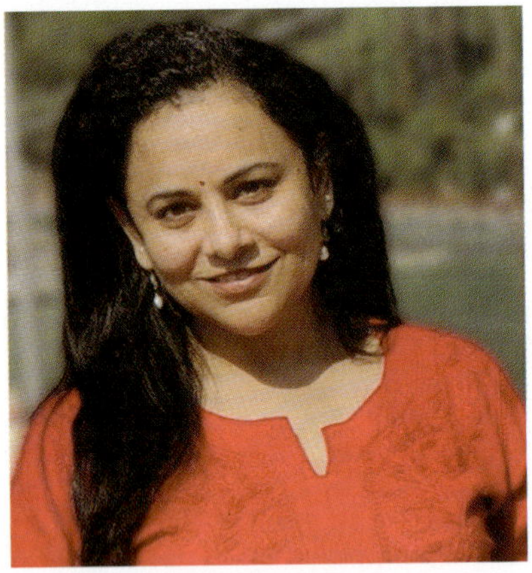

Dr Urvashi Priya Sinha, MBBS, MD, PGDMCH (Hill View Hospital, Discovery Diagnostics, Sharan's Diagnostics, Rad Shine, Jharkhand, India)

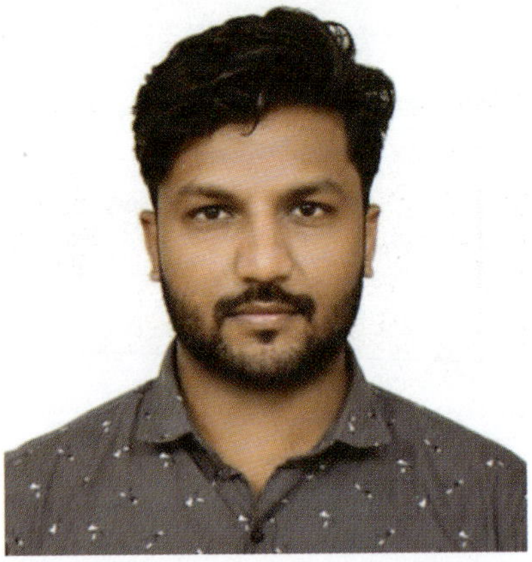

Dr Jaydip Sukhadiya, MBBS, MD (PDU Government Medical College, Rajkot, Gujarat, India)

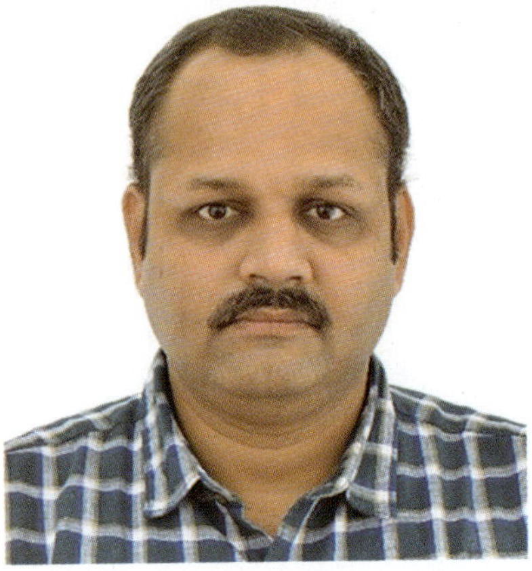

Dr Abanindu Thakur, MBBS, MD (Maldives)

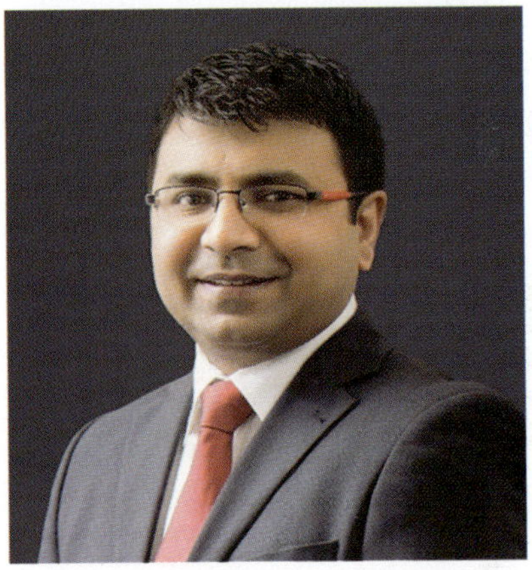

Dr Mitesh Kumar, MBBS, MD, FRCR, Fellowship in Neuroradiology (Singapore)

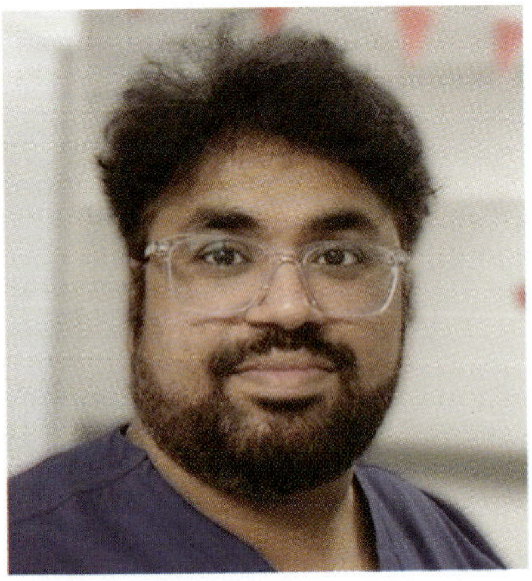

Dr Sateesh Kumar A., MBBS, MD, EdiR, DICR (King Hamad University Hospital, Bahrain)

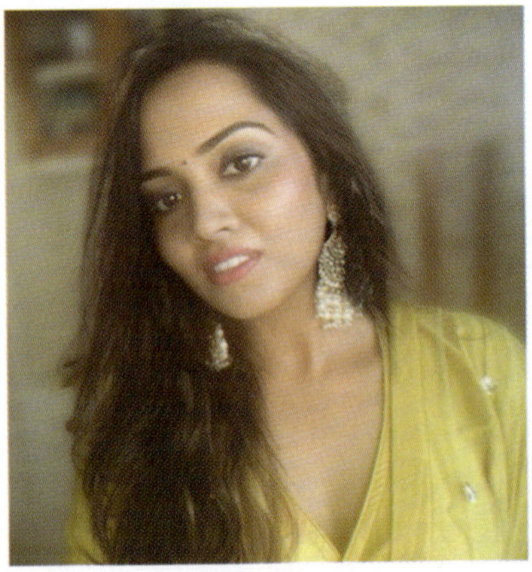

Dr V. Krishnaveni Pillai (Director and CEO, Medline Diagnostics, Trichy and Tanjore, India)

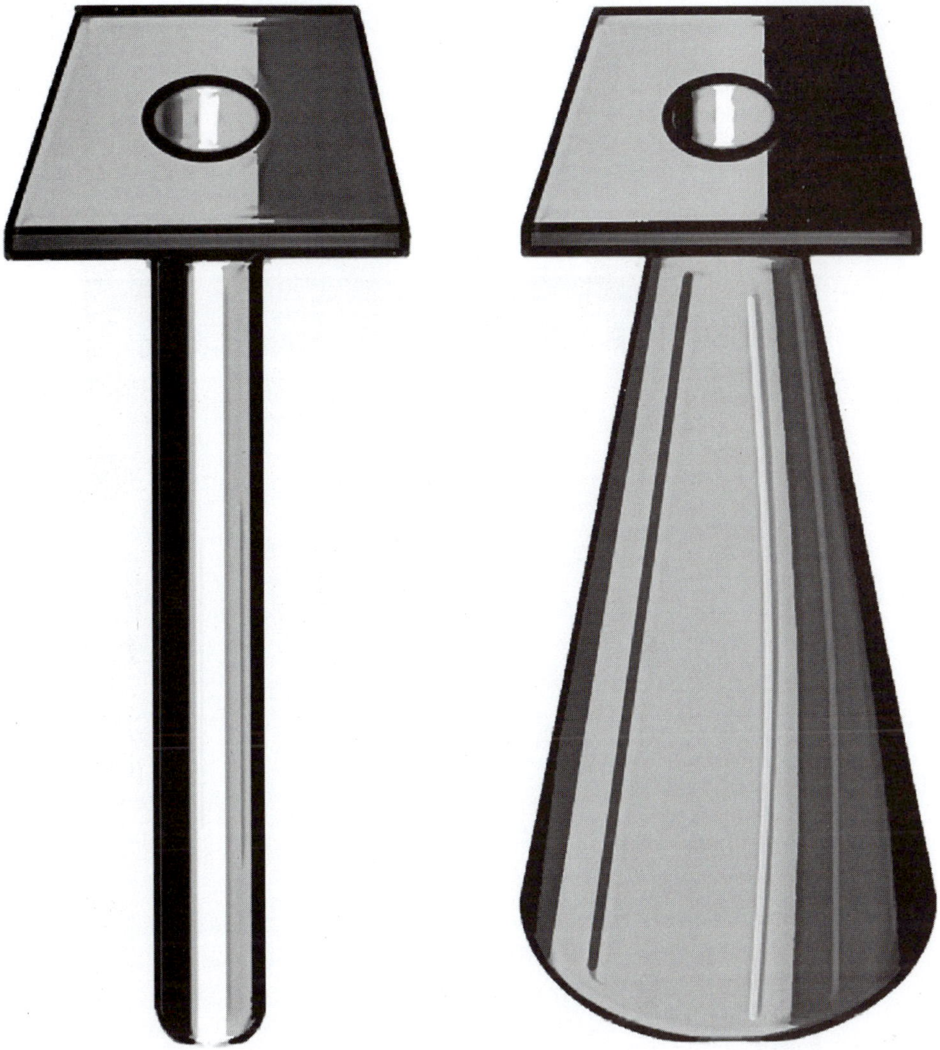

Cylinder and cone type of beam-restricting devices.

Beam-Restricting Devices

- These are beam-restricting devices utilized in radiography to limit the beam size and thereby reducing the scatter radiation. They are attached directly to the X-ray tube and confine the X-ray beam before it enters the body, hence limits the field of view (FOV). Limiting the beam reduces scatter and patient dose.
- They are useful for magnified and focussed view of sella turcica, mastoids, L5–S1, vertebrae and ankle.
- Other beam-restricting devices are as follows:
  1. Aperture diaphragm
  2. Cones and cylinders
  3. Collimators

OSCE

2

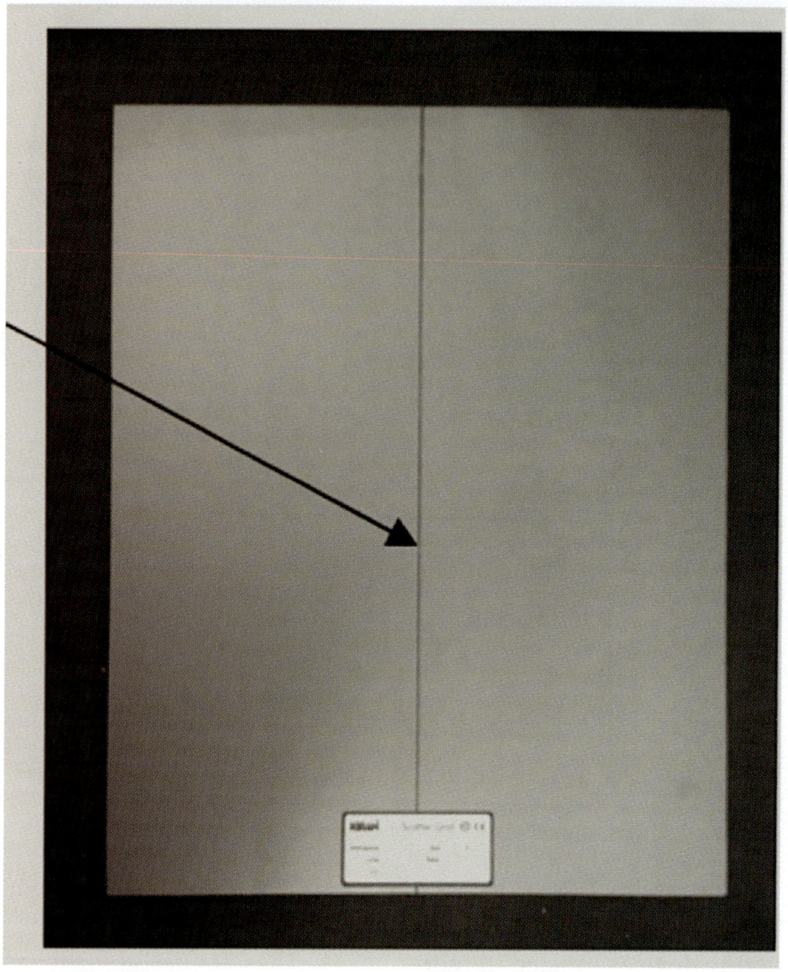

1. Identify the device.
2. What is grid frequency?
3. What does the central line indicate?
4. Write one advantage and disadvantage.

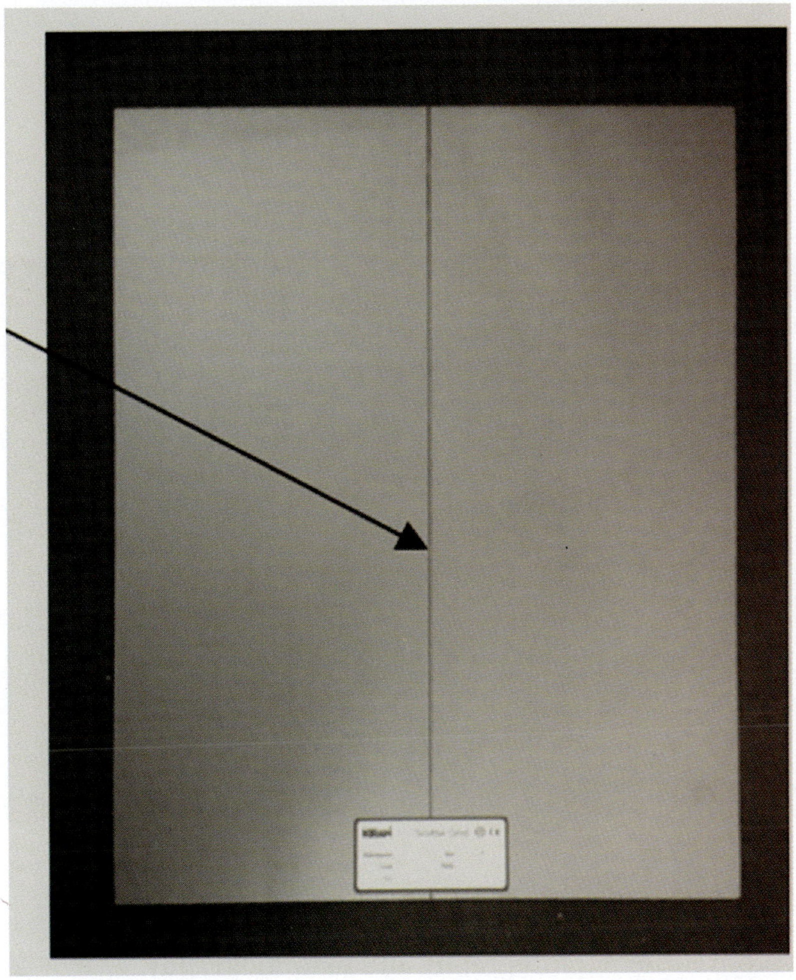

A radiographic grid with arrow at the central line.

Radiographic Grid

- This is a radiographic grid.
- Grid frequency is measured as lines per inch (LPI) and it is the number of lead strips per inch. Generally, the value is 103.
- The central line is the centre of the grid and centre of the cassette and centre of the X-ray beam should align with it. The long axis of the grid is always along the long axis of the table (see the arrows).
- **Advantage:** It reduces scatter radiation and improves image contrast.
- **Disadvantage:** Increased radiographic factors, hence increased patient dose. Also, they are prone for mechanical failure and grid artefacts.

OSCE 3

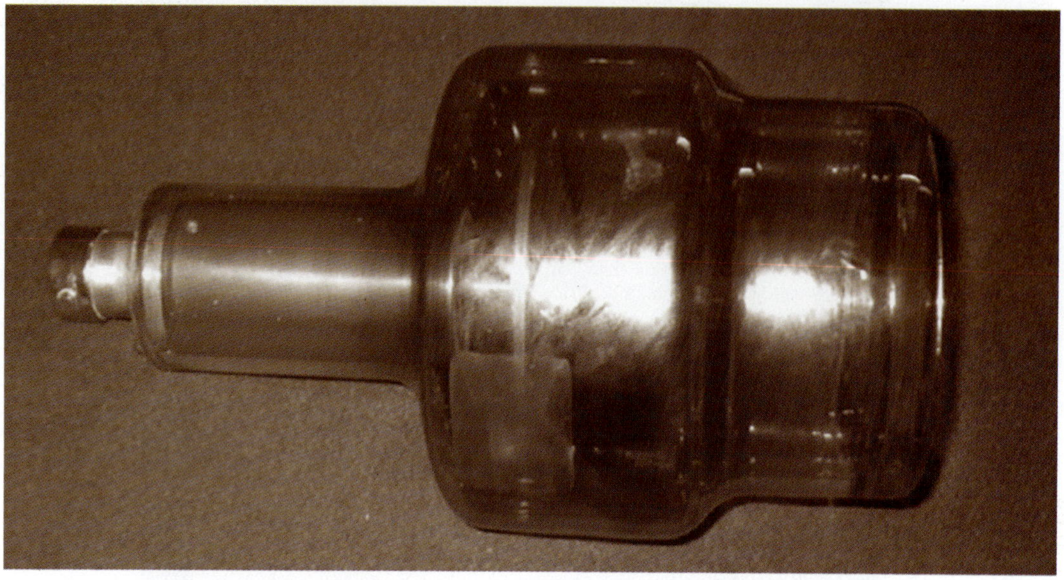

1. What materials are used for anode?
2. Size of focal spot in conventional radiography and mammography.
3. Atomic number of tungsten and barium.
4. Parameters for chest radiography in posteroanterior (PA) view.
5. Dosage of one chest radiograph PA view.
6. Operating kV range of general radiography and mammography.

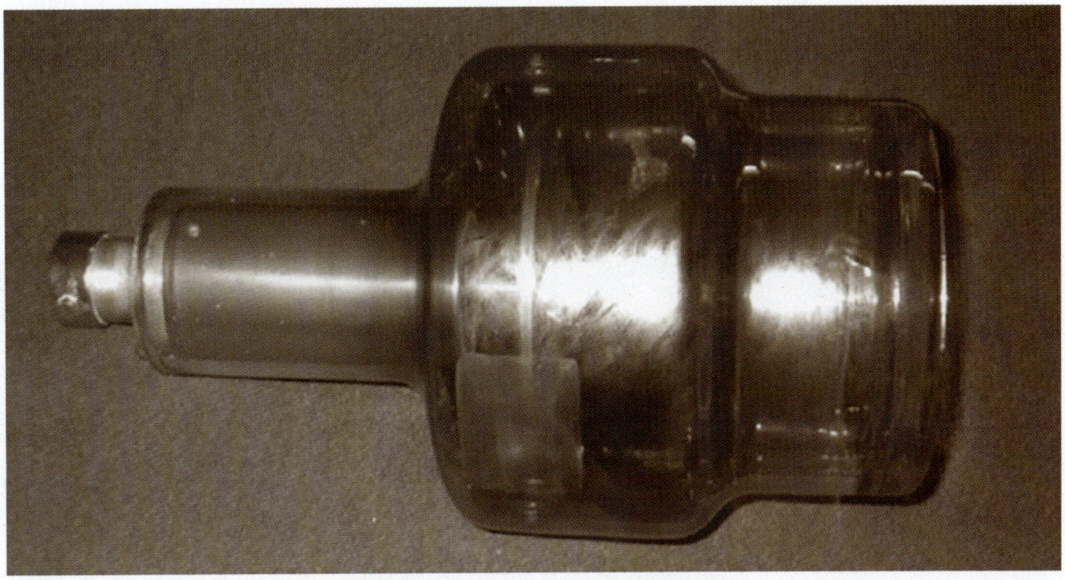

A rotating anode type of X-ray tube.

Rotating Anode Type of X-ray Tube

- Anode disc is made of tungsten-rhenium target track on a molybdenum core backed with graphite.
- Size of focal spot in conventional radiography and mammography: The focal spot sizes commonly employed are 1 and 1.2 mm, usually for general radiography, and 0.3–0.6 mm, usually for mammography.
- Atomic number of tungsten and barium is 74 and 56, respectively.
- Parameters for chest radiography in posteroanterior (PA) view:
  - 55–60 kVp
  - 15–20 mAs
  - SID = 180 cm (6 feet)
- Dosage of one chest radiograph PA view is 0.1 mSv for PA view.
- Operating kV range of general radiography and mammography is in the range of 60–150 kVp and 18–25 kVp, respectively.

OSCE 4

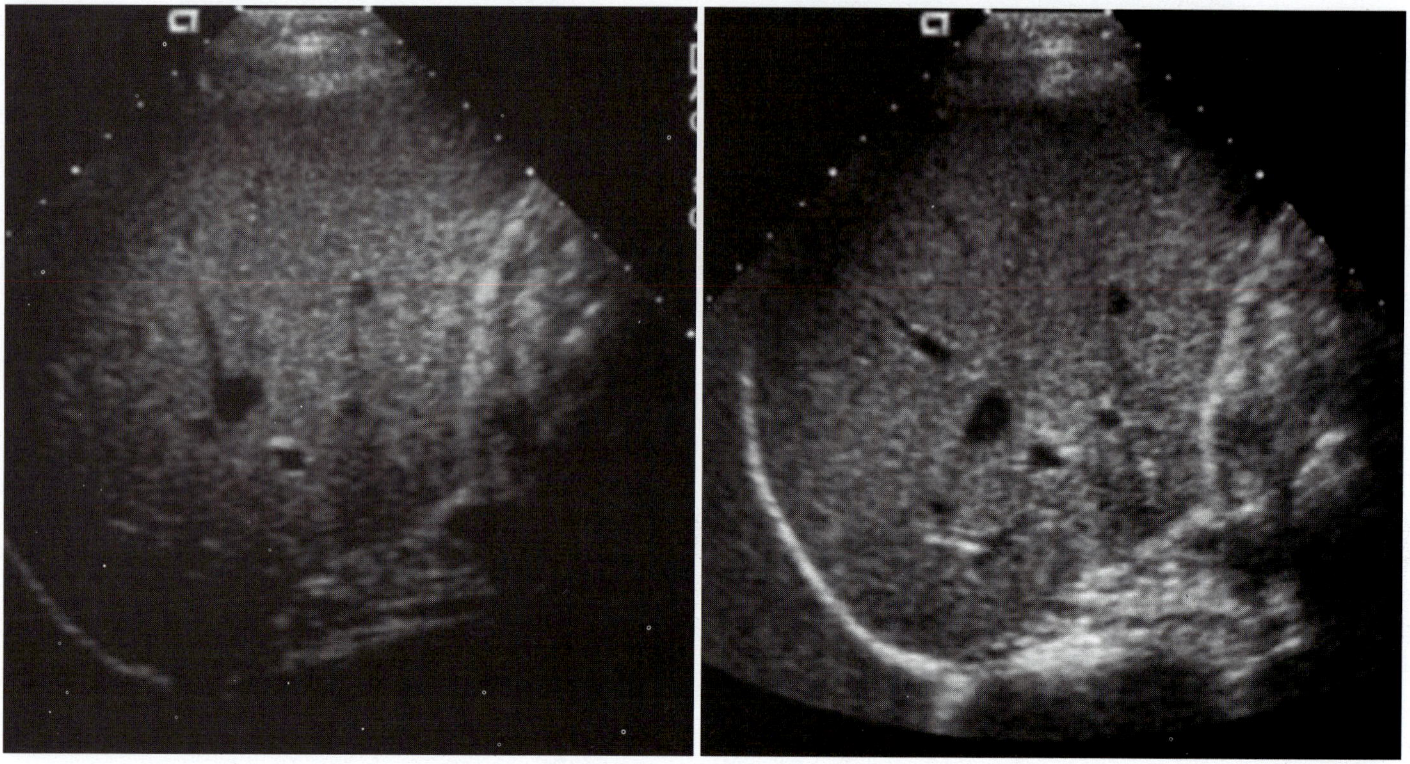

Two views of the liver.

1. **Why is the deep aspect of the liver so hypoechoic on the first image?**
2. **What is the difference between gain and power?**
3. **Should image brightness be controlled first with gain or with power?**
4. **Are gain and power preprocessing or postprocessing controls?**

USG Physics

Distance gain compensation/time gain compensation (TGC):

1. The distance gain compensation curve is inappropriately adjusted on the first image. Increased gain settings were applied to the far field on the second image, and the liver appears normal throughout.
2. Power refers to the strength of the sound pulse that is transmitted by the transducer. Gain refers to the amount of electronic amplification of the signal that returns to the transducer.
3. Increasing the power and the gain both result in brighter images; however, increased power causes greater patient acoustic exposure and can cause artefacts. Therefore, it is best to increase power only when an optimal image cannot be obtained first with adjustment of gain.
4. Preprocessing refers to controls that must be adjusted in real time while the patient is being scanned. Postprocessing refers to controls that can be adjusted on a frozen image. Gain and power are both preprocessing controls.

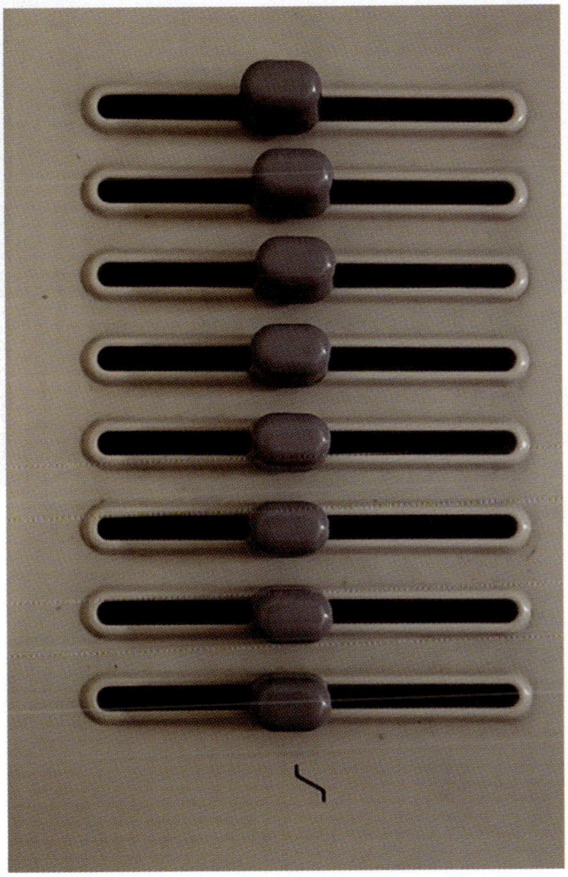

Incorrect time gain compensation settings

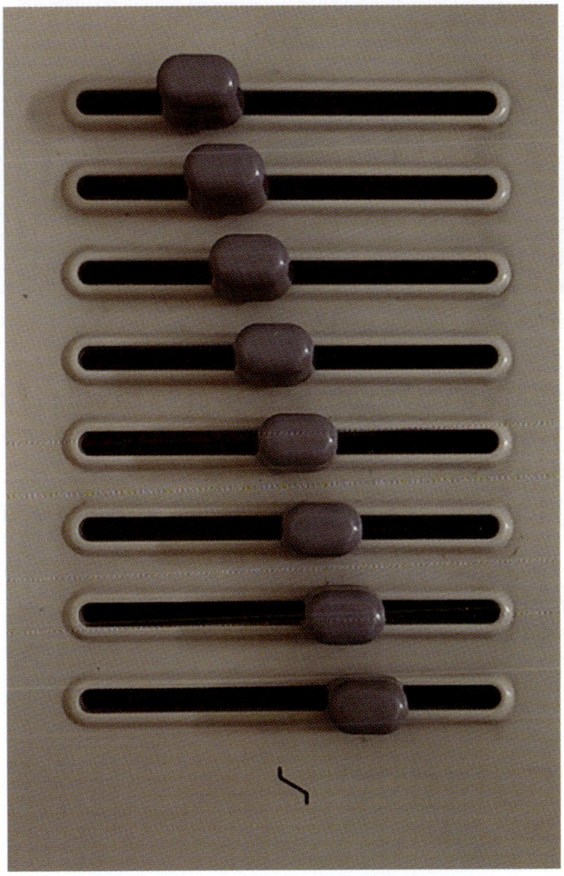

Optimal time gain compensation settings

OSCE 5

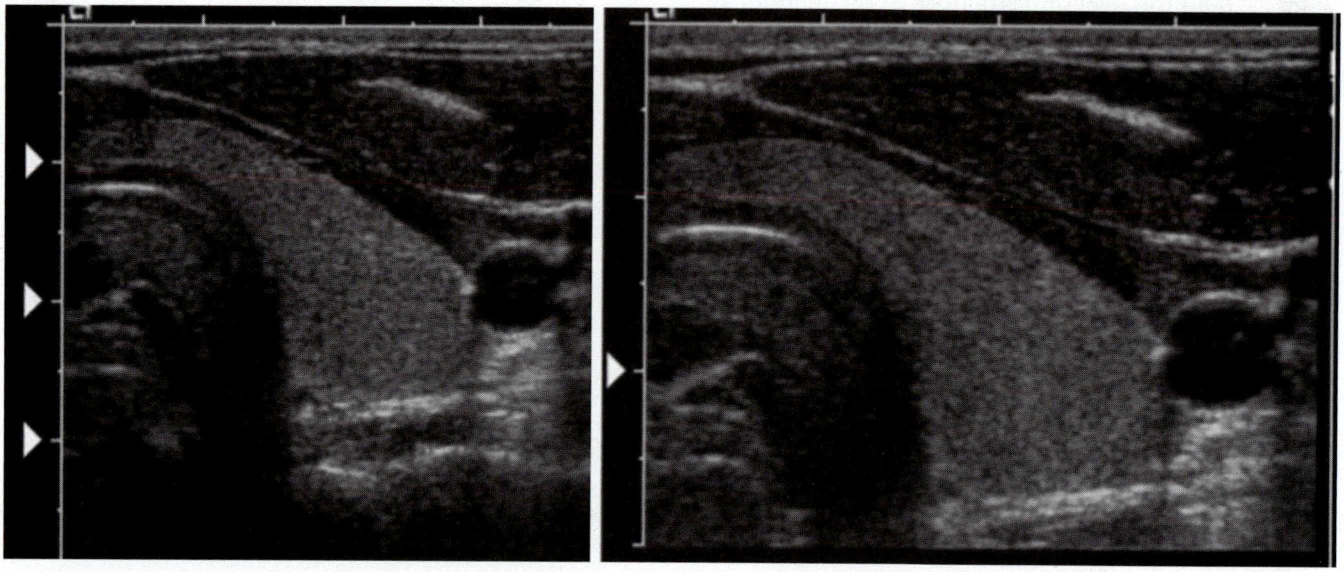

Two views of the thyroid gland ultrasonography.

1. **What do the arrowheads at the left side of the image indicate?**
2. **Which image would you expect to have the higher frame rate?**
3. **What can you do to improve the frame rate while performing real time scans?**
4. **What can you do to improve the resolution while performing real time scans?**

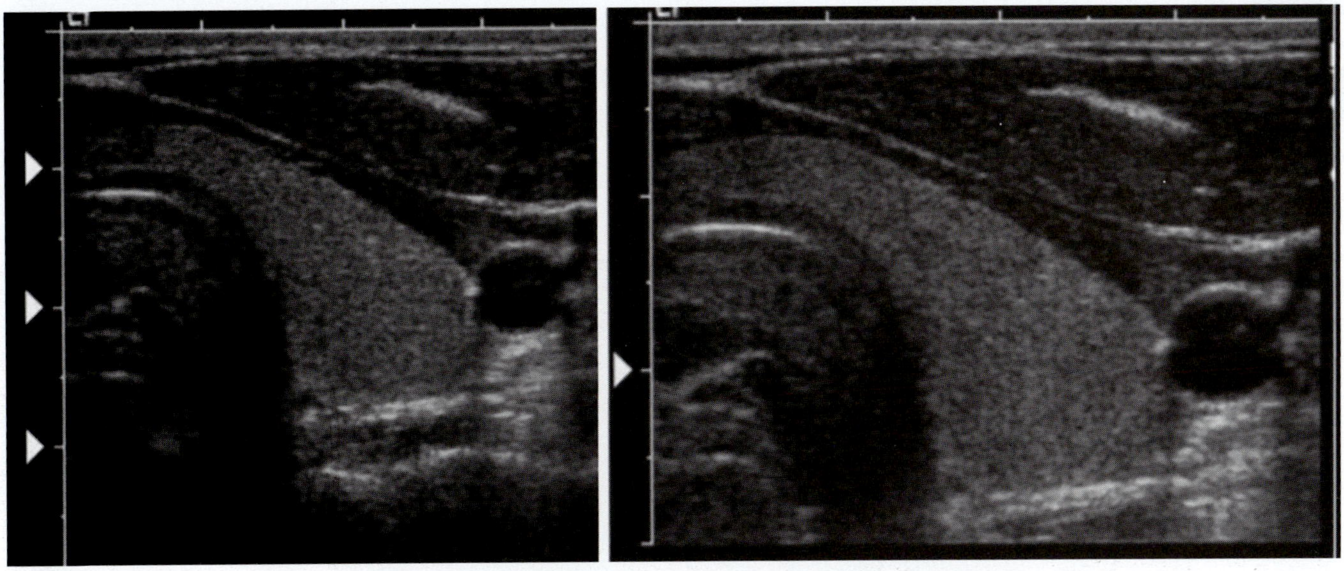

Frame rate and resolution.

ANSWERS:

1. The arrowheads indicate the levels at which the image is focused.
2. The second image, because the field of view (FOV) is smaller and there is only one focal zone.
3. Frame rate can be improved by decreasing the number of focal zones, decreasing the image depth, decreasing the sector width, decreasing the line density and turning off Doppler modes.
4. Resolution can be improved by using a higher frequency transducer, increasing the number of focal zones and increasing the line density.
   - Each ultrasound image is composed of multiple scan lines. The time required to create one frame of a real-time image is calculated by multiplying the speed of sound times the length of the scan lines times the number of lines per image times.
   - Multiplying by 2 is necessary because the sound has to make a round trip from the transducer to the target and back. The longer it takes to generate one frame, the lower the frame rate.
     - Typical frame rates range from 5 to 40 frames per second.
   - Increased frame rates can be obtained by decreasing the length of each scan line (less image depth) or decreasing the number of scan lines (less image width, narrower sector angles and lower line density).
   - In many respects, frame rate and image resolution are competing parameters. As shown in this case, each scan line can be electronically focused at a certain depth. To focus at multiple depths requires multiple pulses for each scan line.
     - In the first image shown in this case, pulses focused in the near field created the superficial aspect of the image, which was pasted to two different images obtained separately with midfield and far-field focusing. Therefore, the improved resolution throughout the FOV that comes with multiple focal zones results in a sacrifice in frame rate. It is also possible to improve resolution by moving the scan lines closer together. This is called increasing line density, and it also has an inverse relationship to frame rate.

OSCE

6

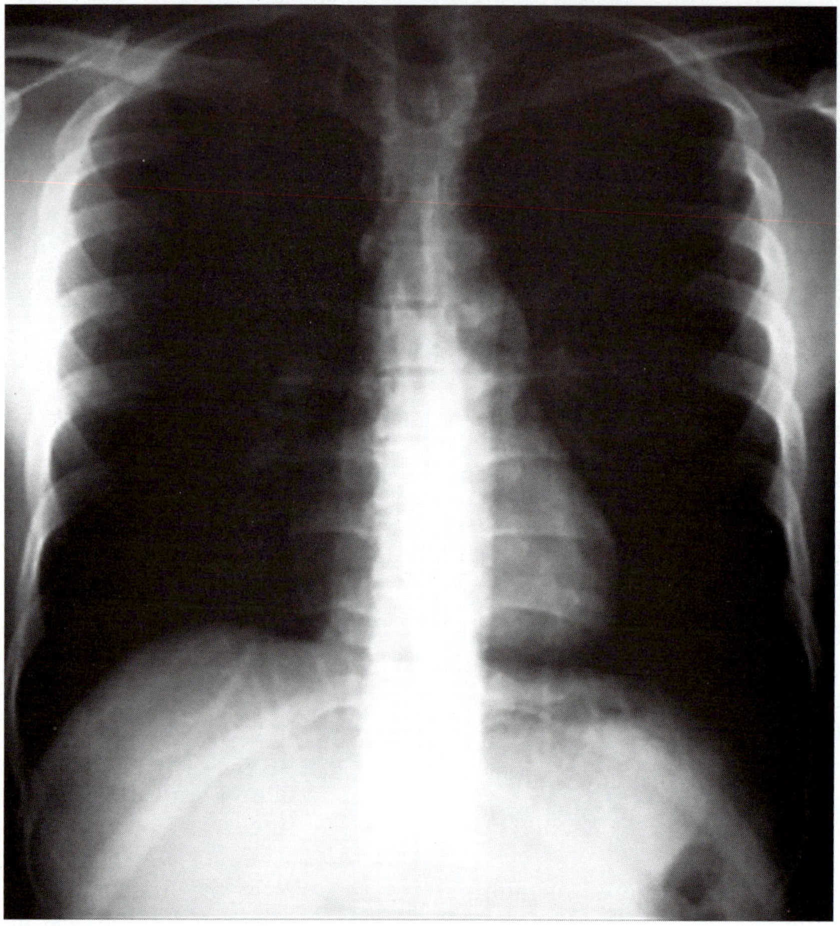

1. **Comment on the penetration of this radiograph.**
2. **What are the radiographic factors for chest posteroanterior (PA) view?**
3. **What is the effect of increasing mAs on patient dose?**
4. **What is the 15% rule?**

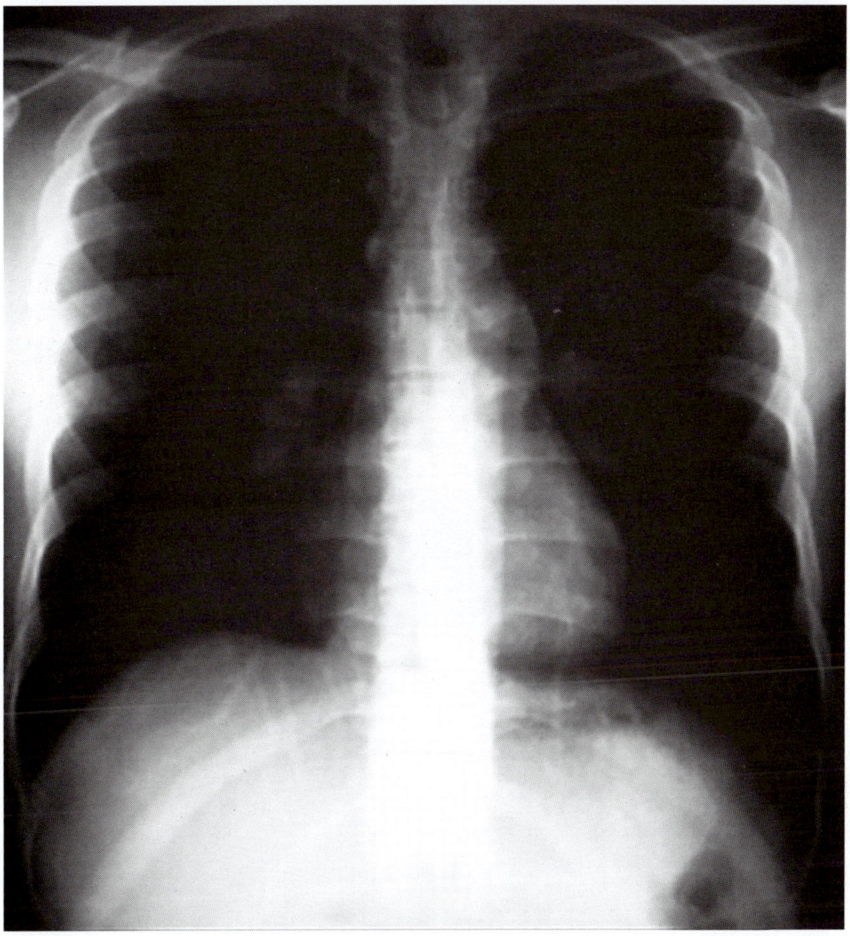

Over-Penetrated Chest Radiograph

- This is an over-penetrated chest radiograph.
- Radiographic factors for chest radiograph postero-anterior (PA) view are as follows:
  - kVp = 55–60
  - mAs = 15–20
- Increasing the mAs results in production of more X-rays and more radiation dose and film blackening. The mean energy of X-rays remains the same, as it depends on the kVp and not the mAs.
- Generally, a high kVp and low mAs technique is employed to limit the radiation dose to the patient. Higher kVp results in more free transmission; therefore, the patient is absorbing less of the dose. Increasing the kVp by 15% will double the density in the radiograph and reduce patient dose in comparison to doubling the mAs. Utilizing the 15% kVp rule provides diagnostic image of similar quality and not adding up to the dose.
- High kVp and very low mAs decrease the image contrast which can result in poor image quality. So, a balance needs to be maintained.
- kVp decides the penetrating power of X-rays.
  - A lower kVp will make the X-ray beam less penetrating.
  - It will result in a more substantial difference in attenuation between the different parts of the subject, leading to higher contrast.
  - A higher kVp will make the X-ray beam more penetrating. It will also result in less difference in attenuation between the different parts of the subject, leading to lower contrast.
  - A very low kVp will result in X-rays which may not even penetrate through the tissues and will not produce any image.

OSCE 7

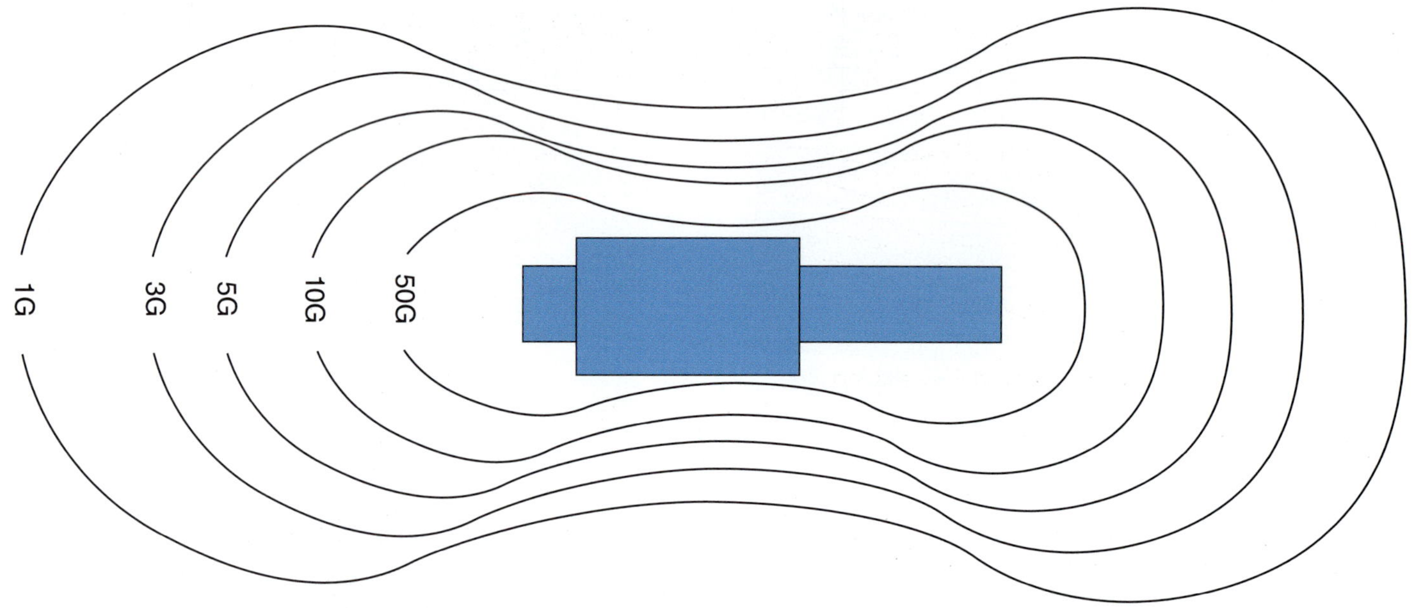

1. What are these lines called?
2. Up to which line, pacemaker can be affected?
3. Up to which field, computers may be affected?
4. Which strength of field can erase your credit card?

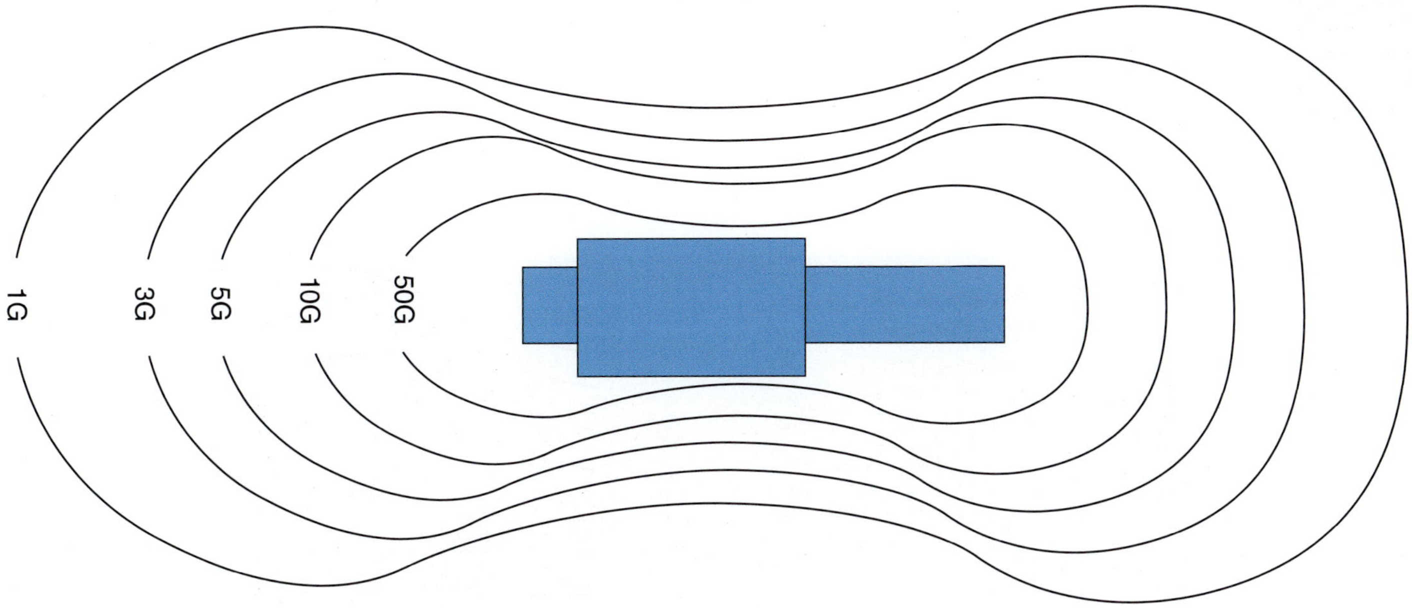

Fringe field lines around a magnet/magnetic resonance imaging (MRI).

Fringe Field Lines

- Fringe field lines are the peripheral magnetic field outside of the magnet core.
- They are important because it can cause interference with nearby electronic devices, such as pacemakers.
  - Up to which line. pace maker can be affected? 5 G line
- Up to which field. computers may be affected? 10 G line
- Which strength of field can erase your credit card? Fields of 30 G

OSCE

8

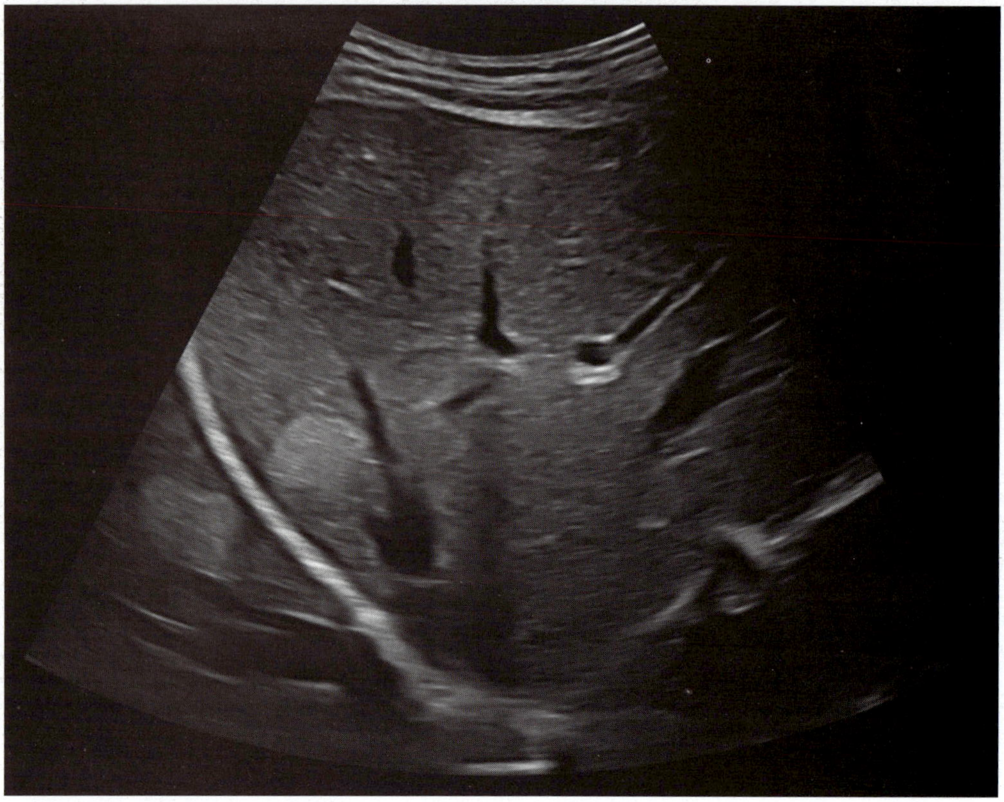

1. Identify the imaging modality and the organ scanned.
2. Which ultrasound artefact is demonstrated here?
3. How can you avoid this artefact?
4. Enumerate two useful ultrasound artefacts.

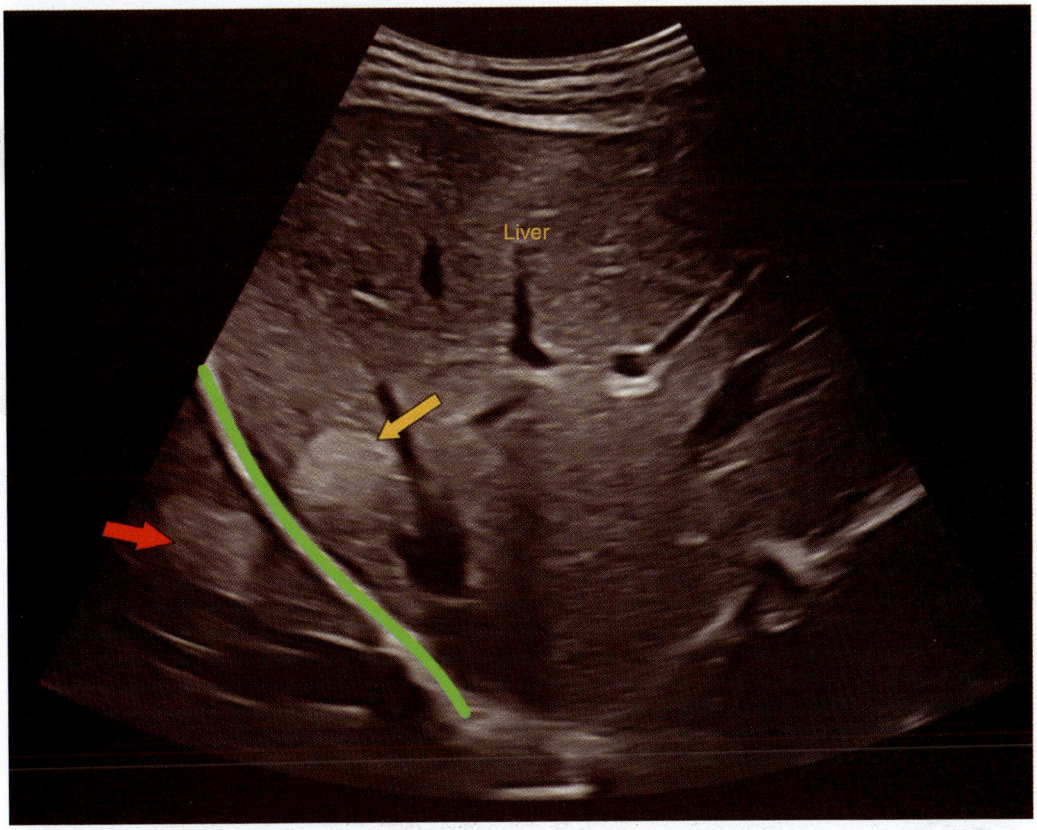

USG of the liver shows a hyperechoic lesion (haemangioma – *yellow arrow*) along with its mirror image (*red arrow*) caused by the highly reflective diaphragm (*green*).

Mirror/Reflection Artefact

- Mirror artefact is a type of artefact in ultrasonography when the ultrasound beam encounters a highly reflective surface such as the diagram or thc wall of a distended urinary bladder. This artefact can be avoided by changing the transducer position and/or angle.
- Acoustic enhancement, acoustic shadowing, comet tail artefact and twinkling artefact are some of the useful artefacts that help in diagnosis.

PART

B

Contrast Agents

OSCE

9

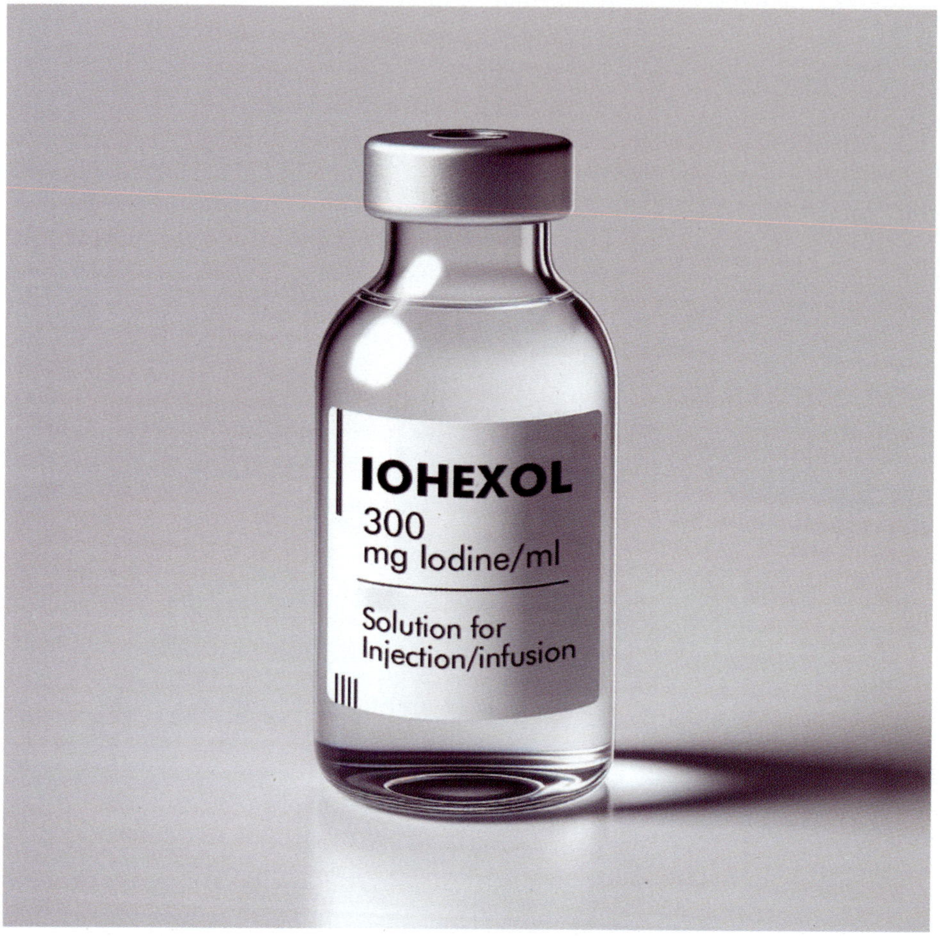

Iohexol

1. **What is the osmolality of this contrast agent?**
2. **What is its serum osmolality?**
3. **Enlist at least two diagnostic criteria for contrast-induced nephropathy (CIN).**
4. **A diabetic patient with a serum creatinine (S Cr) of 1.6 (eGFR of 40) comes for computed tomography (CT). What will you do regarding his metformin?**

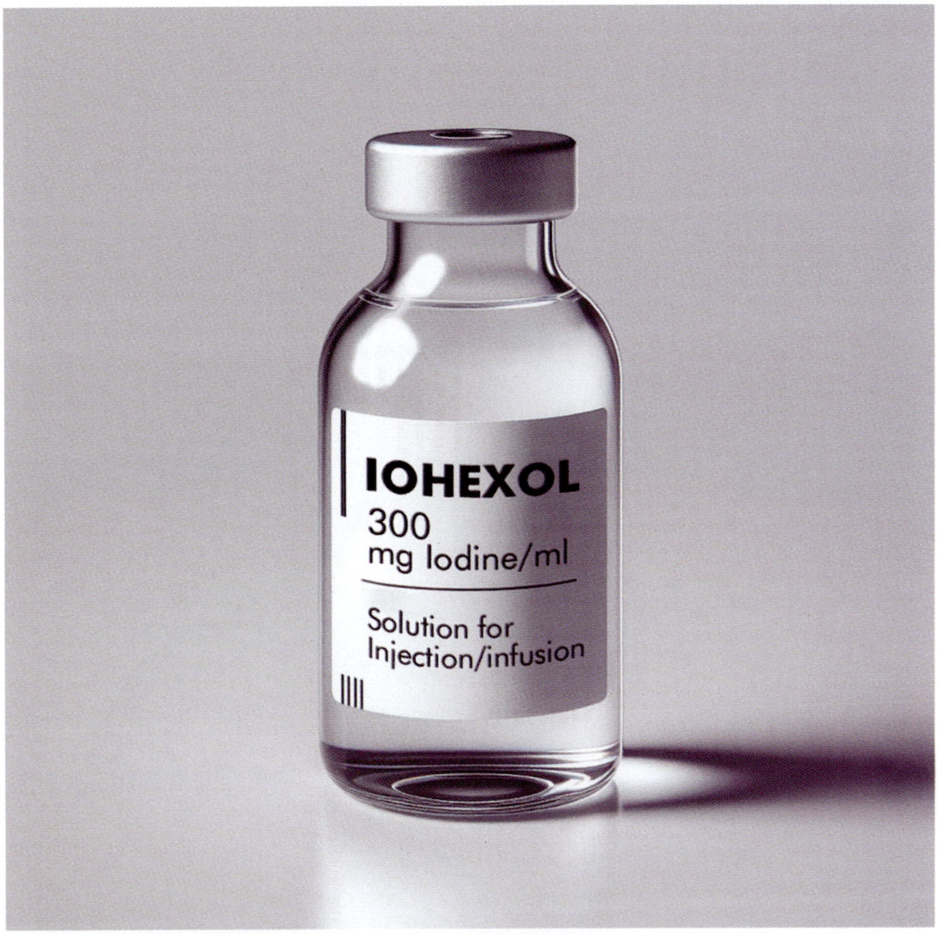

A vial containing iohexol, which is a non-ionic iodinated contrast media containing 300 mg of iodine per mL in this vial.

Non-Ionic Low Osmolar Iodinated Contrast Media

- Iohexol is a low osmolar contrast media; however, its osmolality is still higher than plasma. Osmolality of iohexol-300 is 465 mOsm/L and that of iohexol-350 is 541 mOsm/L.
- Serum osmolality is 290 mOsm/L. Visipaque-320 (iodixanol) is iso-osmolar to serum.
- **Contrast-induced nephropathy (CIN)** is defined as the impairment of kidney function – measured as: Either a 25% increase in serum creatinine (S Cr) from baseline or a 0.5 mg/dL (44 μmol/L) increase in absolute S Cr value within 48–72 hours after intravenous contrast administration.
- When a diabetic patient on metformin with an S Cr of 1.6 (estimated glomerular filtration rate [eGFR] of 40) comes for CT, we need to calculate his eGFR.
    - In patients with good renal function, eGFR > 30 mL/minute, metformin can be continued normally.
    - If eGFR < 30 mL/minute or iodinated contrast is to be given, metformin should be stopped from the time of injection and continued again 48 hours later if renal function remains same.

OSCE 10

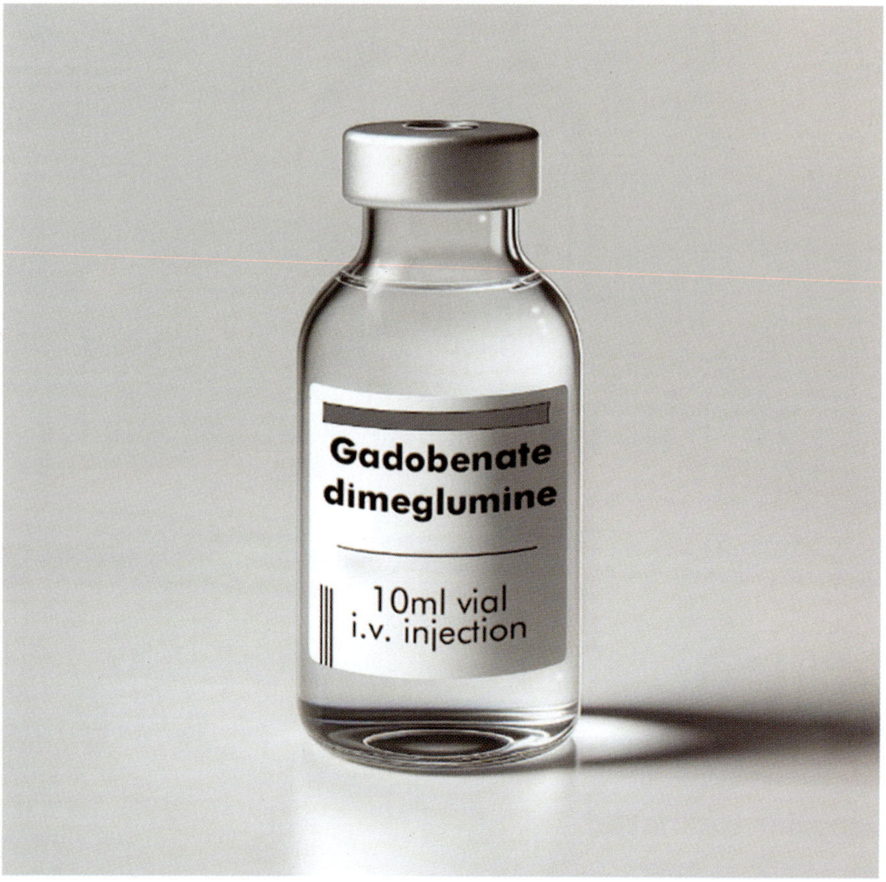

Gadobenate dimeglumine vial (hepatobiliary contrast agent).

1. **Write the classification of gadolinium-based contrast media.**
2. **Name any two hepatobiliary contrast agents.**
3. **What is the most ominous side effect of magnetic resonance imaging (MRI) contrast media in renal patients?**
4. **What is the atomic number of gadolinium?**
5. **What is the mechanism of action of gadolinium-based contrast agent (GBCA)?**
6. **What is earth's magnetic field?**

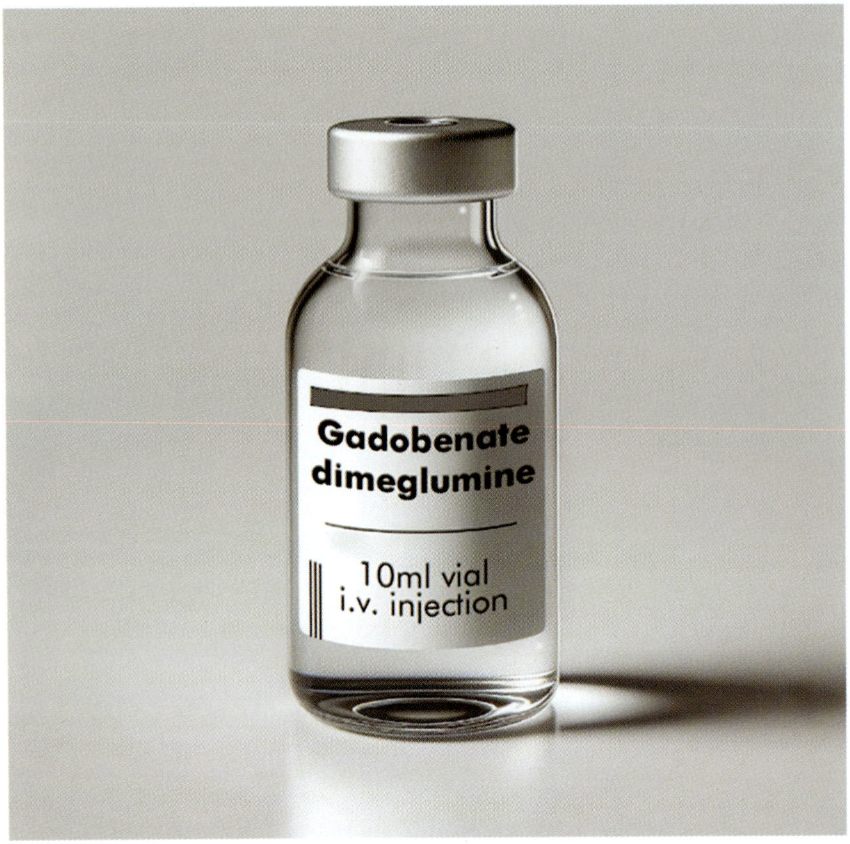

Gadobenate dimeglumine vial (hepatobiliary contrast agent).

Gadolinium-Based MRI Contrast Media

- Gadolinium is a paramagnetic agent and causes reduction in both T1 and T2 of the tissues (i.e. it causes both T1 and T2 relaxation). It leads to increased signal on T1-weighted images and causes negligible reduction of signals on T2-weighted images. Hence, it is primarily used for its T1 shortening effect.
- Gadolinium has an atomic number of 64.
- Magnetic resonance imaging (MRI) contrast media can be classified as:
  - Oral or parenteral contrast media (further as positive and negative)
  - Ionic vs non-ionic
  - Linear vs macrocyclic

Linear	Macrocyclic
• Gadodiamide (non-ionic)	• Gadobutrol (non-ionic)
• Gadopentetate (ionic)	• Gadoteridol (non-ionic)
• Gadobenate (ionic)	• Gadoterate (ionic)
• Gadoxetate (ionic)	• Gadopiclenol (non-ionic)

- Mangafodipir trisodium and gadobenate dimeglumine are the hepatobiliary contrast media.
- Nephrogenic systemic fibrosis is the most ominous side effect of MRI contrast media in renal patients.
- Earth's magnetic field is 25 to 65 microtesla (2.5×10^{-6} T). So, a 1.5 T MRI machine has 60,000 (60 thousand times) stronger magnetic field than the Earth.

PART C

Procedures

OSCE

11

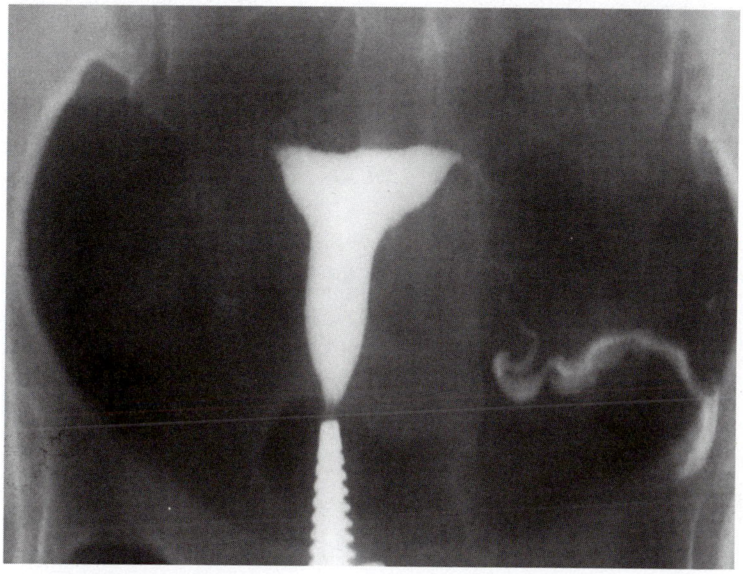

1. Name the above investigation.
2. Write two indications and two contraindications of this study.
3. Identify the abnormality.
4. What is 10-day rule?

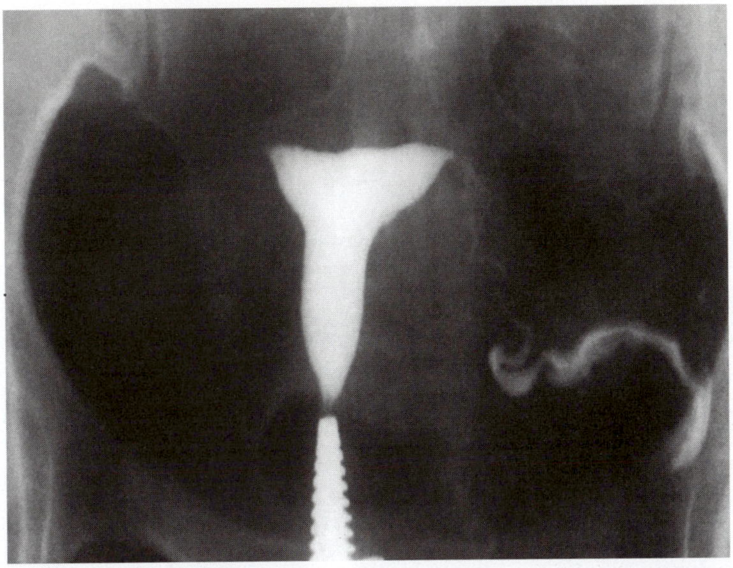

Hysterosalpingography (HSG) study demonstrating a right-sided cornual block.

Hysterosalpingography

- Hysterosalpingography (HSG) is a radiographic contrast study to visualize the endometrial cavity and fallopian tubes and to check their patency.
- Contraindications of this study are pregnancy and active pelvic infection.
- Two indications of this study are infertility to assess uterine morphology and tubal patency.
- The image shows non-opacification of the right-sided fallopian tube suggestive of right-sided corneal tubal block.
- Instruments that can be used in HSG are Sims' speculum, Cusco's speculum, HSG balloon catheter and Leech–Wilkinson cannula.
- **10-day rule:** HSG should be performed within 10 days from the last menstrual period (LMP) to avoid irradiating any unsuspecting pregnancy.

Indications	Contraindications
• Infertility	• Menstruation
• Recurrent abortions	• Pregnancy
• Following tubal surgeries/ fallopian tube recanalization (FTR)	• Pelvic inflammatory disease (PID), recent dilation and curettage (D&C)
• Migrated intrauterine contraceptive devices (IUCD)	• Cervicitis/purulent discharge per vaginal (PV)
• Uterine and tubal lesion	• Last menstrual period (LMP) beyond 10-day rule
	• History of recent D&C
	• Allergy to contrast

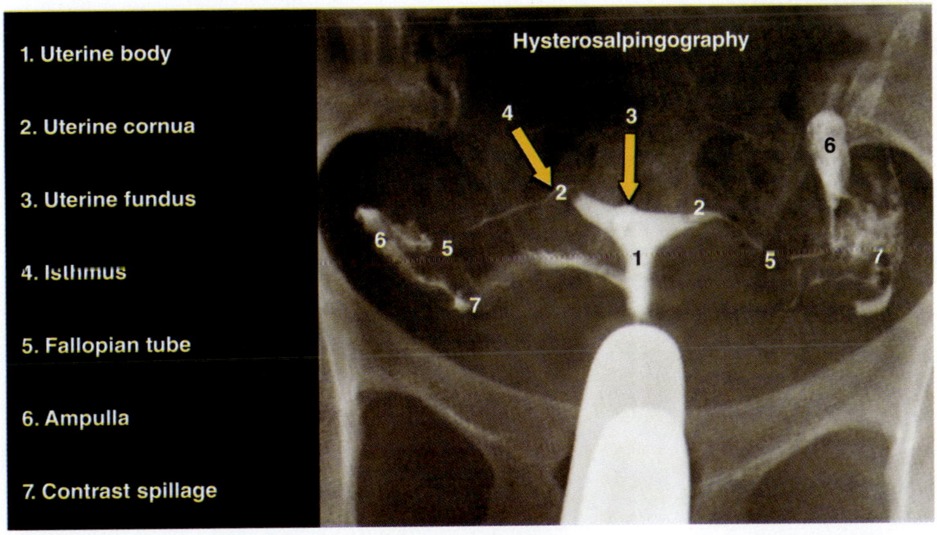

The normal HSG anatomy.

OSCE

12

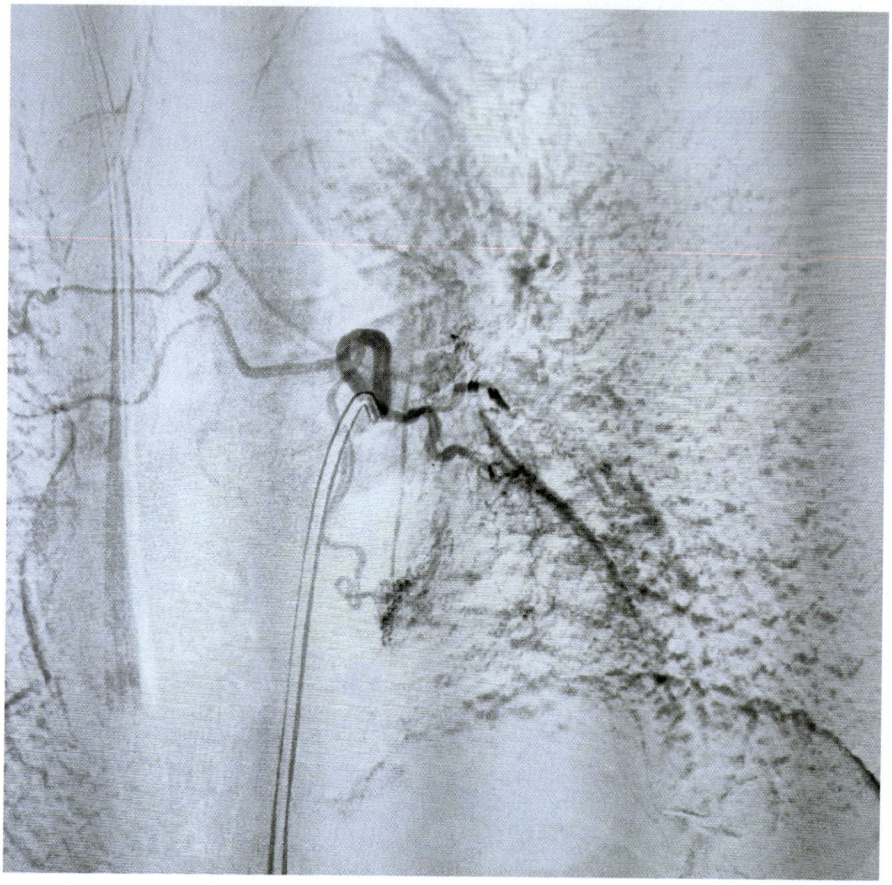

1. Name the procedure.
2. Which catheter is used?
3. What are the complications?
4. What are the common anatomical variants of bronchial artery.

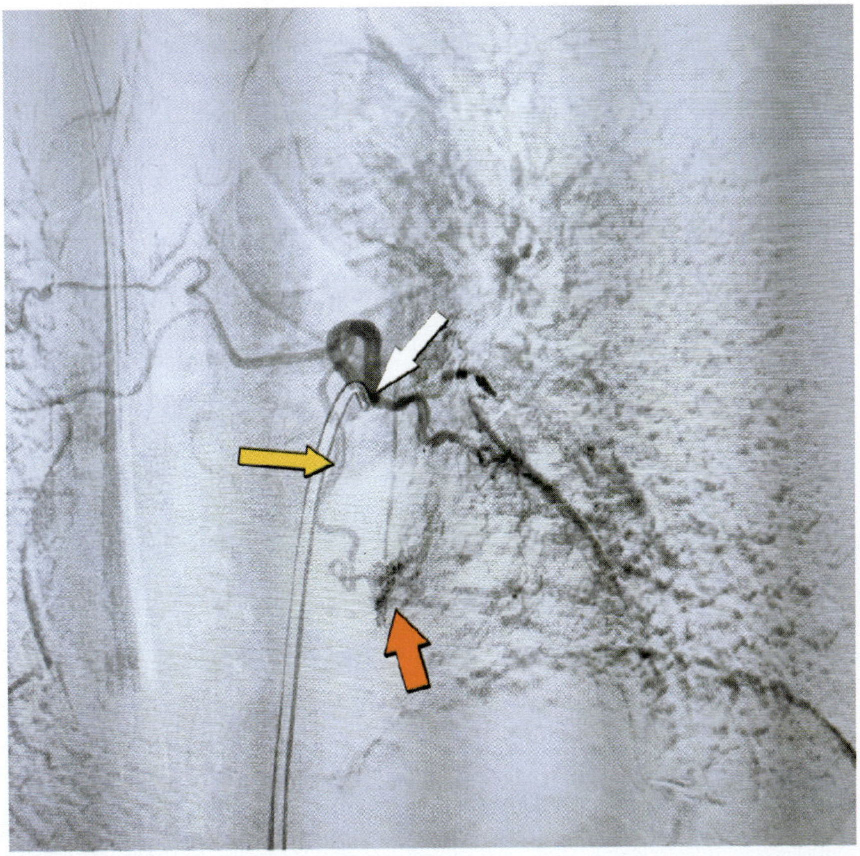

Selective run with a 5 Fr Cobra 1 diagnostic catheter shows the common origin of bilateral bronchial arteries with hypertrophied left bronchial artery (*white arrow*), abnormal contrast blush (*red arrow*) and multiple tiny vessels supplying the left lower lobe (*yellow arrow*).

Bronchial Artery Embolization

- The procedure shown in the image is bronchial artery embolization.
- Commonly used catheters are reverse-curved catheters (Cobra catheter, Sims' or Simmons catheter and Mikaelson catheter).
- Spinal cord ischaemia and transverse myelitis are the potential complications.
- Cauldwell et al. reported four classic bronchial artery branching patterns.

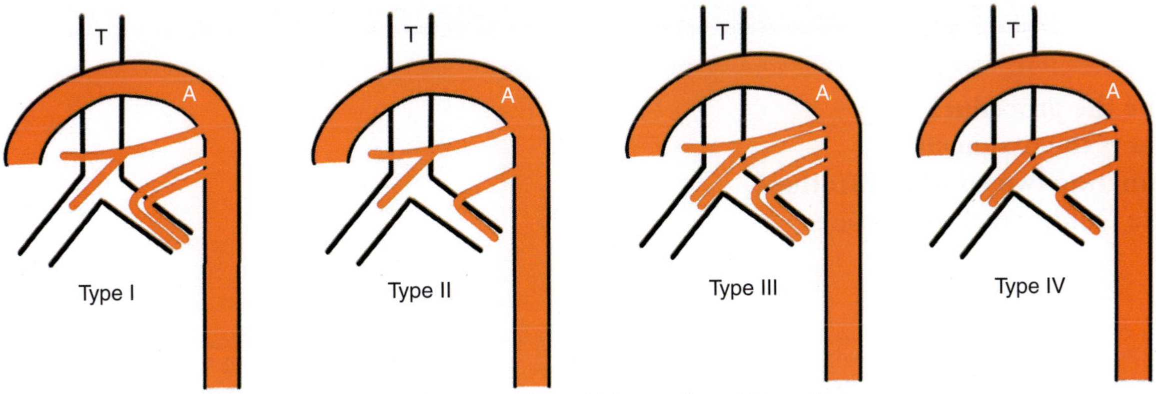

Cauldwell classification of bronchial artery branching pattern.

Variants of bronchial arterial supply:

1. Type I: Two bronchial arteries on the left and one on the right (40.6%) (2-1)
2. Type II: One on the left and one intercostobronchial trunk (ICBT) on the right (21.3%) (1-1)
3. Type III: Two on the left and two on the right (20.6%) (2-2)
4. Type IV: One on the left and two on the right (9.7%) (1-2)

OSCE

13

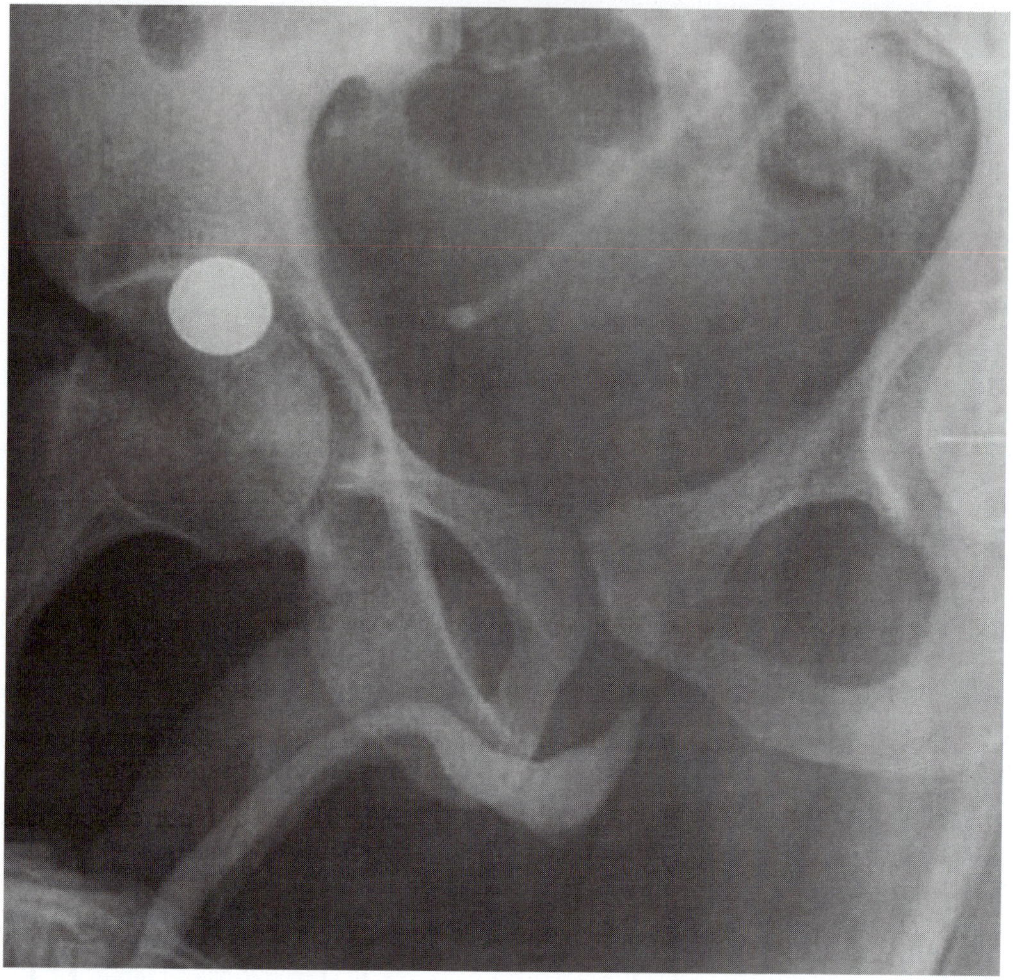

1. Name the procedure.
2. What is the diagnosis?
3. Enumerate two contraindications.
4. Write Goldman classification.

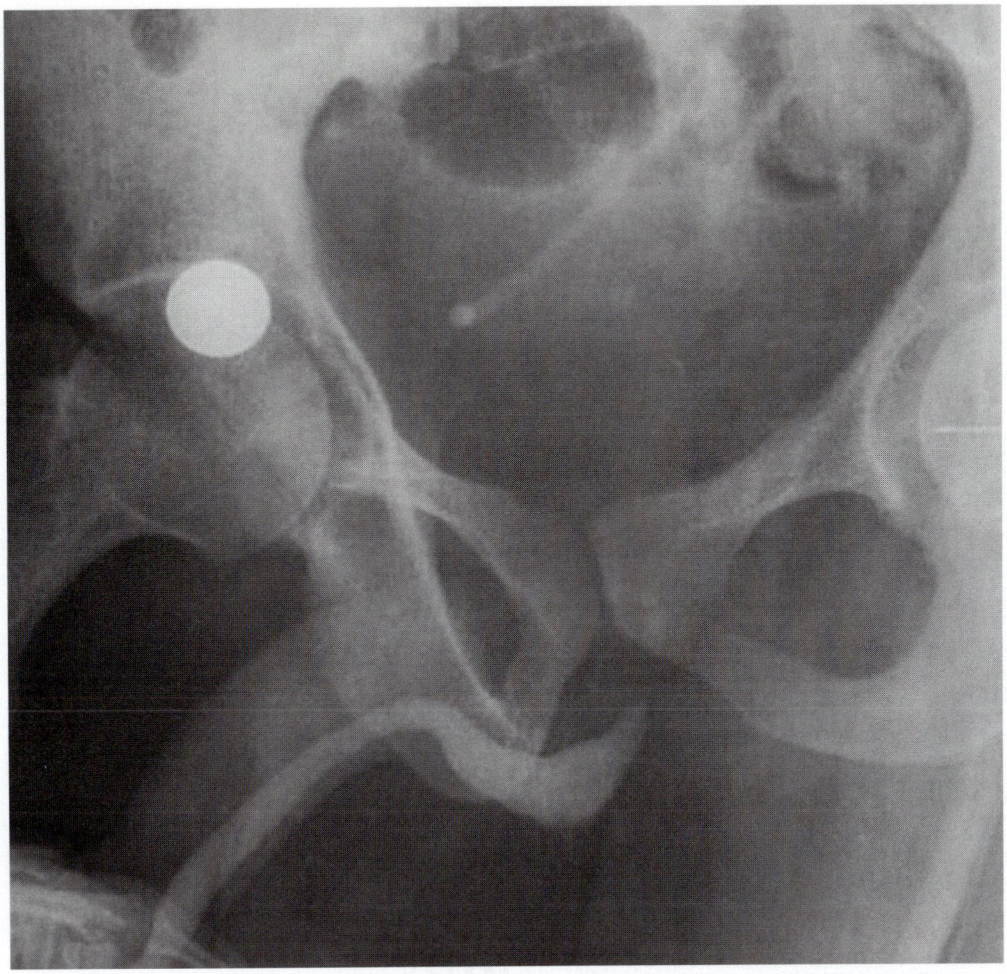

Retrograde urethrography (RGU) study shows the presence of stricture at the bulbomembranous junction.

Retrograde Urethrography

- Retrograde urethrography (RGU) is the radiological procedure to demonstrate the anterior urethra.
- Contraindications for the study are active infection and history of contrast reaction.

- Goldman's urethral injury classification, more widely accepted than the American Association for the Surgery of Trauma's (AAST) classification, categorizes injuries based on anatomical location:
  - Type I: Stretching of the posterior urethra due to disruption of puboprostatic ligaments, with an intact urethra.
  - Type II: Posterior urethral injury above the urogenital diaphragm.
  - Type III: Injury to the membranous urethra, extending into the proximal bulbous urethra with urogenital diaphragm laceration.
  - Type IV: Bladder base injury involving the bladder neck, potentially leading to incontinence if the internal sphincter is affected.
  - Type IVa: Bladder base injury not involving the bladder neck, indistinguishable from type IV radiologically.
  - Type V: Isolated anterior urethral injury.

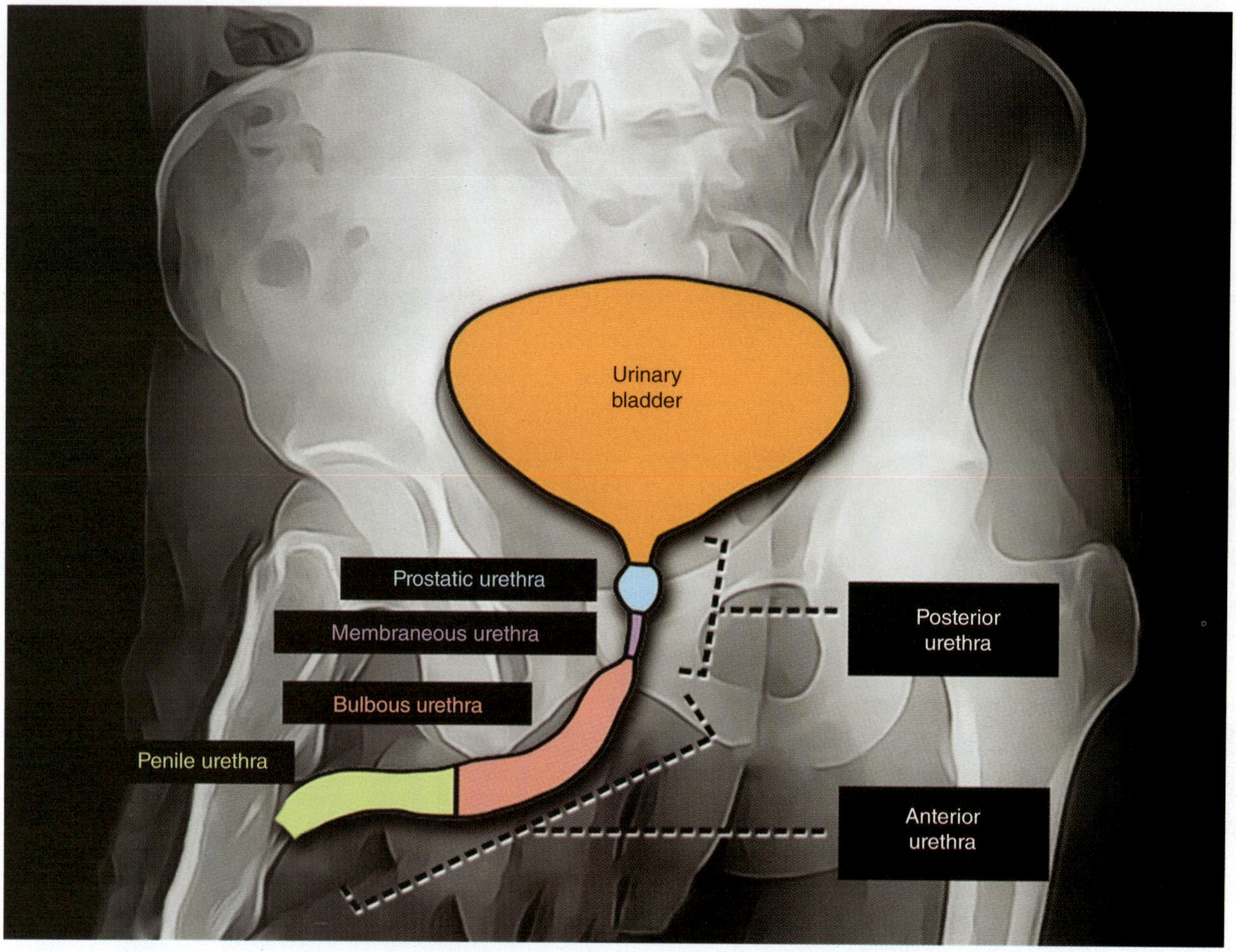

The normal male urethral anatomy.

PART D

Miscellaneous

OSCE 14

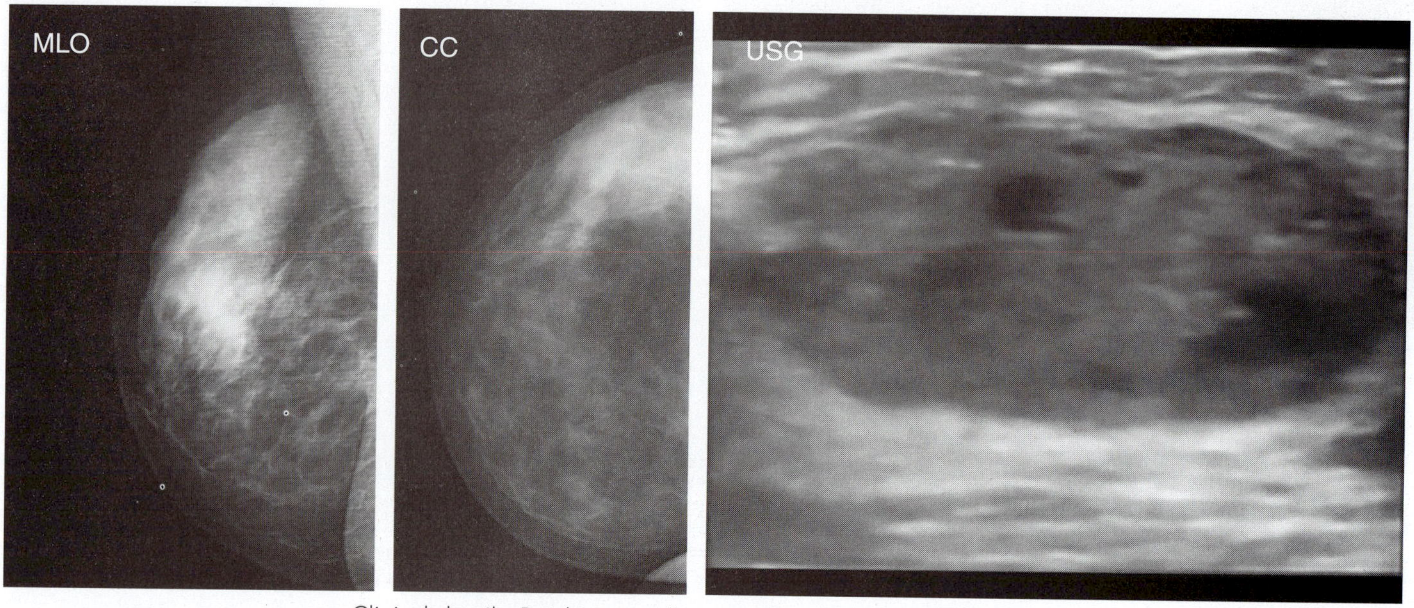

Clinical details: Painless, rapidly growing mass in the right breast.

1. Describe your findings in the mammography and ultrasonography (USG) images. What is the probable diagnosis?
2. Write two imaging features.
3. How does one differentiate between benign and malignant types?
4. Does this mass commonly metastasize?
5. Enumerate differentials for rapidly enlarging breast masses.

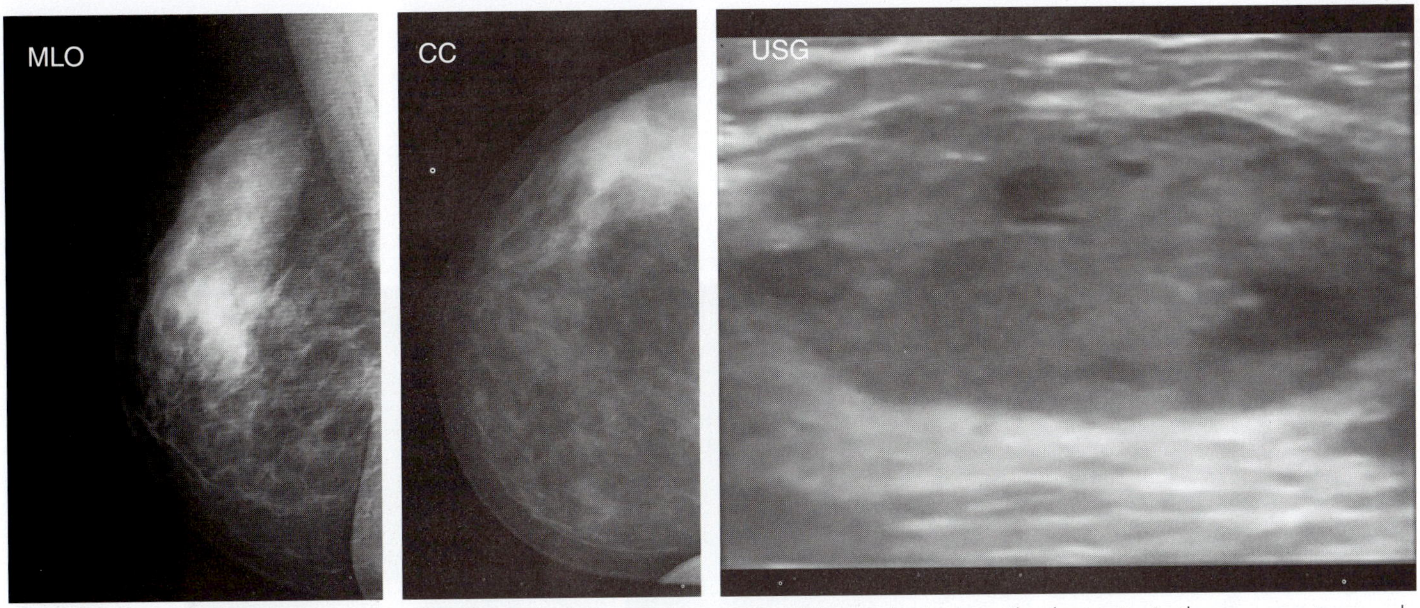

MLO and CC mammography views show a large oval-shaped dense mass with mostly circumscribed margins in the upper-outer quadrant of the right breast. On the ultrasonography (USG) image, it appears as an oval-shaped heterogeneously hypoechoic mass with circumscribed margins, parallel orientation, posterior acoustic enhancement, and some internal rounded and cleft-like cystic areas.

Phyllodes Tumour (Cystosarcoma Phyllodes)

Phyllodes tumour, or cystosarcoma phyllodes, is an uncommon fibroepithelial neoplasm of the breast exhibiting similarities to a fibroadenoma. Typically, it manifests as a large, rapidly growing breast mass. It originates from the periductal stroma of the breast.

Radiological features:

- Mammography: Circumscribed round, oval or lobulated tumour, usually with smooth margins, without spiculation.
- USG: Circumscribed hypoechoic solid-appearing lesions with varying degrees of inhomogeneity and small cystic spaces. Posterior acoustic enhancement is highly suggestive. Vascular areas may be seen. Calcifications are less common than in fibroadenomas.
- Magnetic resonance imaging (MRI):
  - Rounded/oval or lobulated well-circumscribed masses
  - T1: Usually hypointense
  - T2: Variable signal intensity, ranging from homogeneously hypointense to hyperintense
  - T1 post-contrast: Solid components exhibit enhancement post-contrast administration
  - Dynamic contrast: Kinetic curve pattern may exhibit a gradual slow or rapid enhancement
- Differentiation between benign and malignant phyllodes tumours is not possible on imaging.
- They do not commonly metastasize. As they are locally invasive, phyllodes tumours typically necessitate surgical excision for treatment, with larger tumours potentially requiring complete mastectomy. Malignant transformation is observed in 5%–25% of cases (malignant phyllodes tumour).
- Differentials for rapidly enlarging breast masses:
  - Phyllodes tumour
  - Juvenile giant fibroadenoma
  - Abscess
  - Haematoma

OSCE

15

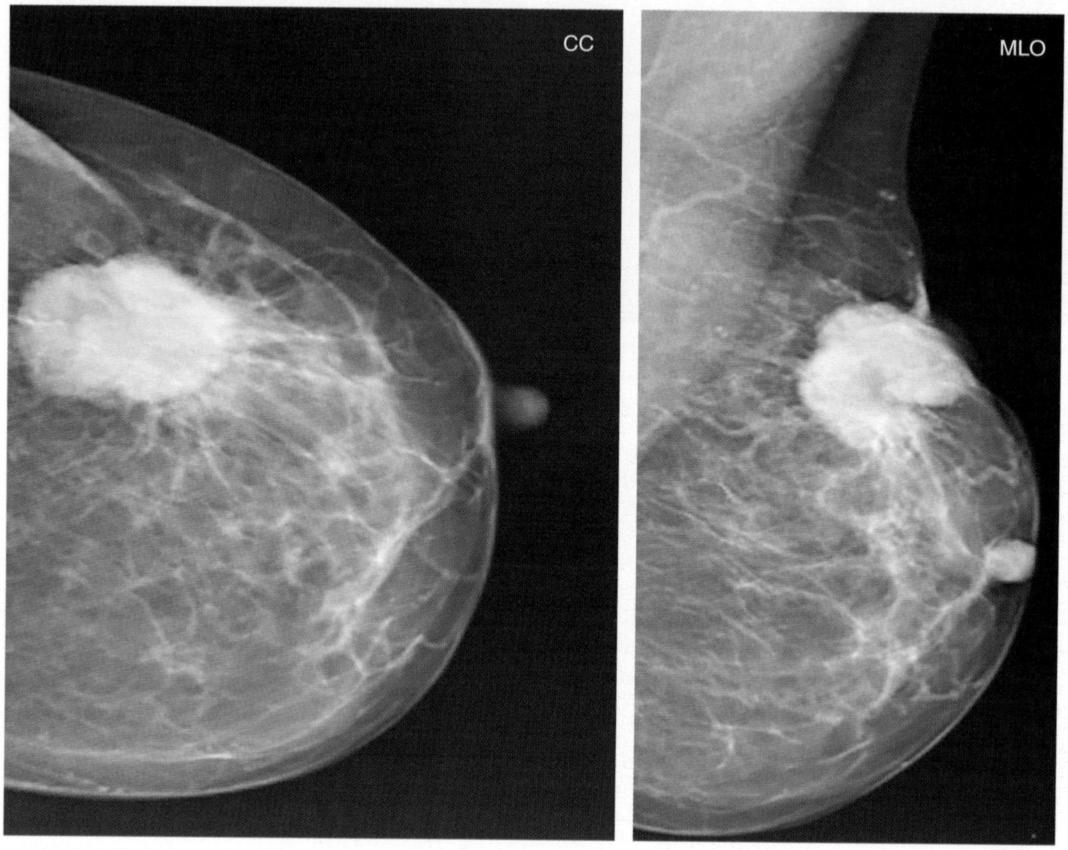

Clinical details: Routine screening mammography.

1. **What is your diagnosis?**
2. **What are the genetic mutations involved?**
3. **What are the risk factors for carcinoma breast?**
4. **What is the density of breast in the given mammography image?**
5. **Classification of density in Breast Imaging Reporting and Data System (BI-RADS) lexicon.**

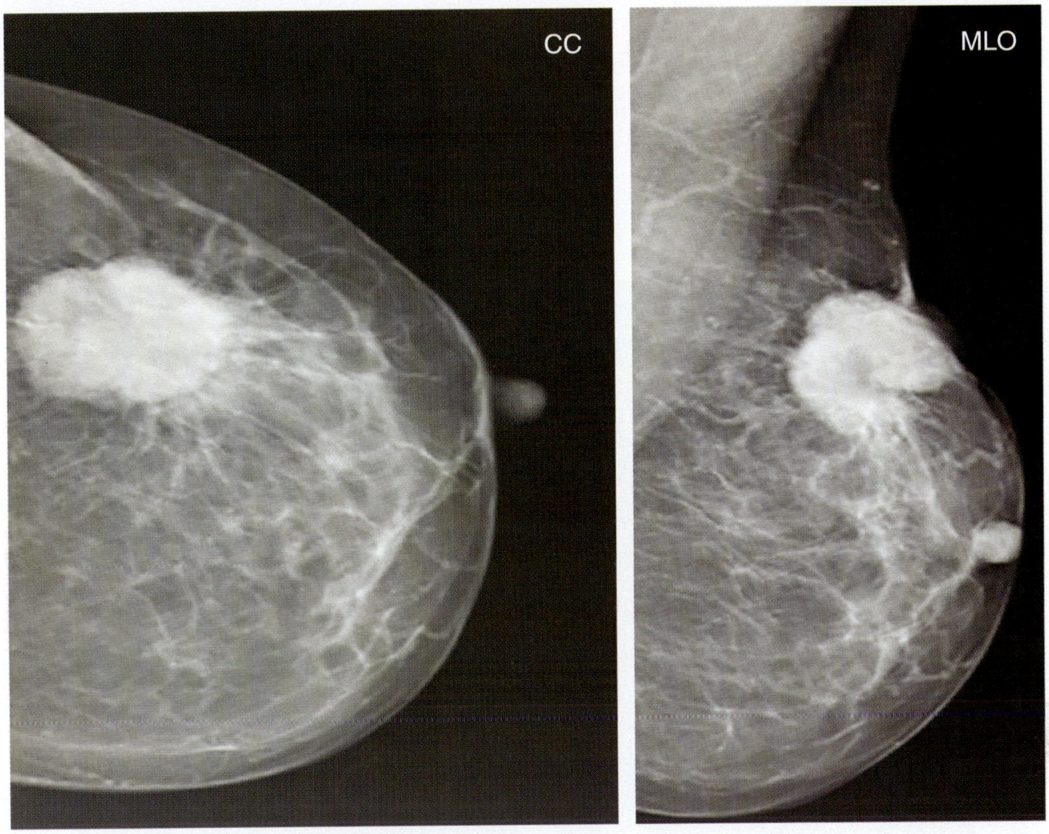

Digital mammography images of the left breast in CC and MLO views demonstrate an oval-shaped dense lesion in the upper-outer quadrant with partially obscured and spiculated margins with resultant nipple retraction.

BI-RADS V

- BI-RADS 5 lesions within the Breast Imaging Reporting and Data System (BI-RADS) indicate breast abnormalities that exhibit a high level of suspicion for malignancy. These cases necessitate prompt intervention, such as biopsy and subsequent management. BI-RADS 5 lesions manifest the morphological features consistent with breast cancer, carrying a probability of malignancy exceeding 95%.
- Genetic mutations involved are BRCA1 and BRCA2 mutations.
- Risk factors for carcinoma breast:
  - Family history
  - Female gender
  - Old age >55 years
  - BRCA1 and BRCA2 mutations

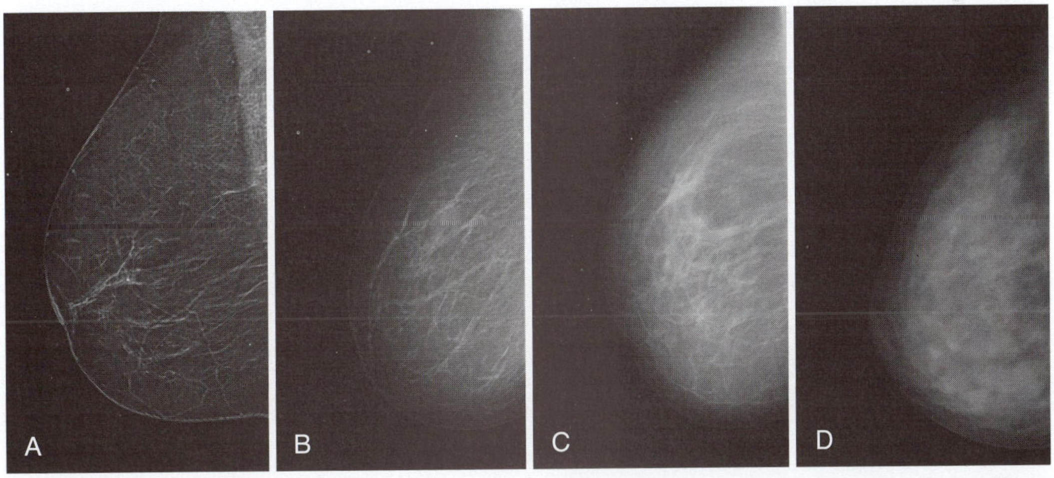

BI-RADS lexicon for breast density categories (a, b, c or d): A, Breasts are almost entirely fatty with minimal fibroglandular density. B, Presence of scattered fibroglandular density throughout the breasts. C, Heterogeneous breast density, which may obscure detection of small masses. D, Extremely dense breasts, significantly lowering mammographic sensitivity.

OSCE

16

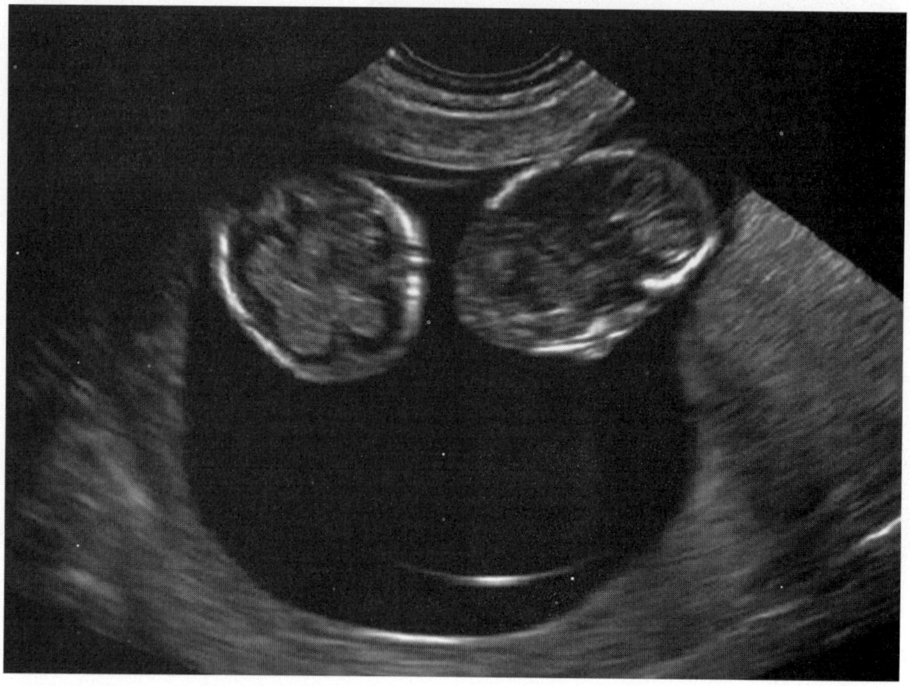

1. What is your diagnosis?
2. Enumerate two complications of such pregnancy.
3. What are the signs to differentiate monochorionic and dichorionic pregnancies?
4. What are the other complications of monochorionic diamniotic (MCDA) pregnancy?

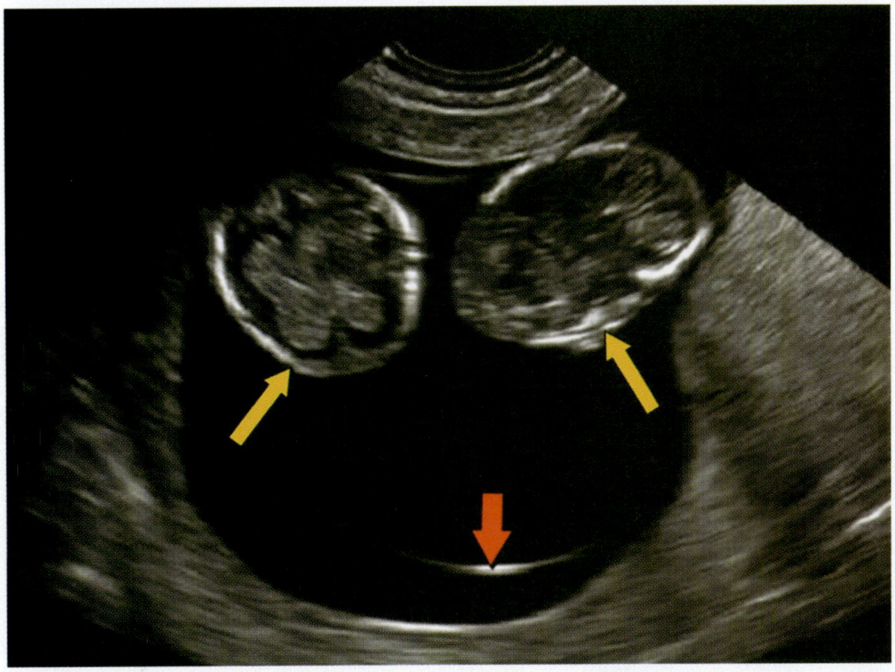

Foetal ultrasound image demonstrates a single amniotic sac (*red arrow*) with presence of twin gestation (*yellow arrows*).

MCMA Twin Gestation

Monochorionic monoamniotic (MCMA) twin gestation represents a specific type of monozygotic twin pregnancies. These embryos are characterized by a single chorionic sac, single amniotic sac and a single yolk sac.

- Complications of such MCMA twin gestation:
  - Twin-to-twin transfusion syndrome
  - Twin embolization syndrome
- Ultrasound (USG) criteria for the diagnosis of dichorionic and diamniotic twins:
  - Two gestational sacs with a thick echogenic chorion surrounding each embryo
  - A thick intertwin membrane (often taken as >2 mm)
  - Twin peak sign (lambda [λ] sign)
- Monochorionic and diamniotic twins:
  - Single gestational sac and almost always two separate yolk sacs
  - Presence of single placenta
  - Thin intertwin membrane
  - T sign of intertwin membrane
- Dichorionic pregnancy has two chorions:
  - So separate gestation sacs, chorion may extend between them
  - Twin peak sign (lambda sign)
  - Thick intertwin membrane (has more than two layers)
  - Presence of two separate placentae
  - Different gender of foetus
- Complications of MCDA pregnancy:
  - Twin-to-twin transfusion syndrome: 15%–30% of cases
  - Twin embolization syndrome
  - Twin reversed arterial perfusion sequence
  - Demise of one twin

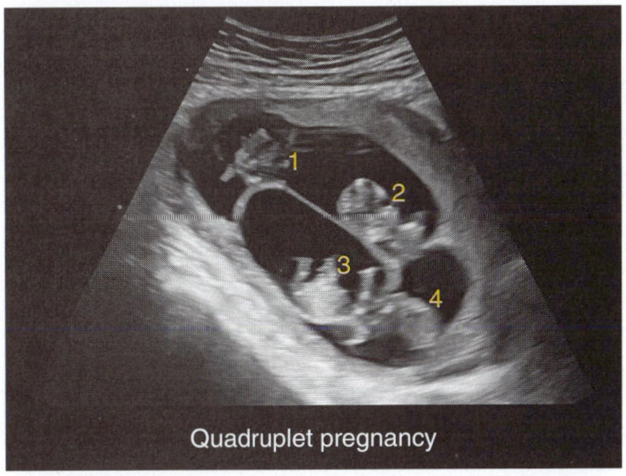

Ultrasound imaging of an early pregnancy demonstrates a quadruplet gestation.

OSCE

17

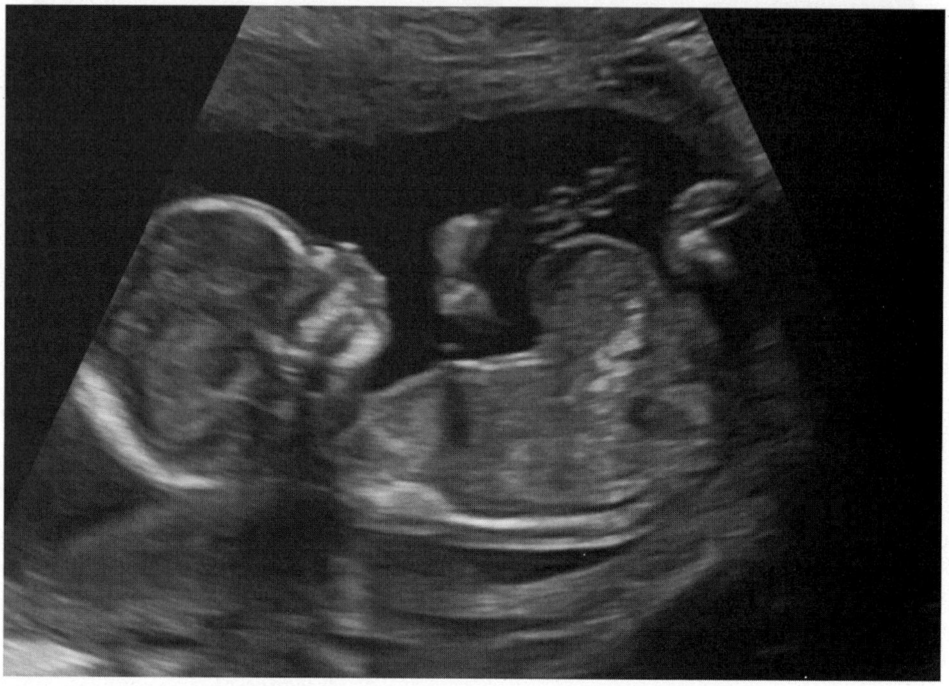

Clinical details: Routine antenatal ultrasound.

1. **What are the imaging findings and the most appropriate diagnosis?**
2. **Which is most commonly associated chromosomal anomaly?**
3. **How would you differentiate Omphalocele from Gastroschisis?**
4. **Name one syndrome in which there is an association of omphalocele with Wilms tumour.**

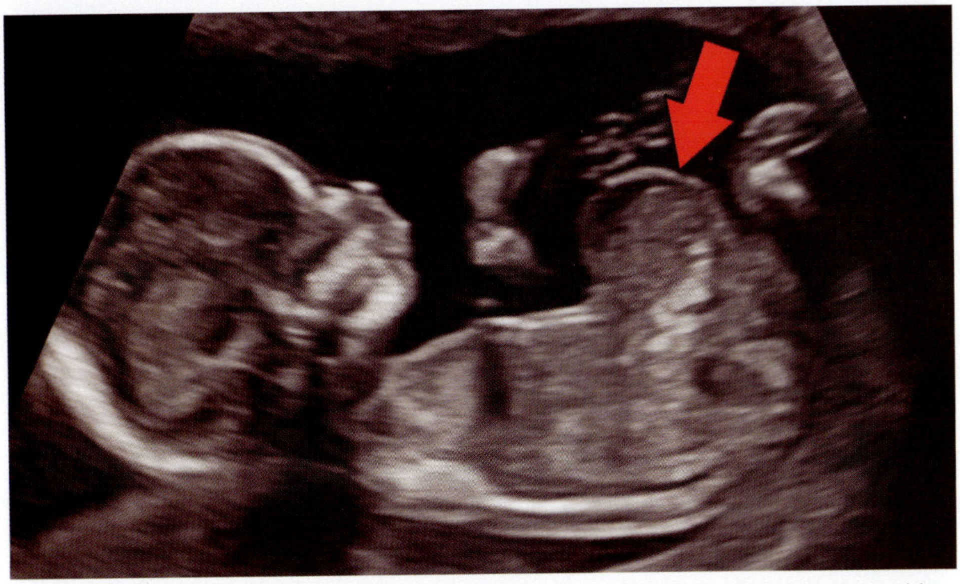

Routine antenatal ultrasound image demonstrates a foetus with abnormal herniation of liver tissue and bowel loops outside the abdominal cavity through a midline abdominal wall defect. There is presence of a covering membrane (*red arrow*) consistent with omphalocele rather than gastroschisis.

Omphalocele

Omphalocele or exomphalos is the most common type of congenital anterior abdominal wall defect, usually diagnosed on foetal sonography. It occurs due to the incomplete formation of the anterior abdominal wall during the gestational period, leading to a congenital midline abdominal wall defect.

It is commonly associated with chromosomal anomalies and syndromes:

1. Trisomy 18 (most commonly associated chromosomal anomaly), trisomy 13, and trisomy 21
2. Turner and Klinefelter syndrome
3. Beckwith–Wiedemann syndrome
4. OEIS complex (Omphalocele, Exstrophy of bladder or cloaca, Imperforate anus and Spinal anomalies like hemivertebrae)
5. Congenital cardiac anomalies

Beckwith–Wiedemann syndrome = hemihypertrophy, macroglossia, omphalocele, localized gigantism and organomegaly

Omphalocele

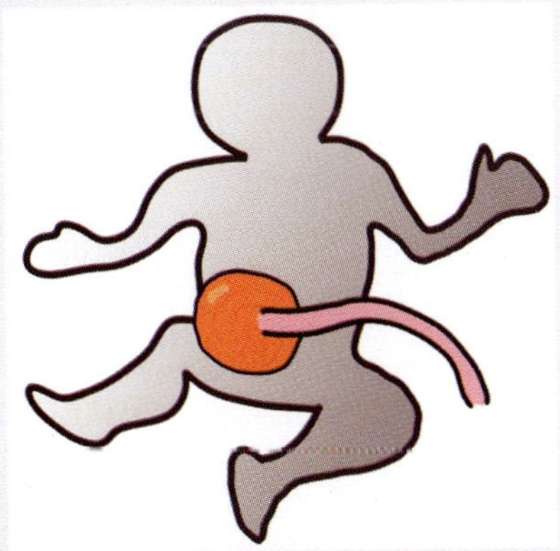

- Hernia contents are covered by a membrane
- Midline defect
- The umbilical cord inserts at the tip of the hernia sac
- May contain bowel loops and/or liver tissue
- More commonly associated with syndromes and chromosomal anomalies

Gastroschisis

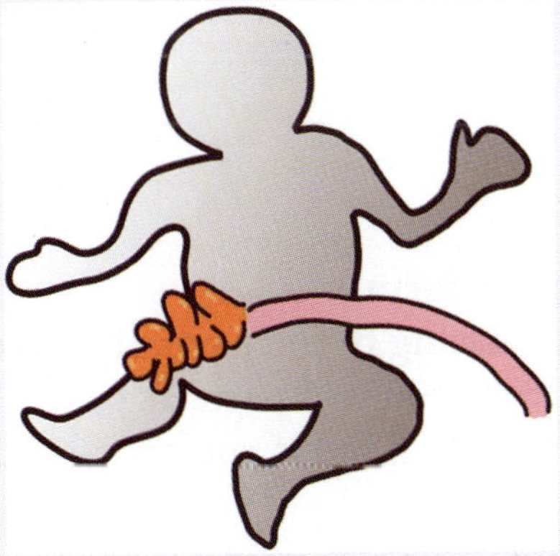

- Free-floating bowel loops with no covering membrane
- Defect is usually on the right side (paraumbilical)
- Umbilical cord insertion is usually on one side of the defect
- Usually contains only bowel loops
- Less commonly associated with other defects; may be associated with intestinal atresia

[See Proviso to section 4(3), Rule 9(4) and Rule 10(1A)]
FORM FOR MAINTENANCE OF RECORDS IN CASE OF A PREGNANT WOMEN BY GENETIC CLINIC/ULTRASOUND CLINIC/IMAGING CENTRE

1. Name and address of Genetic Clinic*/Ultrasound Clinic*/Imaging Centre*:____________
____
2. Registration details:
   i. Registration No. *(Under PC& PNDT Act).*____________
   ii. Registration Expiry Date: ____________
   iii. Make and model number of ultrasound machine used for the pre-natal diagnosis: ________
3. Patient's name ______________________________ Age ________
4. Number of previous children:____________________________
   a) Number of Sons living ________ b) Number of Daughters living ________
5. Husband's/Father's name:____________________________
6. Full address of the patient with Contact Number, if any____________________
____
7. a)Referred by (Full name and address of Doctor(s)/ Genetic Counseling Centre:____________________________
   (Referral note to be preserved carefully with case papers)
   b) Self Referral by Gynaecologist/Radiologist/Registered Medical Practitioner conducting the pre-natal diagnostic procedures: ____________
   Self referral does not mean referral by the Patient) *(Referral note with indications and case papers of the patient to be preserved)*
8. Last menstrual period/weeks of pregnancy:____________________
9. History of genetic/medical disease in the family (specify):____________
   Basis of diagnosis:
   (a) Clinical
   (b) Bio-chemical
   (c) Cytogenetic
   (d) Other (e.g. radiological, ultrasonography etc.-specify)
10. Indication for pre-natal diagnosis
    A. Previous child/children with:
    (i) Chromosomal disorders
    (ii) Metabolic disorders
    (iii) Congenital anomaly
    (iv) Mental Disability
    (v) Hacmoglobinopathy
    (vi) Sex linked disorders
    (vii) Single gene disorder

1. Identify the form.
2. What is missing in the partially filled form?
3. Which form you will paste at your ultrasound centre?
4. Which form is filled if you are performing amniocentesis?

[See Proviso to section 4(3), Rule 9(4) and Rule 10(1A)]
FORM FOR MAINTENANCE OF RECORDS IN CASE OF A PREGNANT WOMEN BY GENETIC CLINIC/ULTRASOUND CLINIC/IMAGING CENTRE

1. Name and address of Genetic Clinic*/Ultrasound Clinic*/Imaging Centre*:__________
2. Registration details:
   i. Registration No. *(Under PC& PNDT Act)*.__________
   ii. Registration Expiry Date: __________
   iii. Make and model number of ultrasound machine used for the pre-natal diagnosis: __________
3. Patient's name __________ Age__________
4. Number of previous children:__________
   a) Number of Sons living ________ b) Number of Daughters living __________
5. Husband's/Father's name:__________
6. Full address of the patient with Contact Number, if any__________
7. a)Referred by (Full name and address of Doctor(s)/ Genetic Counseling Centre:__________
   (Referral note to be preserved carefully with case papers)
   b) Self Referral by Gynaecologist/Radiologist/Registered Medical Practitioner conducting the pre-natal diagnostic procedures: __________
   Self referral does not mean referral by the Patient) *(Referral note with indications and case papers of the patient to be preserved)*
8. Last menstrual period/weeks of pregnancy:__________
9. History of genetic/medical disease in the family (specify):__________
   Basis of diagnosis:
   (a) Clinical
   (b) Bio-chemical
   (c) Cytogenetic
   (d) Other (e.g. radiological, ultrasonography etc.-specify)
10. Indication for pre-natal diagnosis
    A. Previous child/children with:
    (i) Chromosomal disorders
    (ii) Metabolic disorders
    (iii) Congenital anomaly
    (iv) Mental Disability
    (v) Hacmoglobinopathy
    (vi) Sex linked disorders
    (vii) Single gene disorder

Incompletely filled Pre-Conception and Pre-Natal Diagnostic Techniques (Prohibition of Sex Selection) Act (PC-PNDT) form F.

PC-PNDT Form F

- A PC-PNDT form is shown.
- Patient particulars are missing in the partially filled form.
- Form B: Certificate of registration has to be pasted at the ultrasound centre.
- Form G has to be filled for all invasive procedures including amniocentesis.

The enactment of the Pre-Conception and Pre-Natal Diagnostic Techniques (Prohibition of Sex Selection) Act (PC-PNDT) is a crucial legislative measure aimed at addressing the issue of female foeticide, which has contributed to the decline in the female sex ratio in India.

The Indian government enacted the Pre-Natal Diagnostic Techniques (Regulation and Prevention of Misuse) Act (PNDT) in 1994, which took effect on 1 January 1996. Subsequently, amendments were introduced to the Act, leading to its renaming in 2003 as the Pre-Conception and Pre-Natal Diagnostic Techniques (Prohibition of Sex Selection) Act.

FORMS UNDER PC-PNDT

Form A: Registration of imaging centre or renewal of registration

Form B: Certificate of registration (to be displayed at the clinic)

Form C: Rejection of registration of imaging centre

Form D: Form for maintenance of records by genetic counselling centre

Form E: Form for maintenance of records by genetic laboratory

Form F: Form for maintenance of records by genetic clinic/imaging centre

Form G: Consent form for prenatal invasive diagnostic techniques

Form H: Form for permanent maintenance of application for grant/rejection of registration

Under the PC-PNDT Act, offences are characterized as cognizable, non-bailable and non-compoundable. Cognizable means that a police officer has the authority to make an arrest without a warrant. Non-bailable signifies that the police cannot grant bail to the accused. Lastly, non-compoundable indicates that the involved parties cannot reach a settlement and the case cannot be withdrawn or decided not to prosecute.

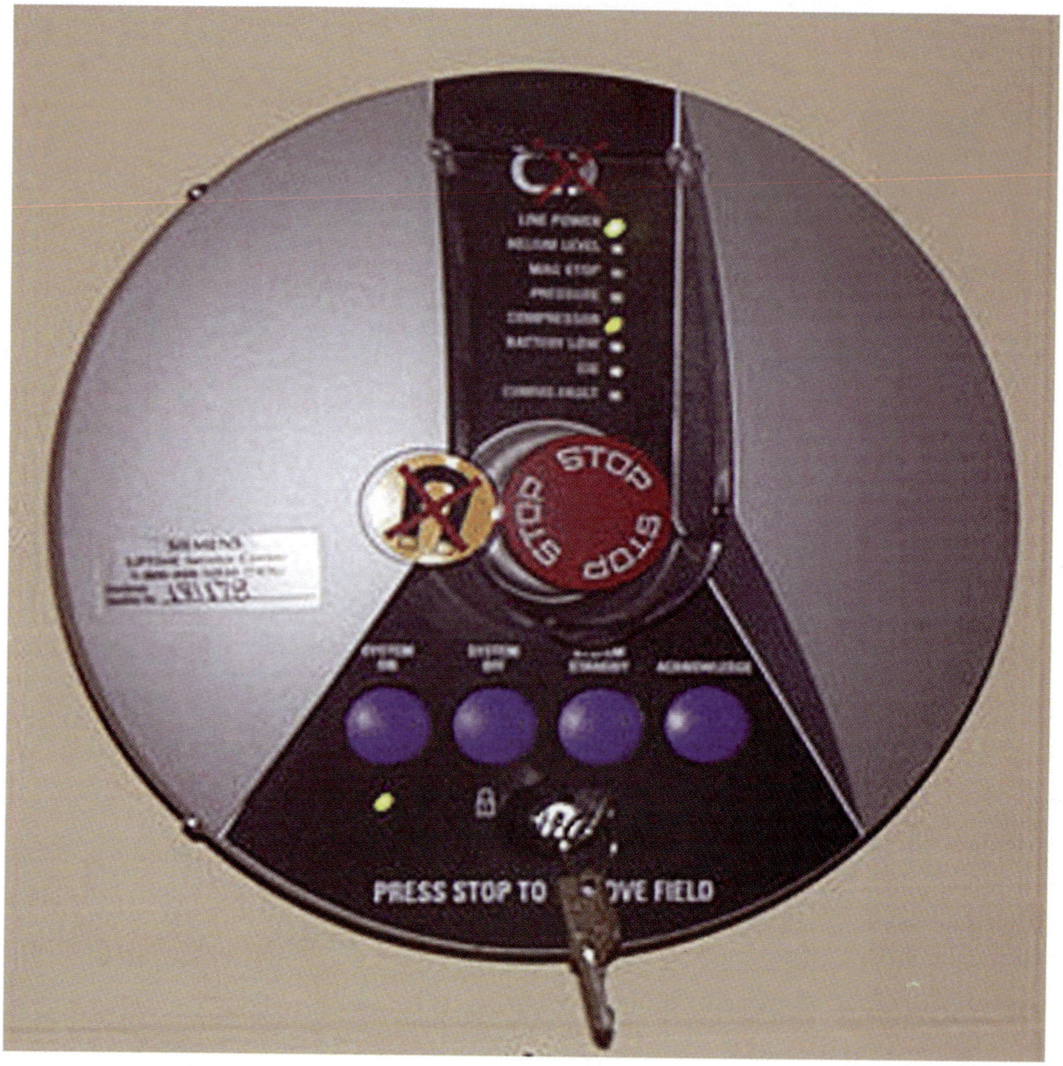

1. What is the use of the red button?
2. What is the role of height and weight in magnetic resonance imaging (MRI) scan?
3. What is the name of this process?
4. Which safety zone is the magnet placed?

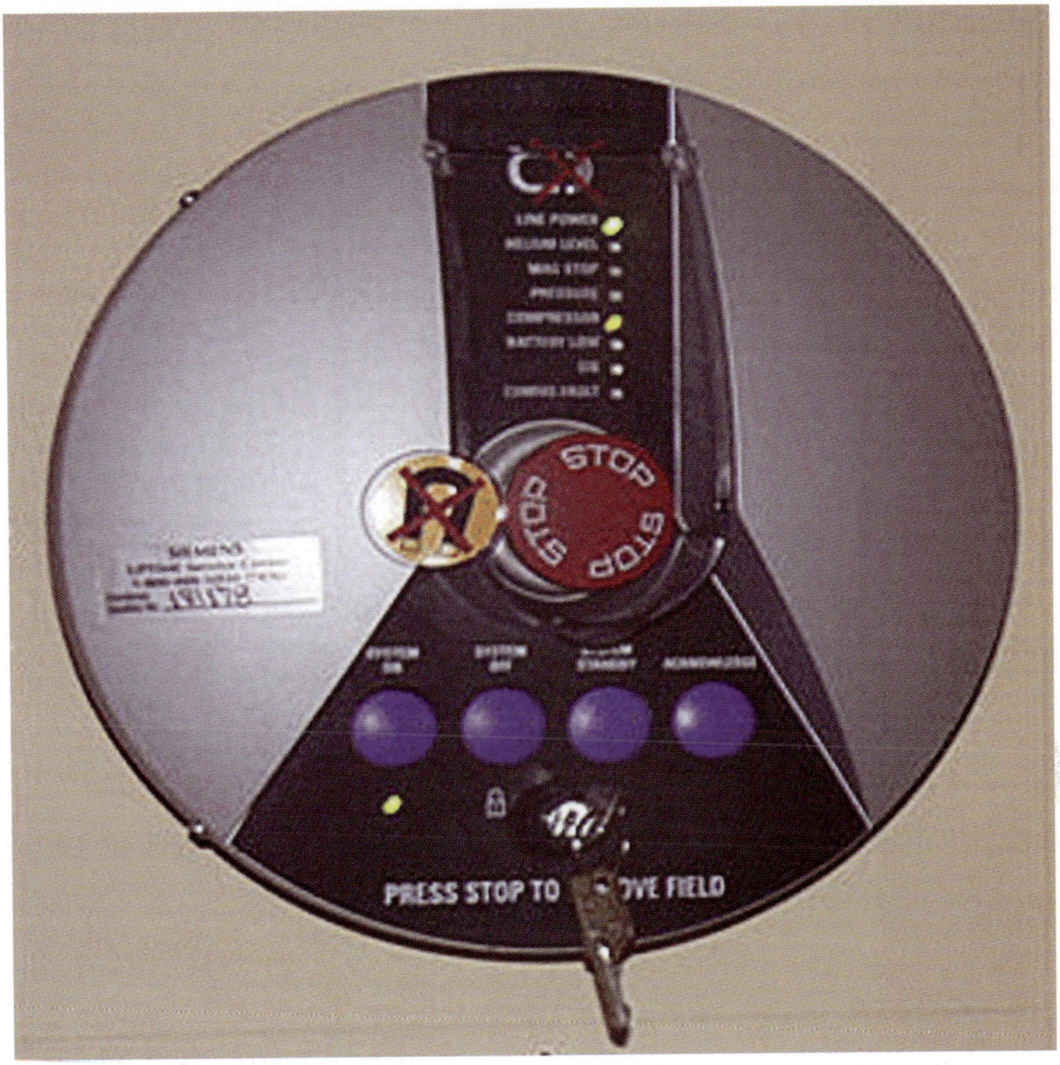

- It is used in emergency situation: Emergency run down/stop magnet
- To determine the length of scan/localizer and the calculation of contrast dose
- Quenching
- Magnetic resonance imaging (MRI) safety zone IV (American College of Radiology safety guidelines):
  - Zone 1:
    - General public area outside the MR environment.
    - This area is the reception and waiting area.
  - Zone 2:
    - Area between zone 1 (public access) and the strictly controlled zone 2 (control room) and zone 3 (magnet).
    - This is the area just outside of the restricted area, zone 3.
    - This is the area of travel in which patients are brought into their procedure.
  - Zone 3: Control room:
    - All access to zone 3 is to be strictly restricted with access to regions within it controlled by and entirely under the supervision of MR personnel.
    - This zone is restricted from general public access by a reliable restricting method that can differentiate between MR and non-MR personnel.
  - Zone 4: Magnet room

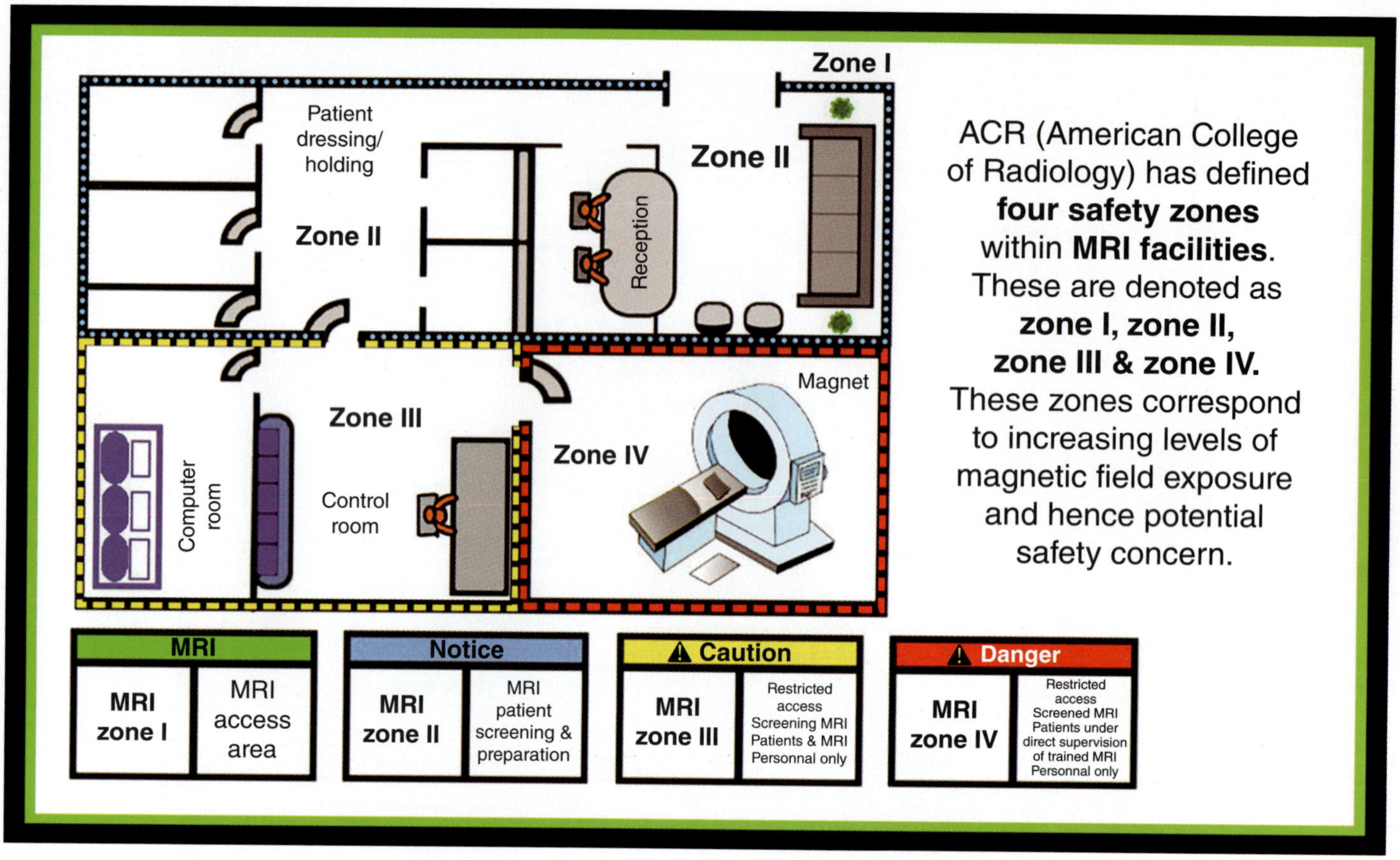
Zone I
Patient dressing/ holding
Zone II
Reception
Zone II
Magnet
Zone III
Zone IV
Computer room
Control room
ACR (American College of Radiology) has defined **four safety zones** within **MRI facilities**. These are denoted as **zone I, zone II, zone III & zone IV.** These zones correspond to increasing levels of magnetic field exposure and hence potential safety concern.
MRI
MRI zone I
MRI access area
Notice
MRI zone II
MRI patient screening & preparation
Caution
MRI zone III
Restricted access Screening MRI Patients & MRI Personnal only
Danger
MRI zone IV
Restricted access Screened MRI Patients under direct supervision of trained MRI Personnal only

PART E

Abdomen

GASTROINTESTINAL AND GENITOURINARY SYSTEM

OSCE

20

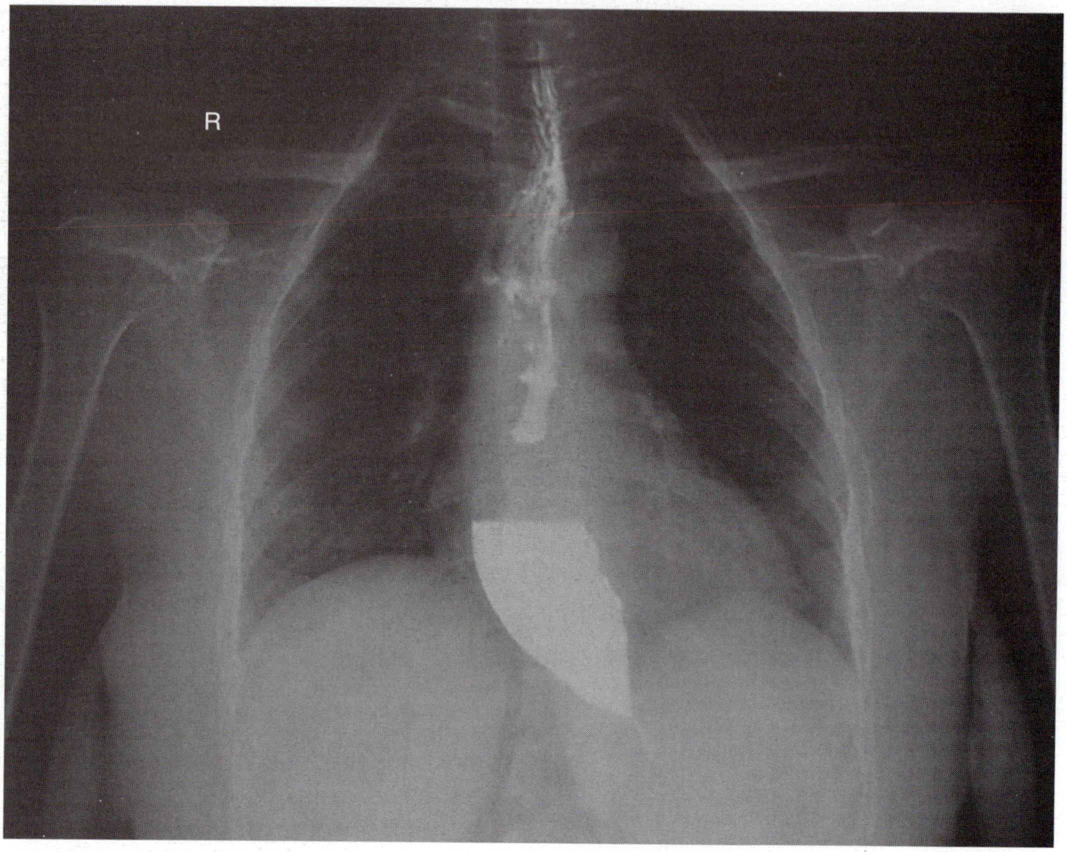

Clinical details: A 35-year-old lady with recent onset dysphagia to both solids and liquids.

1. **Name the investigation and describe your findings.**
2. **What is the most appropriate diagnosis?**
3. **What is the underlying aetiology?**
4. **Name one treatment option.**

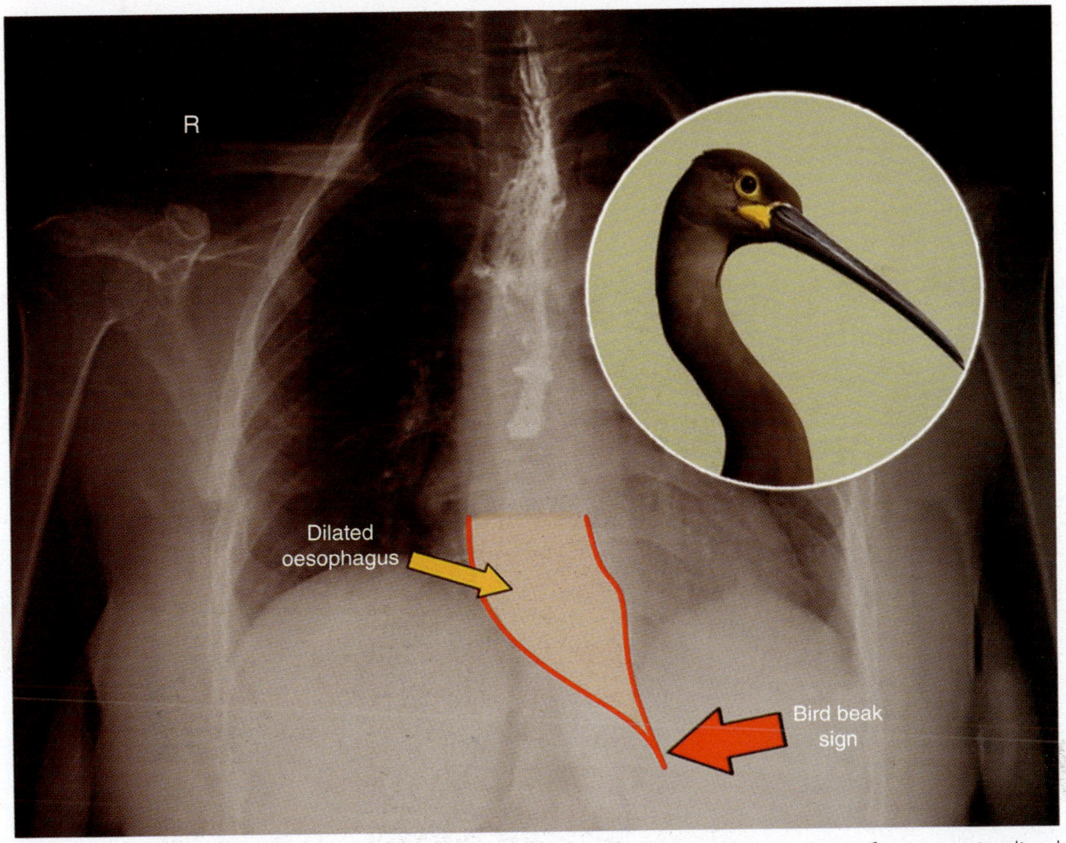

Barium swallow (anteroposterior [AP] view) reveals uniformly dilated oesophagus with pooling of contrast in distal one-third. Fixed abrupt narrowing seen at the gastro-oesophageal junction with a 'bird-beak' configuration – achalasia cardia. Although, the 'bird-beak sign' is often synonymous with the 'rat-tail sign', the latter is traditionally used to signify irregular narrowing related to malignant strictures or pathologies.

Achalasia Cardia

- Achalasia cardia is a type of oesophageal dysmotility disorder characterized by the failure of the lower oesophageal sphincter to relax. Patients complain of dysphagia to both solids and liquids. The underlying aetiology is the loss of ganglion cells in the myenteric (Auerbach's) plexus. It is of two types – primary achalasia (idiopathic cause of loss of Auerbach plexus) and secondary achalasia (pseudoachalasia). Pseudoachalasia may be caused by malignancy, brainstem stroke, strictures due to chronic gastro-oesophageal reflux and Chagas disease.
- Treatment is aimed at relaxing the lower oesophageal sphincter and consists of calcium channel blockers, botulinum toxin injections and surgery (Heller's pyloromyotomy).

OSCE 21

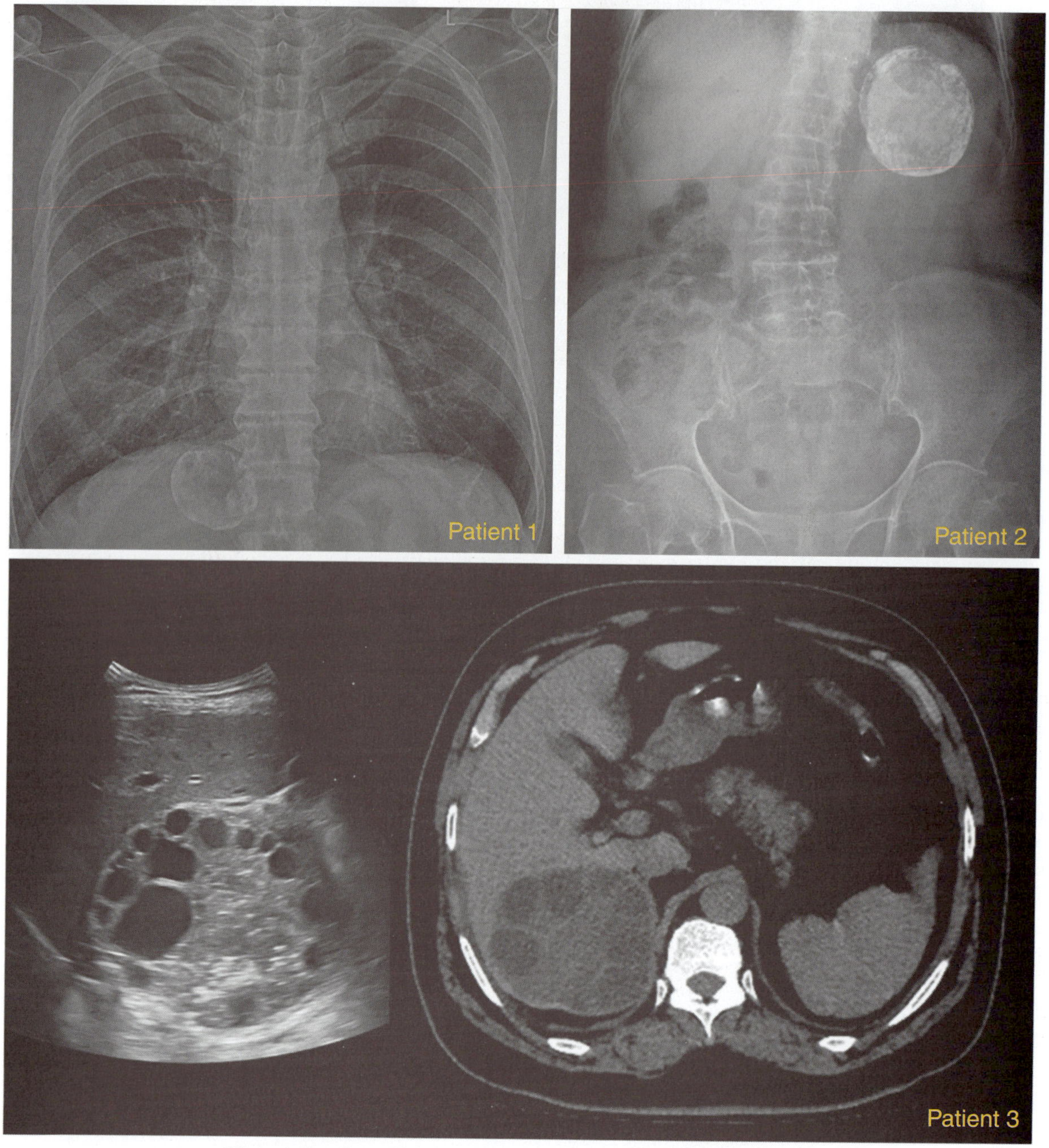

Clinical details: A 40-year-old patient with dull abdominal pain.

1. What is the most appropriate diagnosis in all the three cases?
2. What is the causative organism?
3. Which classification is used in ultrasound diagnosis for patient 3?
4. What should be the treatment in patient 3?

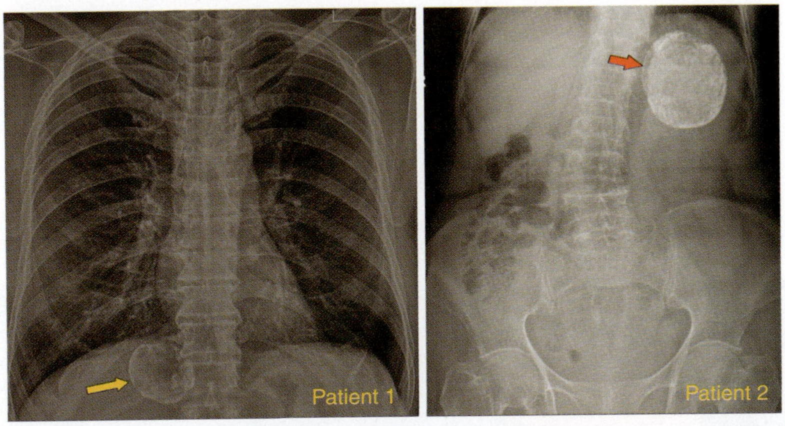

Case 1: Frontal chest radiograph demonstrated a well-defined rounded calcified hydatid cyst in liver (*yellow arrow*) seen just below the right hemidiaphragm in paramedian location.
Case 2: Erect abdominal radiograph shows a calcified splenic hydatid cyst below the left hemidiaphragm (*red arrow*).

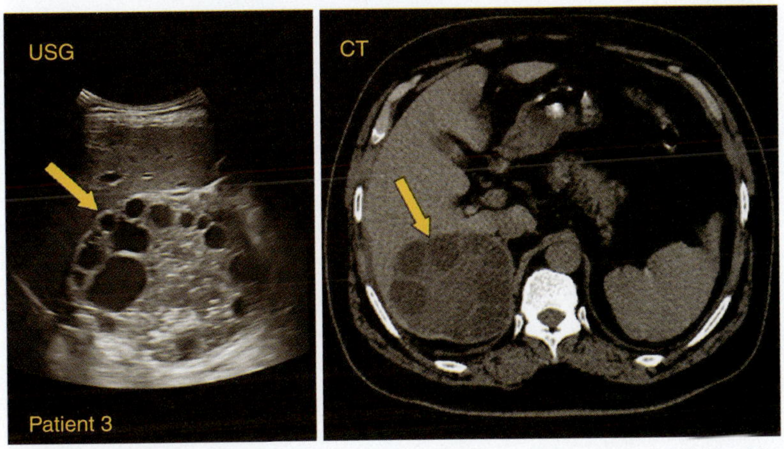

USG abdomen and axial non-contrast CT scan through the upper abdomen reveals a well-defined hypodense cystic lesion in segments VI and VII of liver, showing multiple daughter cysts within – consistent with hydatid cyst.

Hydatid Cyst

- Hydatid cyst is a parasitic infection caused by the tapeworm – *Echinococcus granulosus*. Dogs are usually the definitive hosts, whereas humans are accidental hosts. Infection occurs by ingestion of food which is contaminated by *Echinococcus* eggs. Cyst wall is made up of three layers, namely pericyst, exocyst and endocyst. Liver is the most involved organ. Calcified hydatid cysts can be seen as rounded opacities on radiographs.
- Puncture, Aspiration, Injection and Re-aspiration (PAIR) procedure is usually performed for the treatment of hydatid cyst.

GHARBI CLASSIFICATION IS THE COMMONLY USED ULTRASOUND CLASSIFICATION FOR HYDATID CYST

Type I: Purely cystic (homogenous) fluid collection

Type II: Fluid collection with a membrane/septation

Type III: Multilocular with daughter cysts

Type IV: Heterogenous appearance

Type V: Calcified cyst

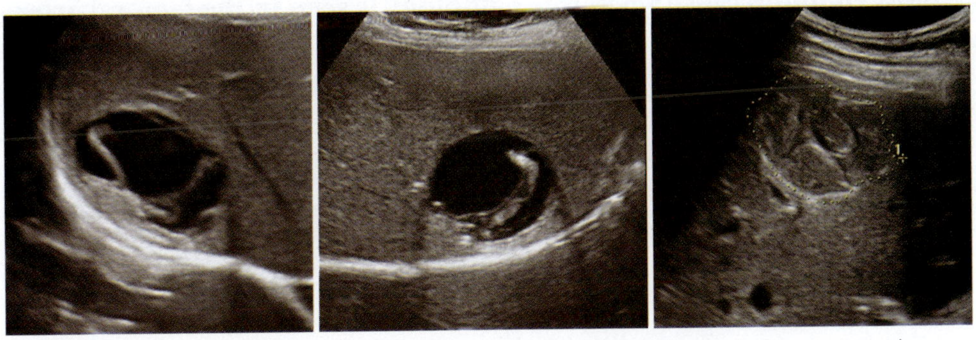

Three different cases of hepatic hydatid cyst seen on abdominal ultrasonography.

OSCE 22

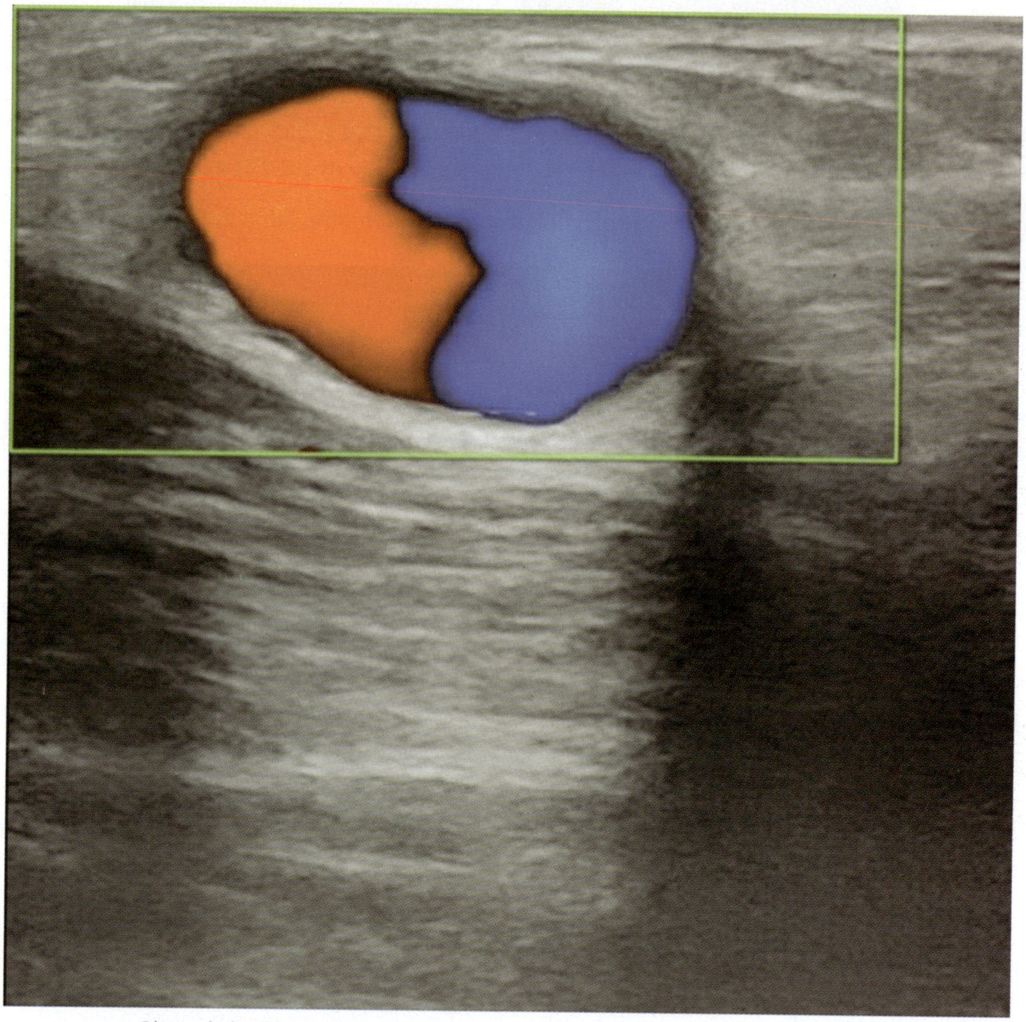

Clinical details: A 55-year-old male without obvious history of trauma.

1. **Identify the modality used.**
2. **What is the classical radiological sign seen here?**
3. **What is the most appropriate diagnosis?**
4. **Which is the most common cause when this pathology is seen in the femoral artery?**

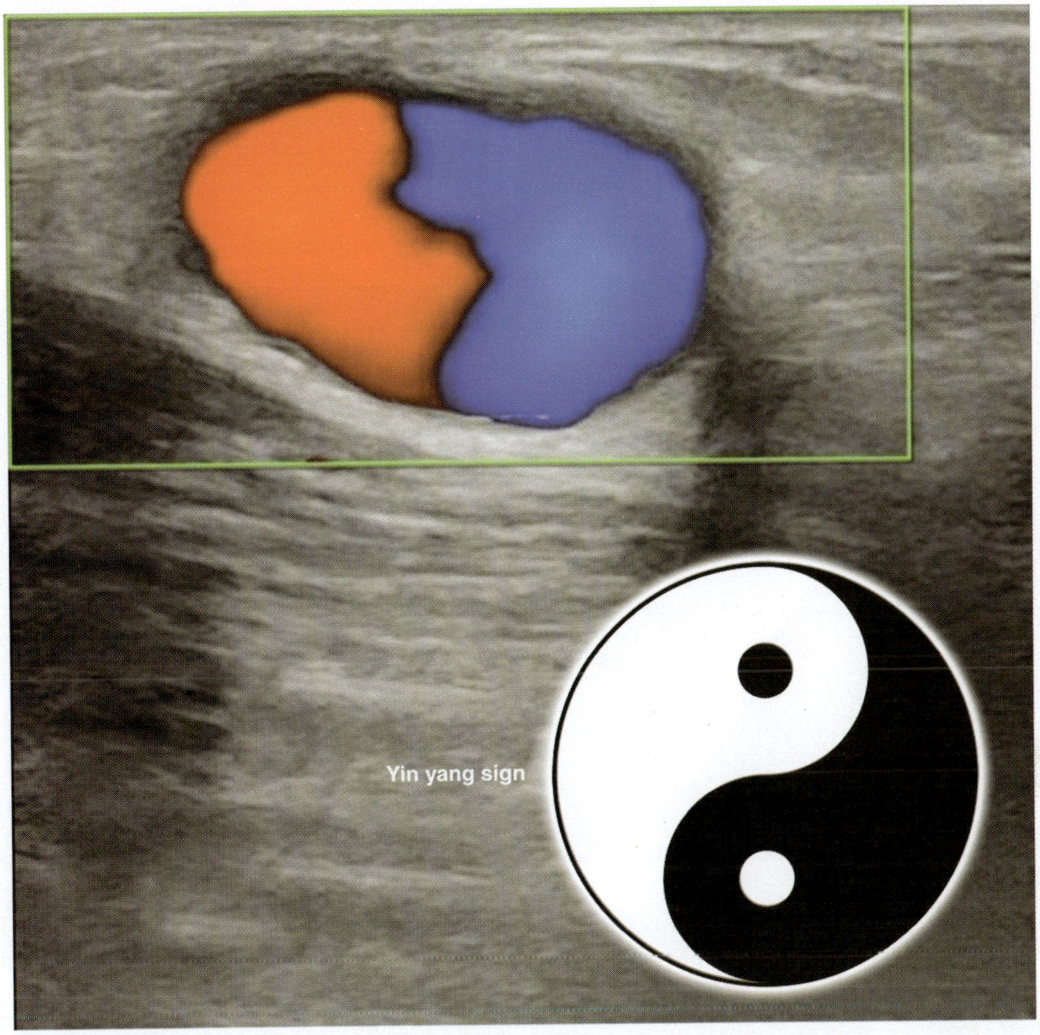

Colour doppler ultrasound image demonstrates the classical 'yin-yang sign' in a sac-like swelling in the right upper arm. It can be likened to the logo of the soft drink Pepsi and is also known as 'Pepsi sign'.

Pseudoaneurysm/Yin-Yang Sign

- A pseudoaneurysm is a false aneurysm which often develops in a blood vessel after accidental or iatrogenic trauma or inflammatory causes. Colour doppler is the most common modality used to evaluate pseudoaneurysms.
- Turbulent/swirling of blood is seen within the pseudoaneurysm due to the high velocity of flow. This causes the characteristic 'yin-yang sign' or 'Pepsi sign'.
- Most common cause of femoral pseudoaneurysm is iatrogenic – commonly due to endovascular procedures.

OSCE

23

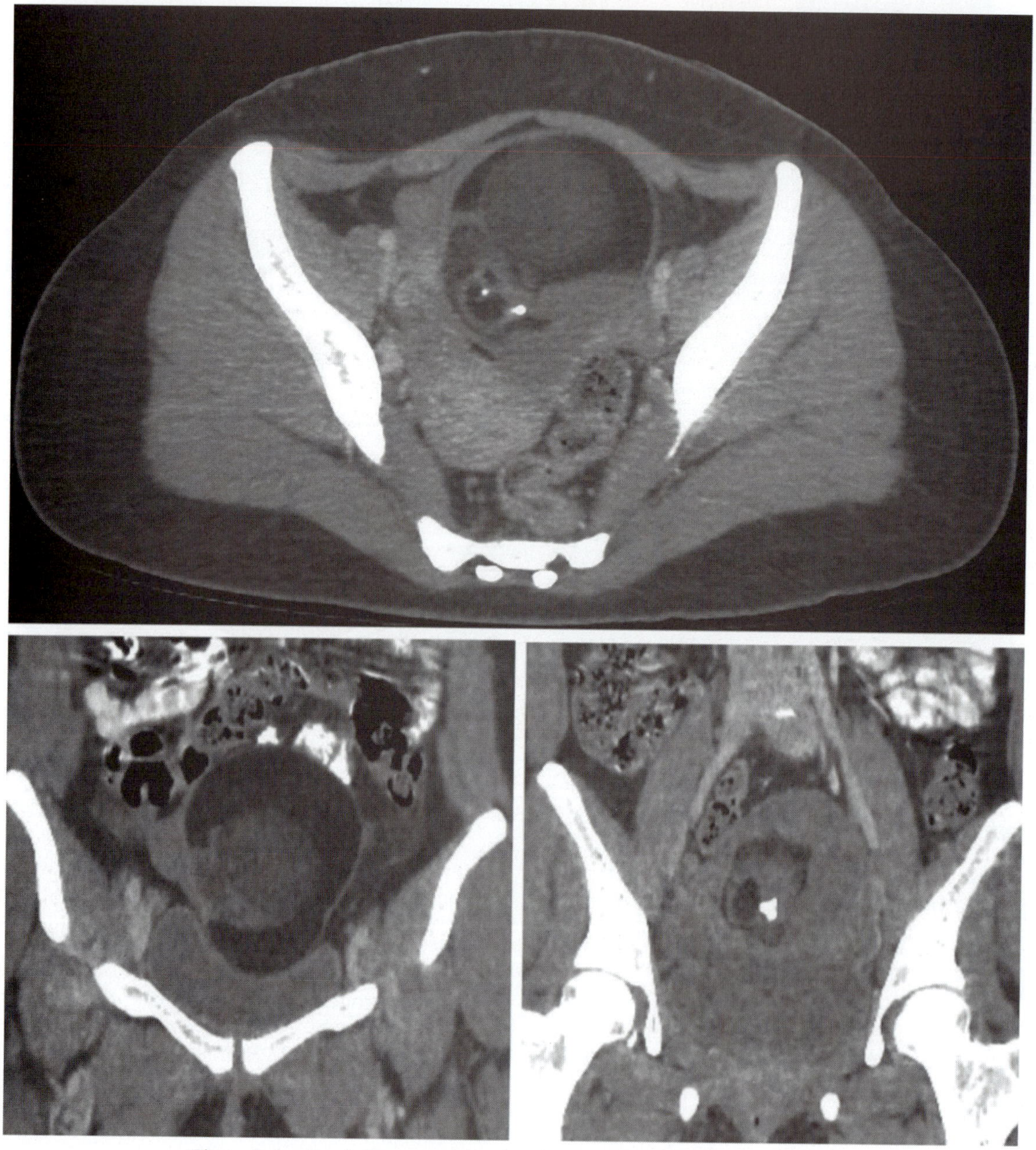

Clinical details: A 20-year-old girl with dull aching abdominal pain.

1. **Describe your findings and give the most appropriate diagnosis.**
2. **What is the most common complication associated with this lesion?**
3. **When should you suspect malignant transformation?**
4. **Enumerate two differential diagnoses of complex adnexal masses.**

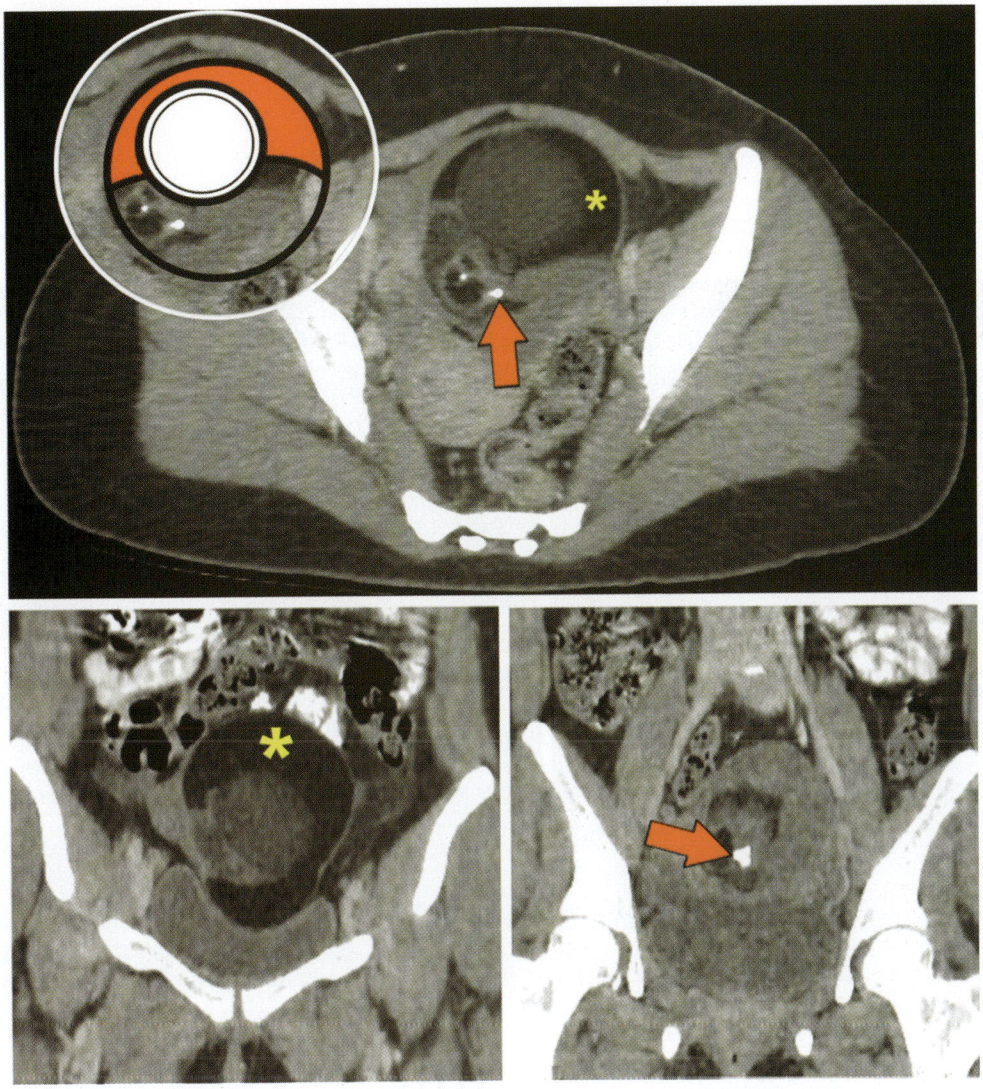

Axial and coronal CECT abdomen: Well-defined heterogenous pelvis mass with fat content (*) (attenuation of -98HU), soft tissue density and calcifications (*red arrows*), suggestive of an ovarian dermoid cyst. The first image demonstrates the classic 'Poké ball sign' of dermoid cyst.

Ovarian Dermoid Cyst

- Ovarian dermoid cyst or mature cystic ovarian teratoma is considered the most common ovarian neoplasm in premenopausal women. It is a slow growing benign neoplasm seen in the adnexal region. Calcifications, adipose tissue, hair and tooth are often seen in addition to fat components.
- **Ultrasonography** findings include cystic mass with echogenic contents (Rokitansky nodule/dermoid plug). Calcifications/tooth may be seen as high reflective components with posterior acoustic shadowing. Fat–fluid or fluid–fluid levels may be evident.
- **CT** is highly sensitive for ovarian dermoid cyst and can demonstrate fat components, calcifications/tooth and fat–fluid levels. Fat-suppressed magnetic resonance imaging (MRI) sequences may be used in the confirmation of fat components.
- **Ovarian torsion** is the most common complication associated with ovarian dermoid cysts. Ovarian torsion is a surgical emergency and should be promptly reported. Rarely, malignant transformation to squamous cell carcinoma has been reported in 1%–2% of cases. Malignant transformation is suspected when the size is more than 10 cm, contains enhancing soft tissue or demonstrated irregular walls. Lesions smaller than 6 cm are followed up annually to monitor growth. Larger lesions are resected surgically.
- Differential diagnoses for complex adnexal masses – cystadenoma/cystadenocarcinoma, haemorrhagic cyst, ectopic pregnancy, endometrioma and tubo-ovarian abscess.

OSCE

24

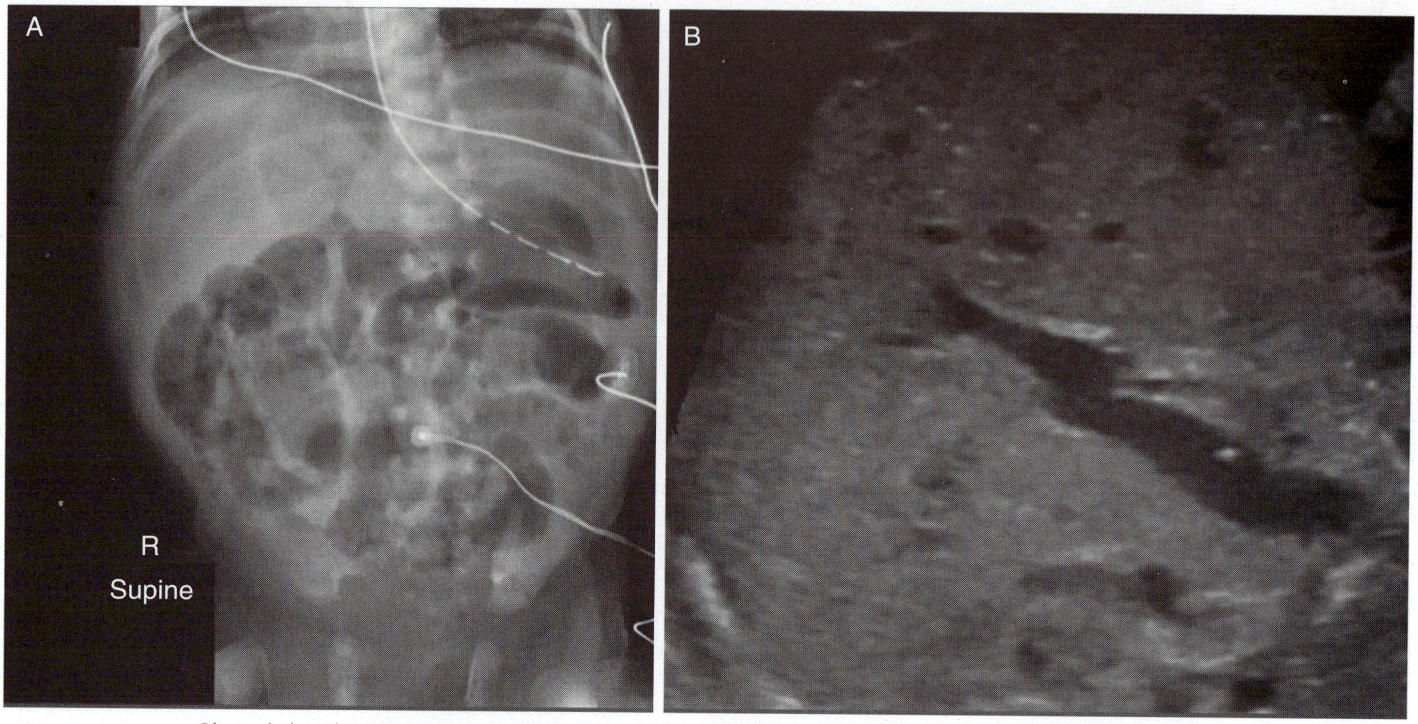

Clinical details: Seven days premature neonate with abdominal distension and bilious vomiting.

1. **What is the appropriate diagnosis?**
2. **Name two risk factors for this entity.**
3. **What are the four classic radiological signs seen here?**
4. **What is the management in this case?**

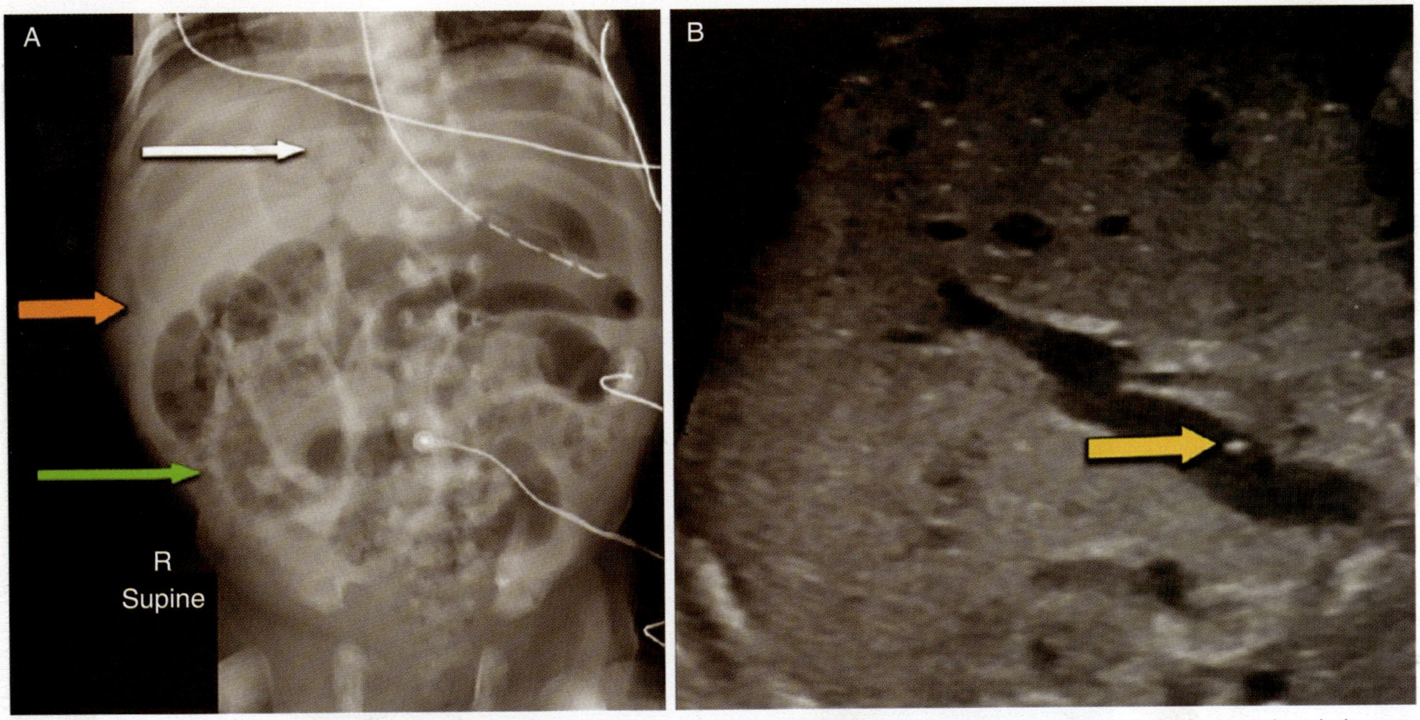

(A) Frontal radiograph of the abdomen: *White arrow* points to portal venous gas. *Orange arrow* points to free air in the abdomen. *Green arrow* points to bubbly lucencies in the bowel wall indicating pneumatosis intestinalis.
(B) Ultrasound of the portal vein: *Yellow arrow* points to echogenic focus in the portal vein indicating portal venous gas.

Necrotizing Enterocolitis

- Necrotizing enterocolitis is the most common gastrointestinal abnormality associated with prematurity. It is characterized by the permeability of the neonatal bowel wall to bacteria with associated inflammation and ischaemia. It is a potentially life-threatening condition with increased morbidity. Risk factors consist of prematurity, congenital heart disease, perinatal asphyxia and decreased umbilical arterial flow in utero.
- **Classic radiological signs:** On abdominal radiograph, bubbly lucencies in the abdomen indicating pneumatosis intestinalis are seen. Bowel wall oedema, portal venous gas and free air in the abdomen are also seen indicating pneumoperitoneum. Ultrasonography shows portal venous gas as echogenic mobile foci within the portal vein.
- **Management:** Necrotizing enterocolitis can be managed both medically and surgically and appropriate patient selection is essential in optimizing the outcome. A clinical staging system has been developed, with stages I and II receiving medical therapy and stage III undergoing surgery. Medical management consists of supportive measures and cessation of oral feeding, along with broad-spectrum antibiotics and gastric aspiration. Surgery is usually reserved for patients with evidence of perforation and entails resection of clearly necrotic bowel and the creation of a proximal enterostomy. Other relative indications for surgery include portal venous gas, a fixed dilated loop on serial X-rays and abdominal wall erythema on laparoscopy. Re-anastomosis is usually delayed until the infant has completely recovered.

OSCE

25

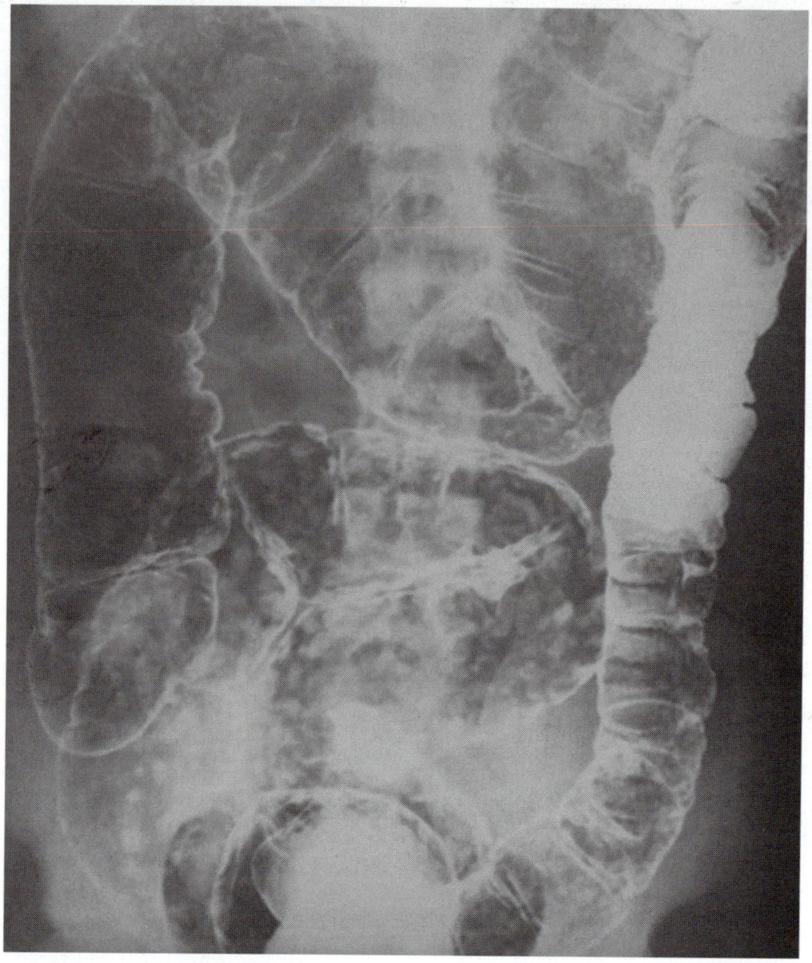

Clinical details: A 55-year-old with iron deficiency anaemia secondary to chronic painless rectal bleeding.

1. **Describe your findings.**
2. **What is the most appropriate diagnosis?**
3. **What another investigation/s would be recommended?**
4. **Name two hereditary polyposis syndromes.**

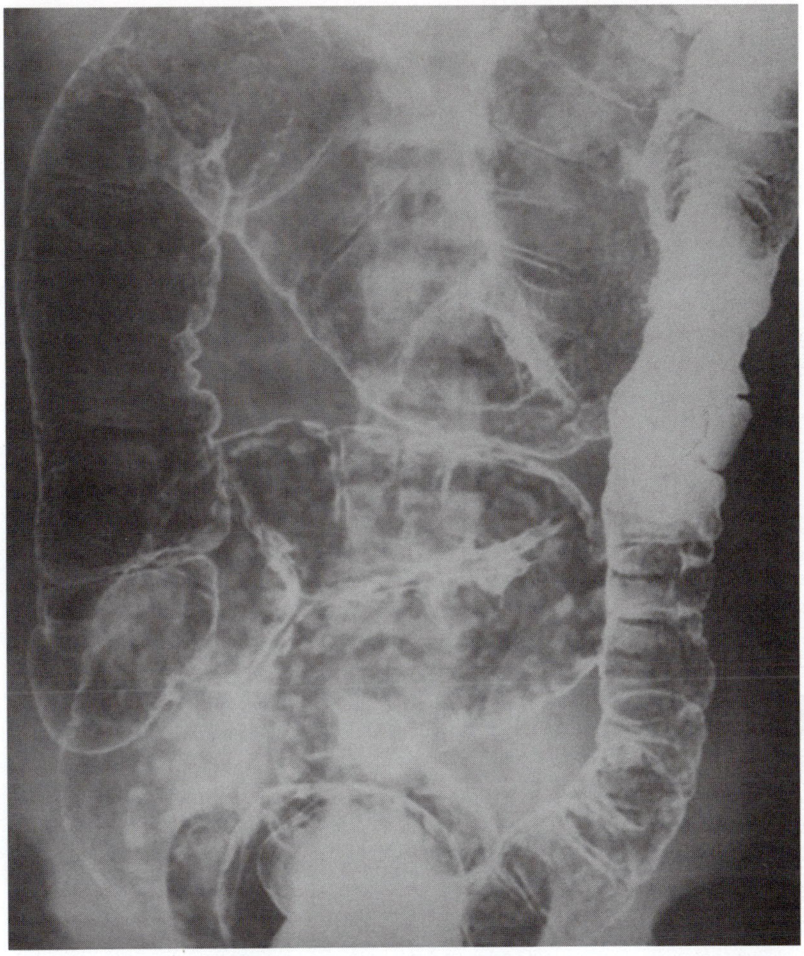

Double contrast barium enema image showing presence of multiple filling defects throughout the colon suggestive of polyposis. No evidence of mass lesion/external compression/stricture/contrast extravasation.

Colonic Polyposis

- **Colonoscopy** is the 'gold standard' method of detecting intra-luminal colonic lesions. Other investigations of value include 'CT colonography' or 'virtual colonoscopy', **magnetic resonance colonography** (MRC) and capsule endoscopy.
- **Hereditary polyposis syndromes** are as follows:
    - Hereditary non-polyposis colorectal cancer (HNPCC)
    - Familial adenomatous polyposis (FAP) syndrome
    - Gardner syndrome
    - Turcot syndrome
    - Cowden syndrome
    - Peutz–Jeghers syndrome
    - Juvenile polyposis syndrome (~25% are familial and autosomal dominant)
- **Non-hereditary polyposis syndromes:**
    - Serrated polyposis syndrome (SPS), also known as hyperplastic polyposis syndrome
    - Cronkhite–Canada syndrome
    - Juvenile polyposis syndrome (~75% are non-hereditary)

OSCE

26

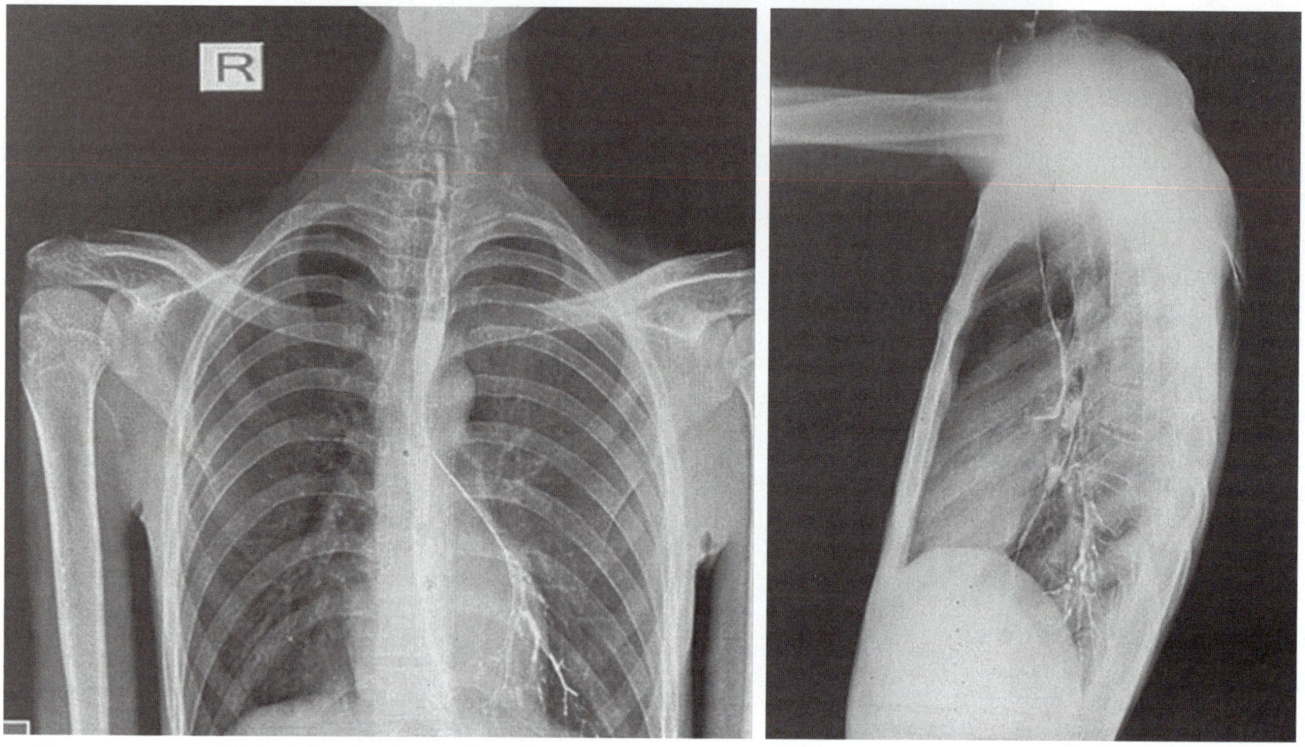

Clinical details: A patient undergoing barium swallow develops severe coughing.

1. **What is the most appropriate diagnosis?**
2. **What are the complications?**
3. **Who is prone to it and what are the predisposing factors?**
4. **What is the management?**

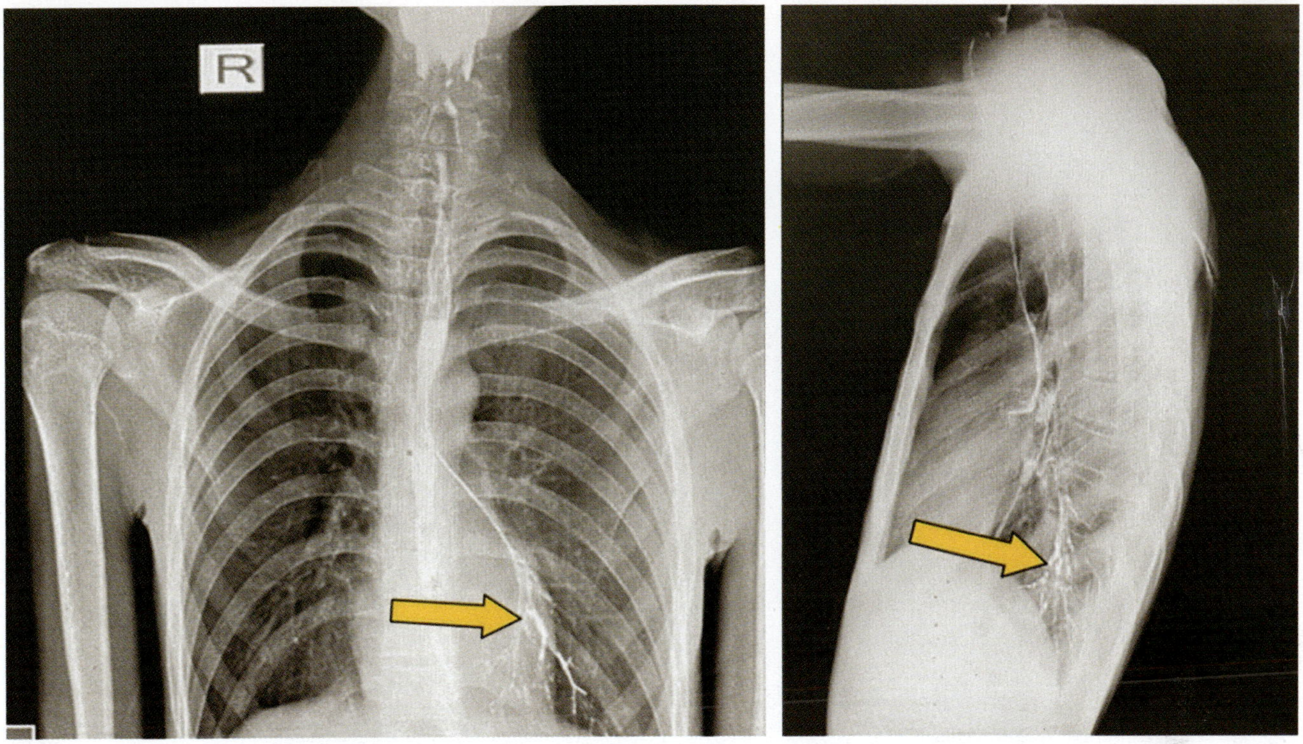

Frontal and lateral radiographs of the chest obtained following a barium swallow study. The larynx and peripheral tracheal lumen are opacified with barium. There is also abnormal opacification of the left lower lobe bronchi with barium (*yellow arrow*). These imaging findings are consistent with barium aspiration.

Barium Aspiration

- Barium studies are commonly performed in individuals with digestive tract disorders and barium swallows are indicated in patients with swallowing difficulty.
- Barium is an inert substance but its aspiration may cause consequences varying from patient been asymptomatic (microaspiration), morbidity to death.
- Microaspiration is usually asymptomatic and hence not detected.
- Complications are observed in cases with moderate amount of barium being aspirated and symptoms vary from cough, respiratory distress, hypoxia and even death.
- Barium is inert but can cause chemical pneumonitis and mechanical compromise of the alveolar system of the lungs by mechanical obstruction.
- Underlying aetiologies which raise the occurrence of aspiration include oesophageal motility disorders, altered level of consciousness and malignancies in the elderly age group.
- Moderate to large amount of barium aspiration should be managed with resuscitation and bronchoscopy with suction followed with physiotherapy and antibiotic cover to prevent secondary aspiration pneumonitis.
- Most severe complication is acute respiratory distress syndrome and is lethal even after mechanical ventilatory support.

OSCE

27

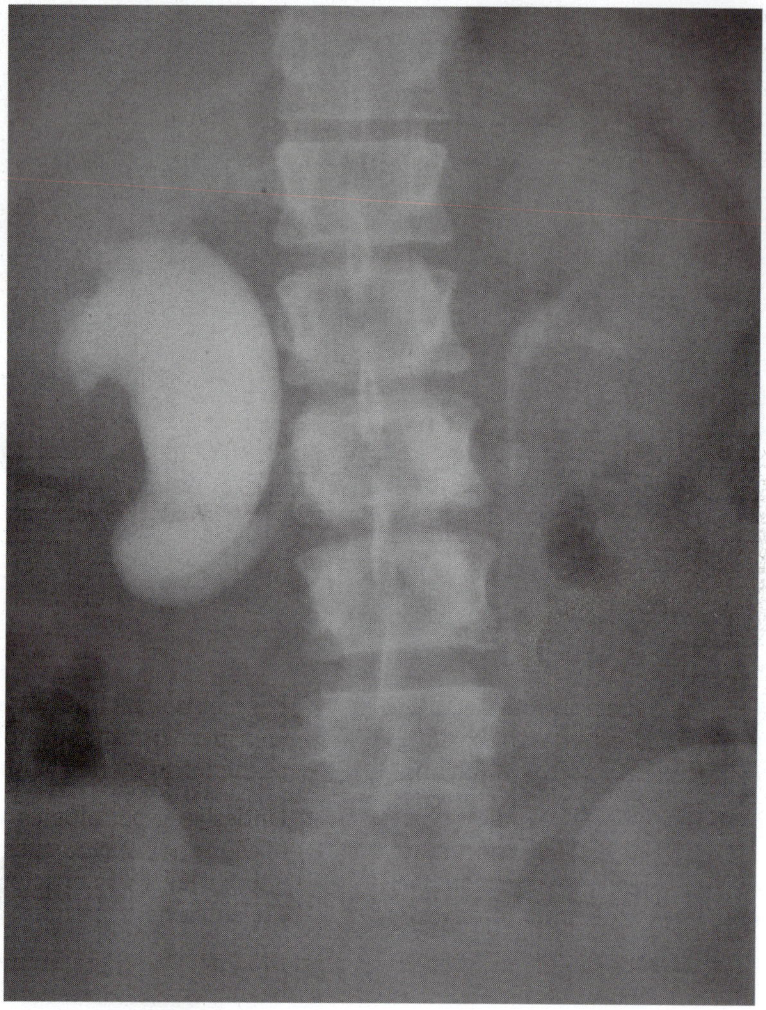

Clinical details: Patient with chronic right lumbar pain.

1. **Identify the investigation performed.**
2. **Describe your findings.**
3. **What is the most appropriate diagnosis?**
4. **How many types are there?**

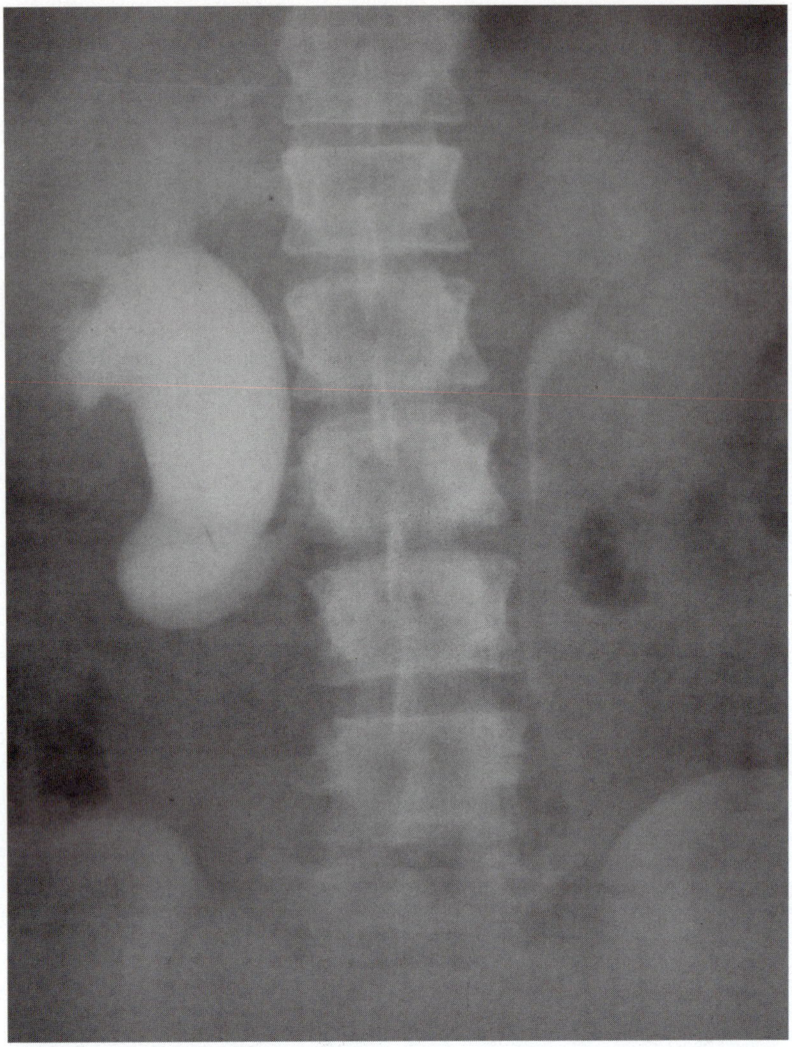

Spot film taken during intravenous pyelogram (IVP) shows right hydronephrosis with 'reverse J'-shaped right ureter in a case of retrocaval ureter.

Retrocaval Ureter

- Retrocaval ureter is an abnormal ureteric course which results due to a developmental anomaly of the inferior vena cava. It is also known as circumcaval ureter. This develops when the right supracardinal system fails to develop.
- Two types are known: Type I or low loop type and type II or high loop type. Type I is more common and is usually associated with moderate to severe hydronephrosis.
- On intravenous urography or intravenous pyelogram (IVP), the ureter is seen as a fishhook shaped or reverse J shaped/S shaped. Surgical management is recommended in symptomatic cases and severe hydronephrosis.

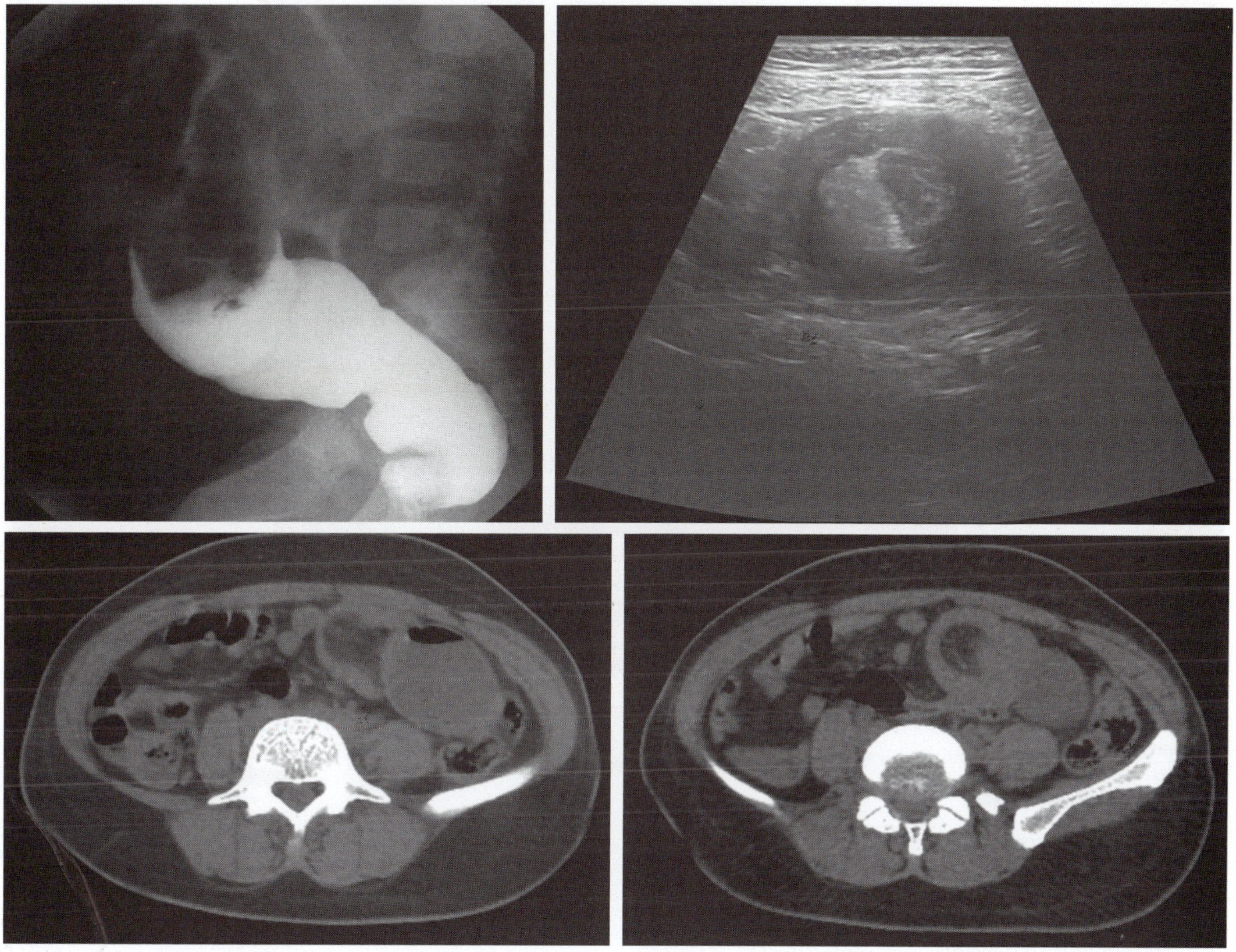

Clinical details: Child with red jelly-like stool with 'sausage-shaped' mass felt upon palpation of the abdomen.

1. Identify the investigations and describe your findings.
2. What is the most appropriate diagnosis?
3. Name two common lead points in adults.
4. Which is the most common subtype?

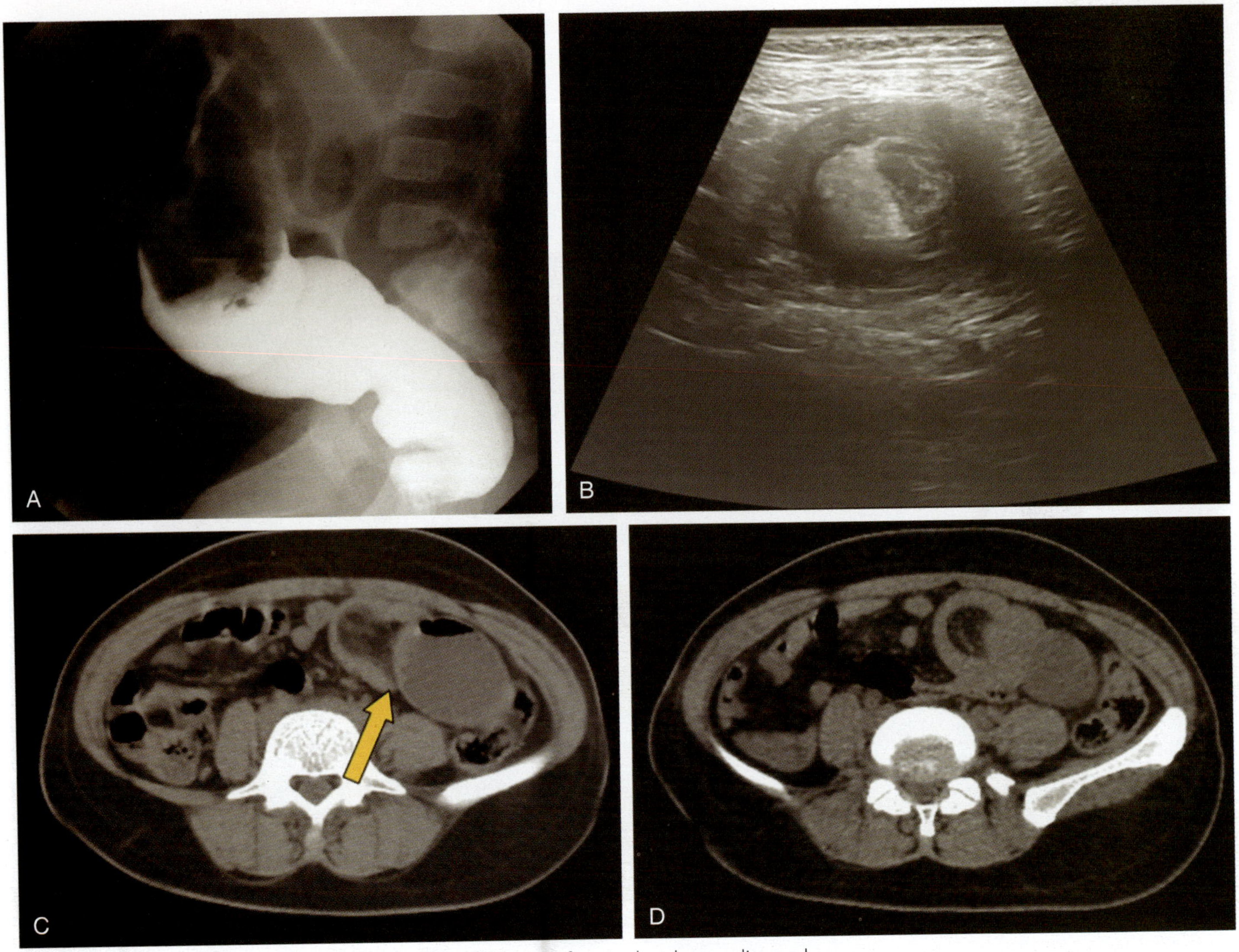

(A) Barium enema: Shows the typical claw-shaped filling defect in the descending colon.
(B) Transabdominal ultrasound shows the target sign (or doughnut sign) of telescoping of a bowel loop within adjacent bowel loop.
(C) and (D): Axial NCCT abdomen reveals the bowel-within-bowel configuration of intussusception.

Intussusception

- Intussusception is the telescoping of one segment of bowel loop into another adjacent segment of bowel loop. The 'receiving' bowel loop is called intussuscipiens, while the bowel loop 'prolapsing' is called intussusceptum.
- It is commonly seen in children and usually occurs without a lead point in children. In ~5% of cases, lead points may be observed – lymph nodes, Meckel's diverticulum, polyps and duplication cysts.
- In adults, a lead point is seen in majority of cases and include: GI malignancy (colorectal carcinoma, gastrointestinal [GI] lymphoma or metastases), benign neoplasms like GIST and polyps.
- The most common type of intussusception is the ileocolic type. Other types are ileoileocolic, ileoileal and colocolic.
- In children, it is usually managed by hydrostatic reduction or air enema. In adults, surgery is usually required (laparotomy).

OSCE

29

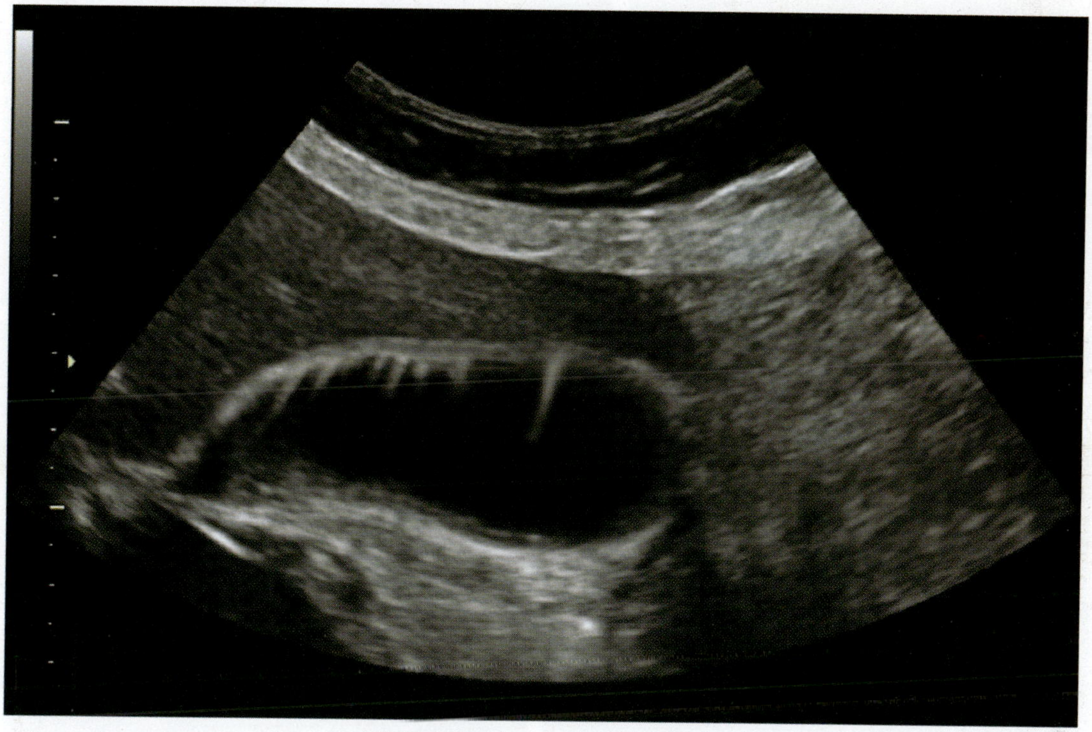

Clinical details: Incidental finding.

1. **Describe the findings in the provided image.**
2. **What are the three morphological types?**
3. **What classical artefact is observed in this case?**
4. **What is the pearl necklace sign?**

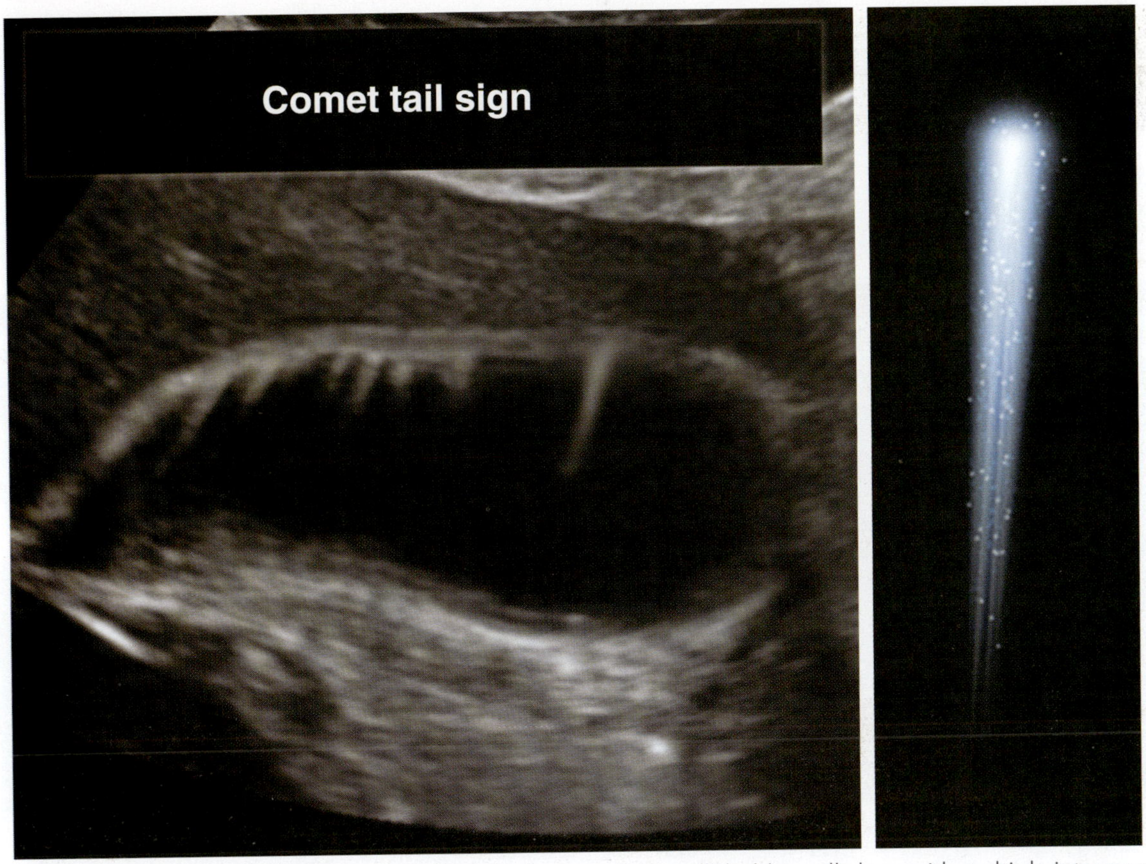

Selected ultrasound image of gallbladder reveals diffuse thickening of the gallbladder wall along with multiple intramural echogenic foci with comet-tail artefacts, suggestive of adenomyomatosis of the gallbladder.

Adenomyomatosis of the Gallbladder

- Adenomyomatosis of the gallbladder is a common benign condition of the gallbladder in which there is diffuse or focal hyperplasia of the gallbladder wall, along with the formation of multiple Rokitansky–Aschoff sinuses, which are exaggerated epithelial invaginations in the gallbladder wall forming intramural diverticulae.
- It is usually asymptomatic and is found incidentally on abdominal ultrasonography scans and usually requires no treatment. However, it can also be associated with biliary pathology such as gallstones.

RADIOLOGICAL FEATURES

- Ultrasound is the investigation of choice for diagnosing gallbladder adenomyomatosis. On ultrasound, adenomyomatosis of the gallbladder shows gallbladder wall thickening with associated intramural echogenic foci showing comet-tail artefacts. It may be focal, segmental or diffuse (generalized).
- **Comet-tail artefact** is a type of reverberation artefact where repetitive reflections occur within tiny structures, such as the echogenic intramural foci in the wall of the gallbladder in gallbladder adenomyomatosis.
- On MRI, gallbladder wall thickening is readily demonstrated, and Rokitansky–Aschoff sinuses appear as intramural lesions with low signal intensity on T1, high signal intensity on T2-weighted images and lack enhancement.
- The 'pearl necklace sign' refers to the unique curvilinear arrangement of numerous rounded intraluminal cavities appearing as hyperintense signal on T2-weighted MR imaging and MR cholangiopancreatography in gallbladder adenomyomatosis.
- Gallbladder adenomyomatosis usually requires no treatment in asymptomatic patients, absence of gallstones or any other pathology. However, a cholecystectomy may be necessary in certain cases where it may be difficult to differentiate focal adenomyomatosis from gallbladder malignancy.

OSCE

30

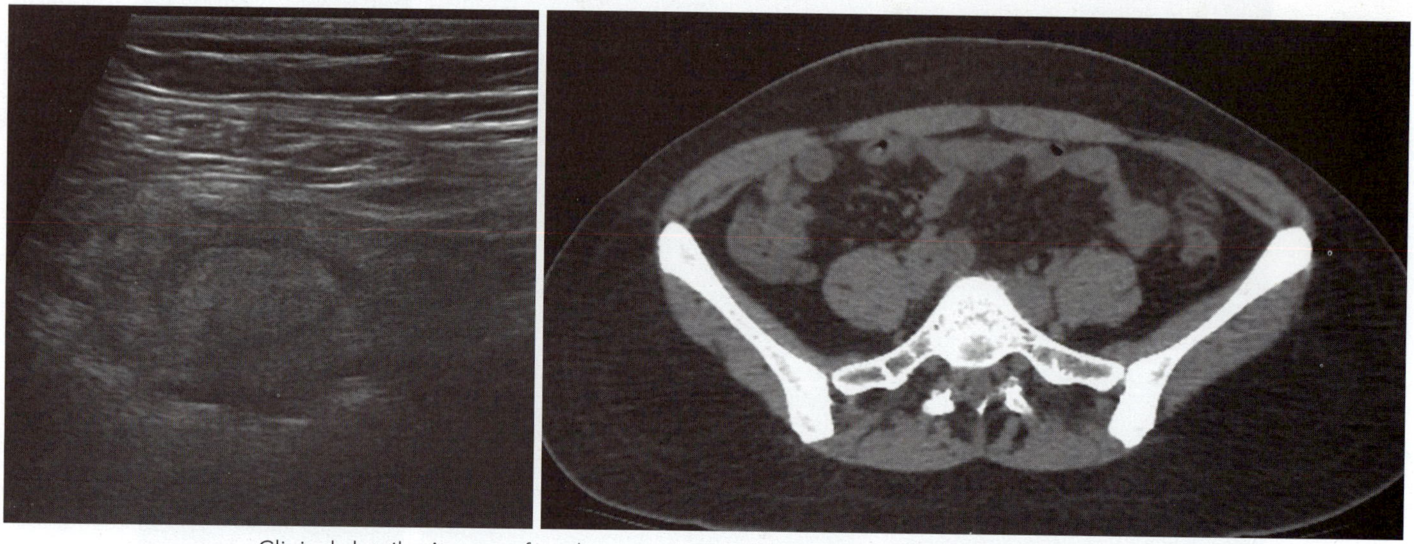

Clinical details: A young female presented with left lower quadrant pain for 3 days.

1. **Describe the findings shown on ultrasound and CT.**
2. **What is the most appropriate diagnosis?**
3. **Enumerate two points to differentiate it from omental infarct.**
4. **What is the treatment protocol?**

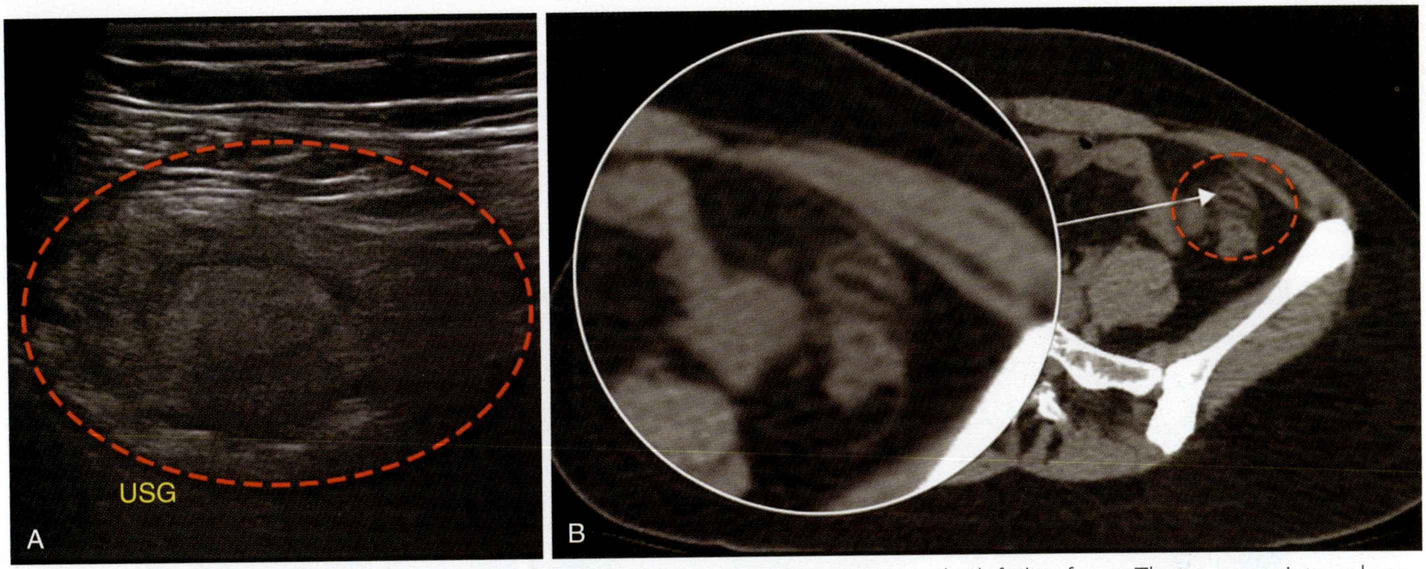

(A) Ultrasound abdomen reveals an ovoid mass like area of increased echogenicity in the left iliac fossa. There was no internal vascularity on colour Doppler (not shown in image). (B) NCCT of the lower abdomen shows an ovoid structure of fat density in the left iliac fossa, with a thin high-density rim. There is slight inflammatory fat stranding surrounding the lesion. There was no adjacent colonic wall thickening.

Epiploic Appendagitis

- Epiploic appendagitis is a benign condition which can clinically mimic diverticulitis. It usually manifests with acute pain in the lower quadrant, with similar features to acute diverticulitis. It is caused by either torsion of the appendage or spontaneous thrombosis of the blood vessel supplying it, leading to ischaemia and inflammation.
- Patient is usually present with localized pain and tenderness in the abdomen, most commonly in the left iliac fossa.

RADIOLOGICAL FEATURES

- On ultrasound, epiploic appendagitis is seen as a non-compressible, rounded or oval hyperechoic mass like lesion, without showing any internal vascularity. It is usually surrounded by a thin hypoechoic line or rim. It is usually less than 3 cm in size.
- Features on CT are rather characteristic:
  - Ovoid fat density structure in the left iliac fossa with a thin high-density rim (hyperattenuating ring sign) and surrounding inflammatory fat stranding
  - A hyperdense dot may be seen in the centre, which represents a thrombosed vascular pedicle
  - Little to no adjacent colonic wall thickening
  - Most commonly seen in the left iliac fossa

Differential diagnosis includes (1) diverticulitis, (2) omental infarction, (3) mesenteric panniculitis and (4) acute appendicitis if the pain is right sided.

Epiploic appendagitis is usually treated conservatively with oral anti-inflammatory drugs. It is usually self-limiting and does not require any surgical treatment. Most patients recover within 10 days with conservative anti-inflammatory medication.

Epiploic Appendagitis	Omental Infarction
• Usually less than 3 cm in size (smaller)	• Usually more than 5 cm in size (larger)
• More common on the left side	• More common on the right side
• Hyperattenuating ring sign is present	• No hyperattenuating ring sign

OSCE

31

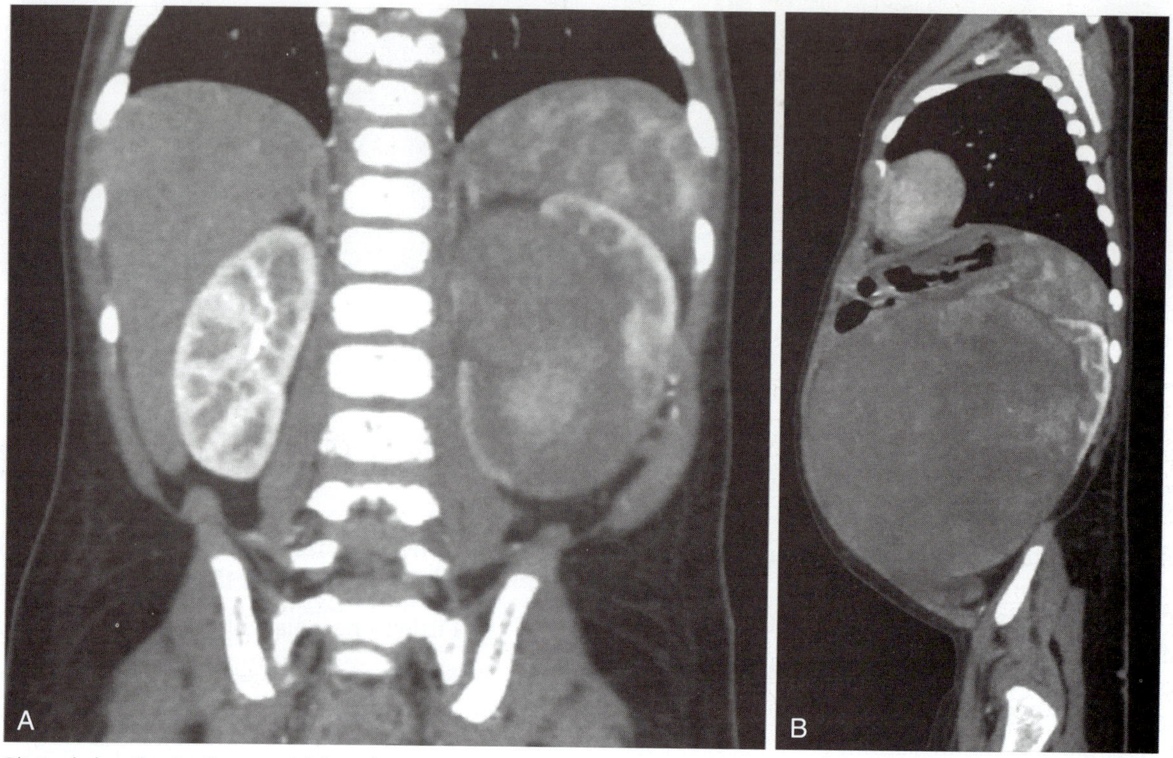

Clinical details: An 8-year-old female presented with left upper quadrant abdominal mass with hypertension.

1. **Describe the findings in the provided images?**
2. **What is the most appropriate diagnosis?**
3. **Name two associated syndromes.**
4. **List four differentiating points between this pathology and neuroblastoma.**

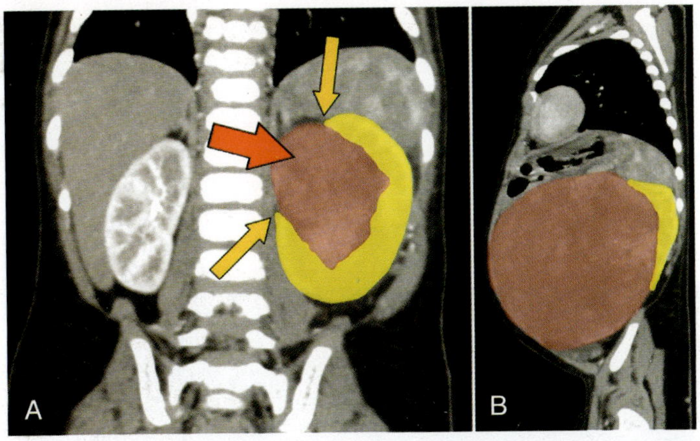

Coronal and sagittal contrast-enhanced computed tomography (CT) scan shows a large heterogeneously enhancing mass lesion (*red*) arising from the left kidney (*yellow*). *Yellow arrows* demonstrate the claw sign.

Wilms Tumour

Wilms tumour, or nephroblastoma, is the most common renal malignancy of childhood. The peak incidence is between 3 and 4 years of age, with the majority of patients presenting before the age of 5 years. It may occur earlier, especially with syndromic associations.

SYNDROMES ASSOCIATED WITH WILMS TUMOUR

- WAGR syndrome (Wilms, Aniridia, Genitourinary abnormalities and Mental retardation)
- Beckwith–Wiedemann syndrome (hemihypertrophy, macroglossia, omphalocele, localized gigantism and organomegaly)
- Denys–Drash syndrome (Wilms, male pseudohermaphroditism and glomerulonephritis)
- Perlman syndrome
- Sotos syndrome

It usually presents as a painless abdominal mass in the upper quadrant. Haematuria is seen in one-fifth of the cases. Due to the excess production of renin, hypertension may be present.

Claw sign: The 'claw sign' is a useful indicator in determining whether a mass arises from a solid organ or is just located adjacent to it, causing its compression. When the adjacent organ forms sharp angles around the mass, then claw sign is positive, signifying that the mass is arising from that particular organ.

RADIOLOGICAL FEATURES

X-ray abdomen	A large Wilms tumour may be seen on a plain radiograph as a large soft tissue opacity displacing the adjacent bowel loops.
Ultrasound	USG is usually the primary investigation done in suspected paediatric renal tumours. On USG, Wilms tumour is seen as a solid mass with heterogeneous echotexture (haemorrhage, necrosis and/or calcifications). IVC examination is necessary to detect tumour invasion. The 'claw sign' may be seen on ultrasound.
CT	CT demonstrates a heterogeneous soft tissue mass with or without haemorrhage, necrosis and calcifications. Enhancement is usually heterogeneous, though less than that of the adjacent renal parenchyma. 'Claw sign' helps differentiate it from a neuroblastoma. Other important findings which must be reported are tumour invasion into the renal veins and inferior vena cava, synchronous contralateral mass, lymph nodes or hepatic metastatic deposits and lung metastasis.
MRI	MRI is often used for staging and for assessing IVC invasion. Wilms tumour appears hypointense on T1, hyperintense on T2 and enhances heterogeneously post-contrast.

Treatment of Wilms tumour usually involves nephrectomy and chemotherapy.

An important imaging differential is neuroblastoma.

Wilms Tumour	Neuroblastoma
• Age group = 3–4 years	• Younger age group = below 2 years
• It displaces the adjacent structures	• It encases vascular structures without invasion
• Calcification is uncommon (10%)	• Calcification is common (90%)
• It is usually well marginated	• Poorly marginated
• Claw sign with kidney is positive	• No claw sign with kidney
• It extends into renal vein or IVC	• Causes elevation of aorta away from the vertebrae
• Lung, liver metastases; does not usually metastasize to bones (unless clear cell Wilms variant)	• Bone metastases

OSCE

32

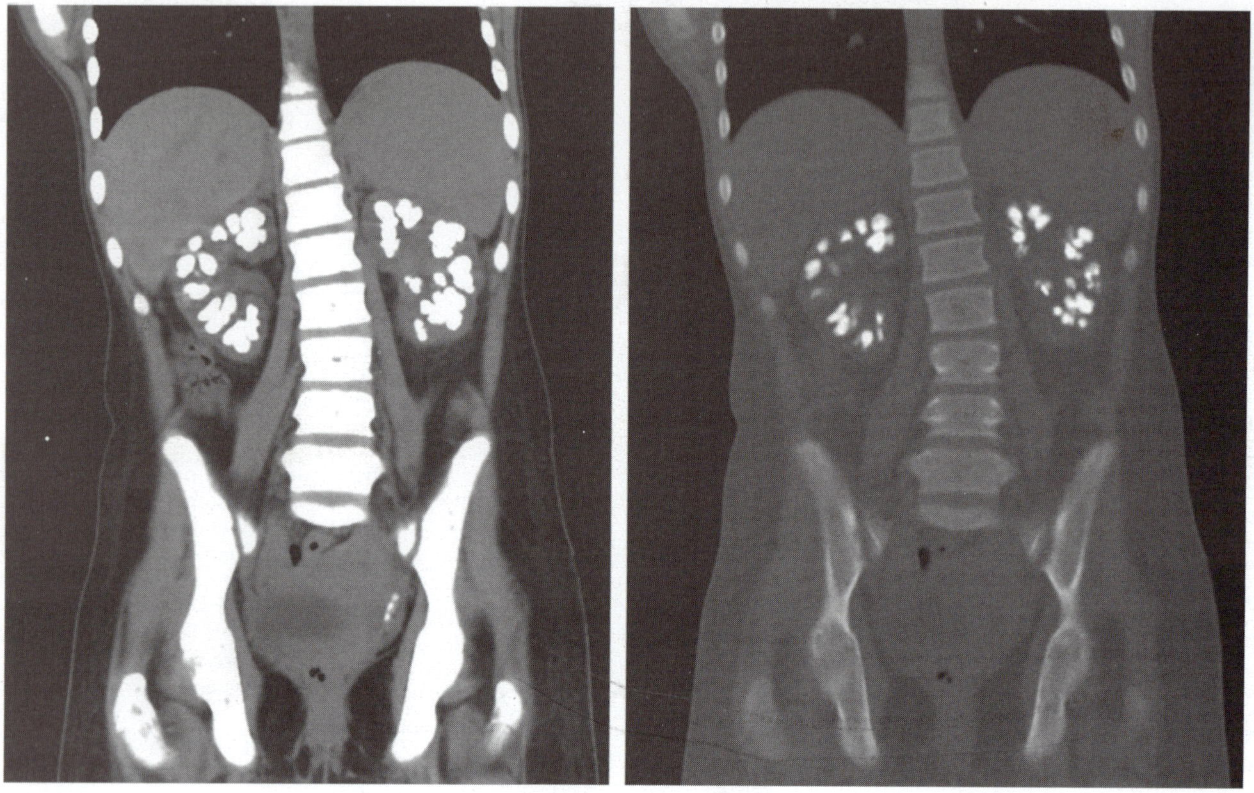

Clinical details: History withheld.

1. **Describe the findings in the provided images.**
2. **What is the most appropriate diagnosis?**
3. **List four causes for the above imaging picture. Which is the most common cause?**
4. **List two causes of cortical nephrocalcinosis.**

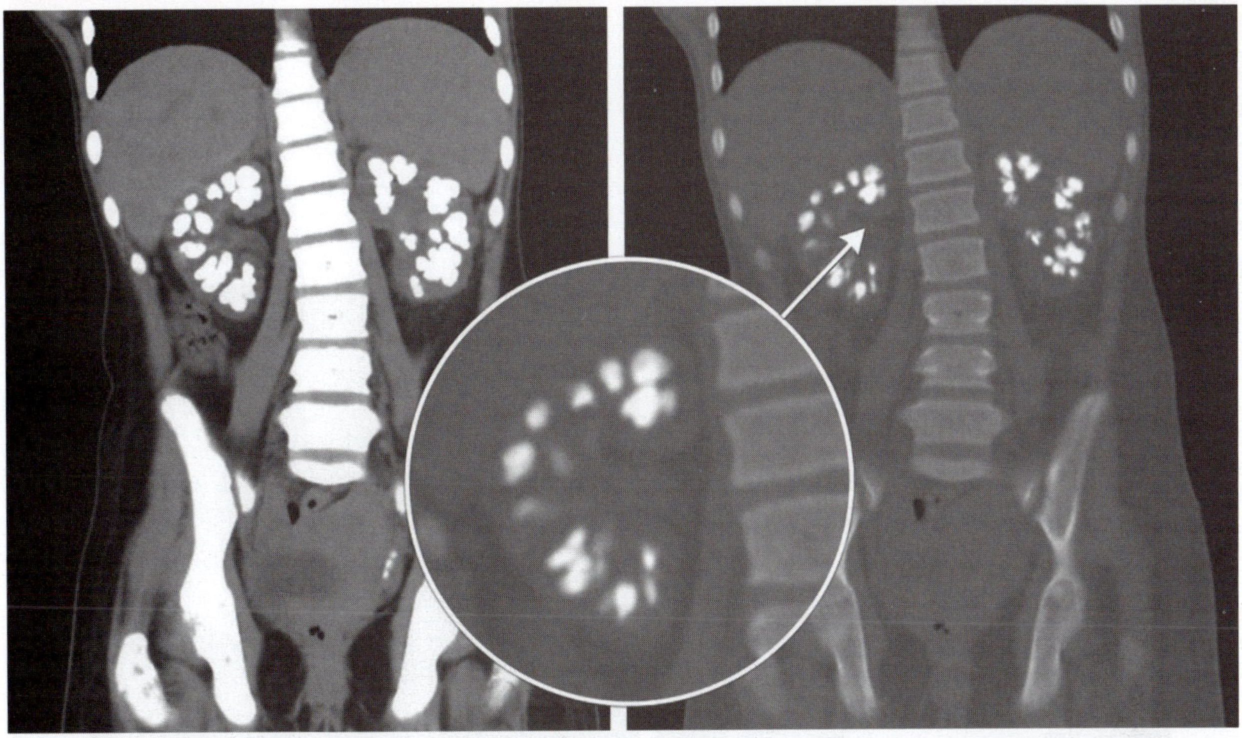

Coronal computed tomography (CT) images of the abdomen in soft tissue and bone window demonstrate multiple foci of dense calcifications in the medullary region of bilateral kidneys. There were no renal tract stones in the collecting system, ureter or urinary bladder.

Nephrocalcinosis

The abnormal deposition of calcium salts in renal parenchyma is termed as 'nephrocalcinosis'. It is divided into two types, namely:

1. Medullary nephrocalcinosis (more common): Deposition of calcium salts in the medulla of the kidneys; usually bilateral and diffuse type of deposition.
2. Cortical nephrocalcinosis: Deposition of calcium salts in the cortical regions of the kidneys; patchy type of deposition.

Causes of each type are as follows:

Medullary Nephrocalcinosis	Cortical Nephrocalcinosis
Hyperparathyroidism (most common cause)	Cortical necrosis
Medullary sponge kidney	Hyperoxaluria or oxalosis
Renal tubular acidosis (type 1)	Chronic glomerulonephritis
Papillary necrosis	Alport syndrome
Hypercalcaemia or hypercalciuria	
Renal tuberculosis	

OSCE

33

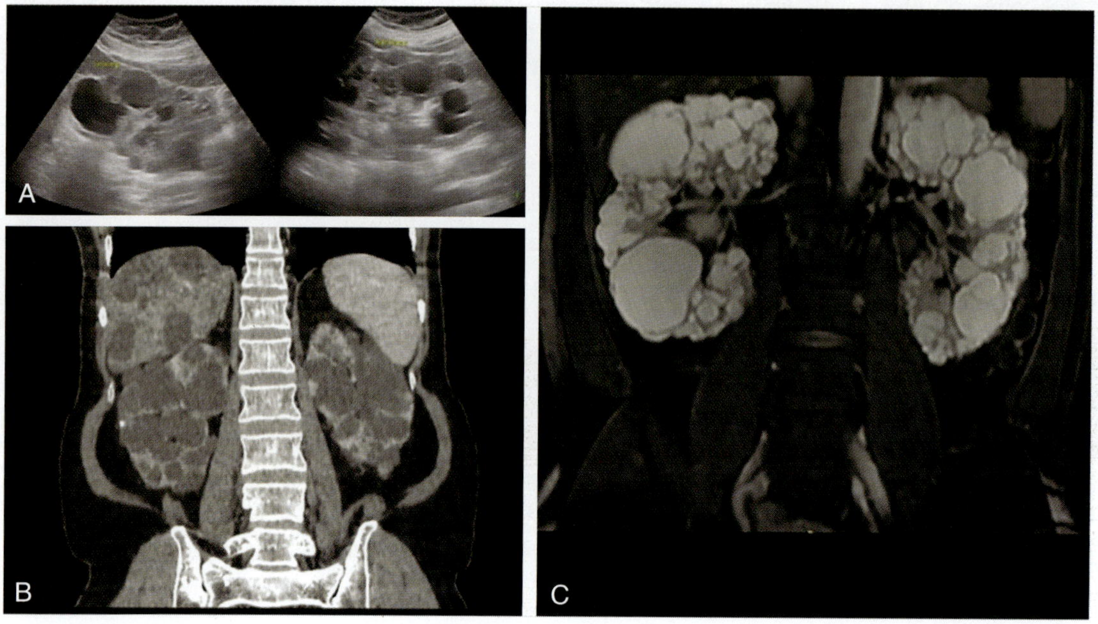

Clinical details: A young male presented with chronic dull pain in the bilateral flanks with haematuria.

1. **Describe the findings in the provided images.**
2. **What is the most appropriate diagnosis?**
3. **What is the concerning intracranial lesion associated with this condition?**
4. **List three possible complications of this pathology.**

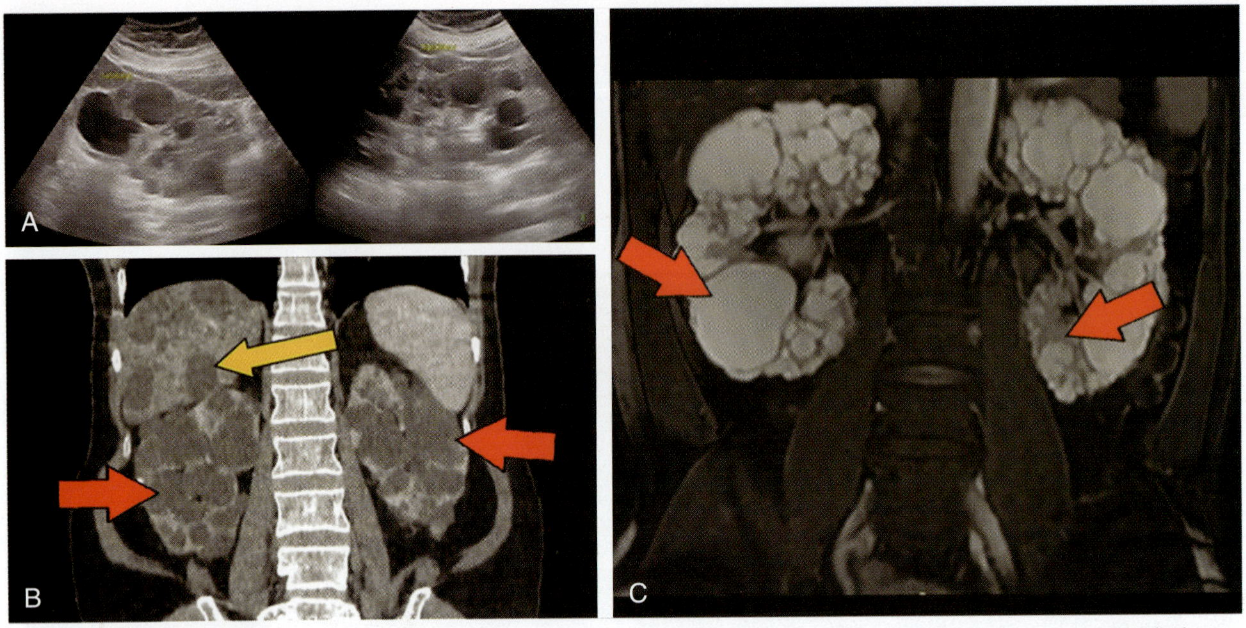

(A) Ultrasound, (B) coronal CECT abdomen and (C) coronal T2-weighted (T2W) magnetic resonance imaging (MRI) kidneys demonstrate innumerable cysts (*red arrows*) of varying sizes in the bilateral kidneys with distorted renal architecture. Additionally, CECT abdomen (B) shows multiple hepatic cysts (*yellow arrow*).

Autosomal Dominant Polycystic Kidney Disease

- Autosomal dominant polycystic kidney disease (ADPKD) is characterized by bilaterally enlarged kidneys with multiple cysts of varying sizes. Additionally, cysts are also seen in the liver, spleen and/or pancreas. Polycystic kidney disease 1 (PKD1) and polycystic kidney disease 2 (PKD2) genes are implicated in ADPKD.
- Clinically, patients may present with dull flank pain, haematuria, hypertension, abdominal mass or renal failure.
- ADPKD can be associated with a number of other conditions such as:
  1. Cerebral berry aneurysm
  2. Bicuspid aortic valve
  3. Mitral valve prolapse
  4. Multiple biliary hamartomas (von Meyenburg complexes)

RADIOLOGICAL FEATURES

Intravenous pyelography (IVP)	• 'Swiss cheese nephrogram' = bilateral enlarged kidneys with stretched renal calyces
Ultrasound	• Bilateral enlarged kidneys with distorted renal architecture and multiple cysts of varying sizes scattered in the bilateral kidneys • Posterior acoustic enhancement in the simple cysts • Cysts with complications such as haemorrhage, show increased echogenicity within the cysts • Cysts in liver, spleen and pancreas may be seen
Computed tomography (CT)	• Simple cysts appear hypodense with internal fluid attenuation and thin walls • Cysts with haemorrhage show increased density within them • Cyst wall calcifications may be seen
Magnetic resonance imaging (MRI)	• Simple cysts appear hyperintense on T2, hypointense on T1, without any solid enhancing components • Solid enhancement within the cysts raises the possibility of malignancy (RCC)

Complications include following:

1. Recurrent UTI
2. Haemorrhage or infection within the cysts
3. Calculus formation due to urinary stasis
4. Renal failure

OSCE

34

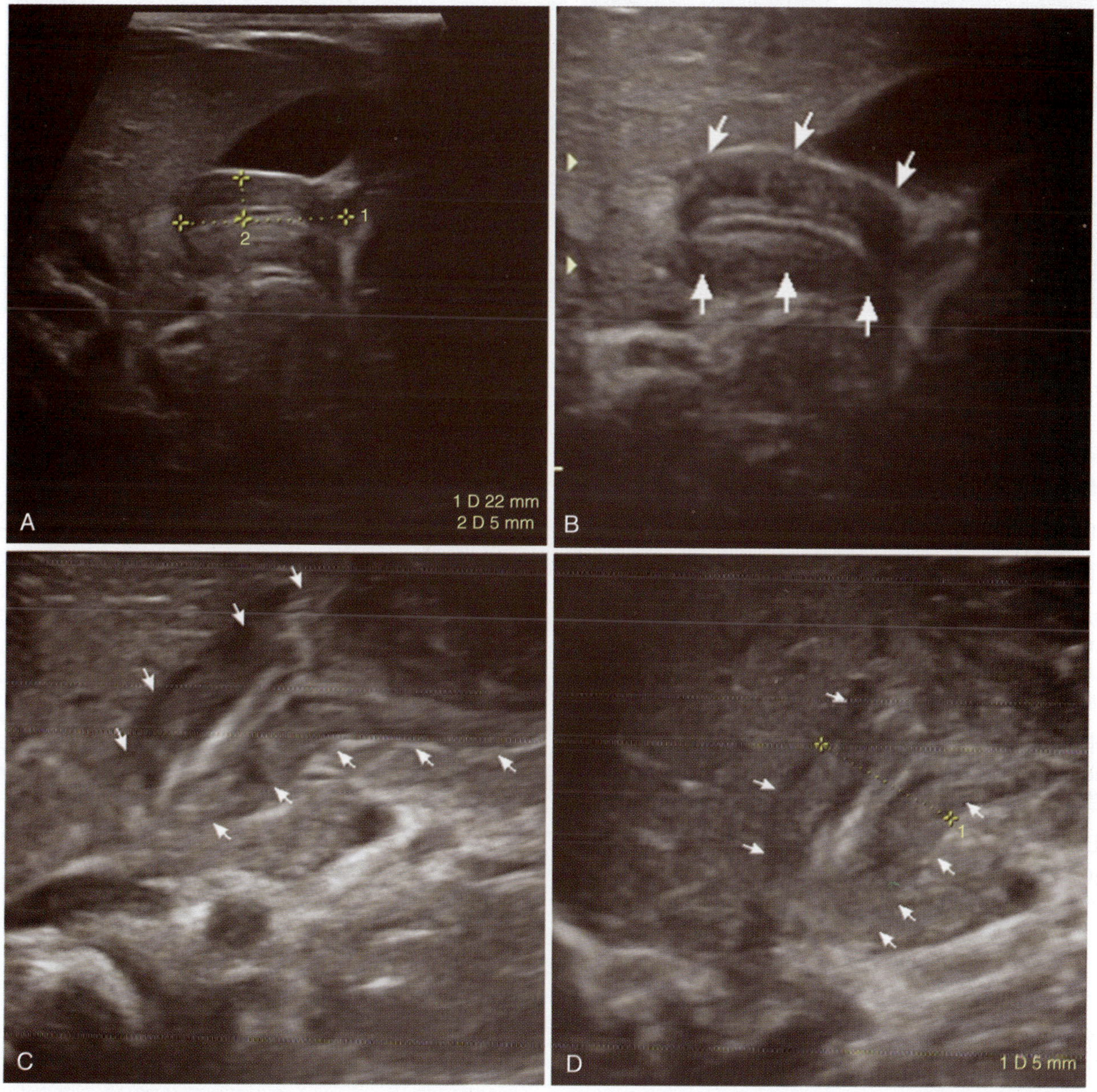

Clinical details: A 1-month-old infant was brought to the emergency with recurrent vomiting.

1. **What is the most appropriate diagnosis?**
2. **What is the characteristic type of vomiting seen in this condition?**
3. **What kind of electrolyte imbalance would you expect this infant?**
4. **Enumerate two sonographic signs of this condition.**
5. **List two other causes of upper gastrointestinal (GI) obstruction in the paediatric age group.**

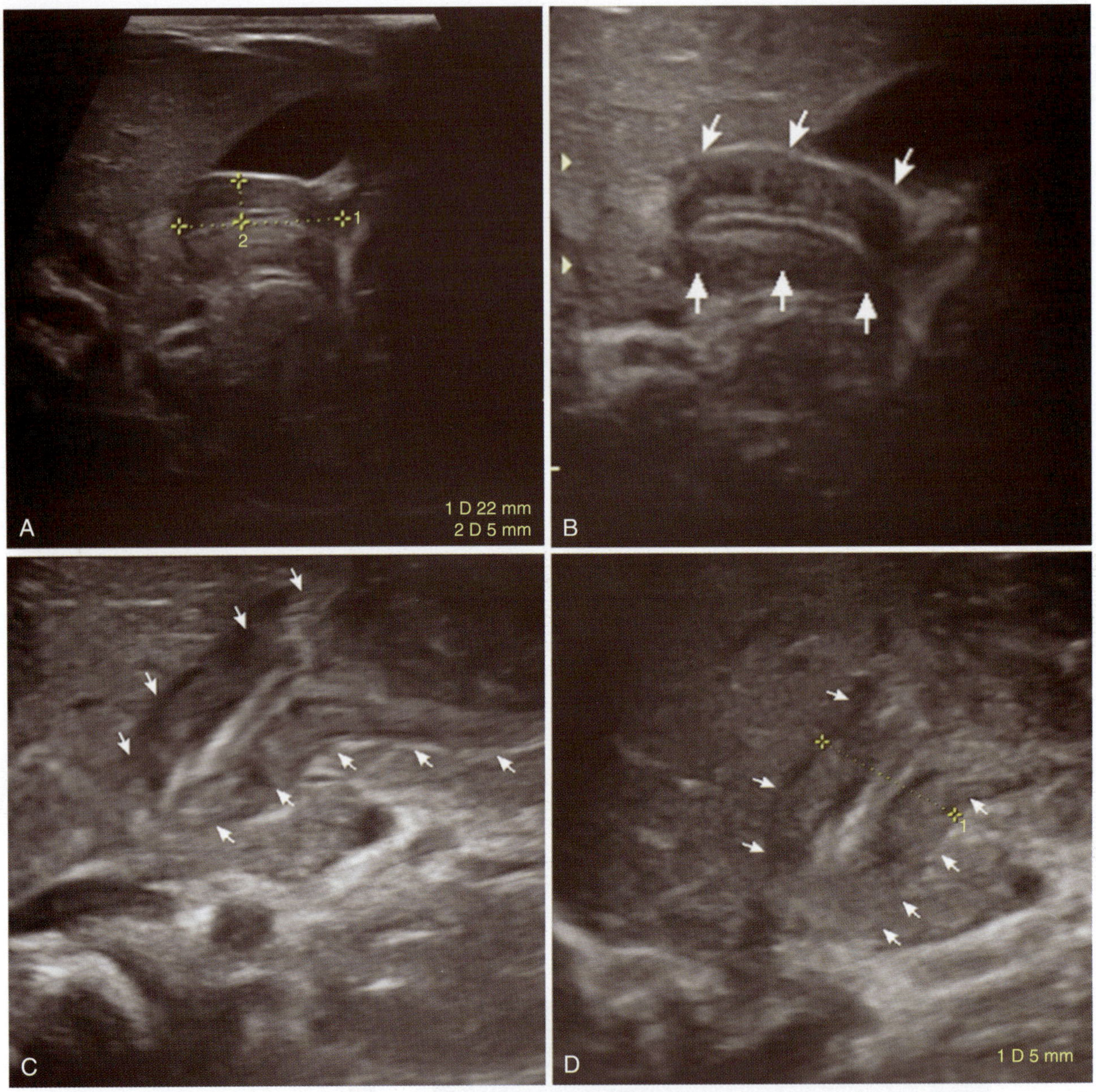

Ultrasound of the pylorus demonstrates increased thickness of the muscular walls (5 mm) and increased length (20 mm) of the pylorus, consistent with hypertrophic pyloric stenosis (HPS).

Hypertrophic Pyloric Stenosis

- Hypertrophic pyloric stenosis (HPS) is defined as idiopathic hypertrophy and hyperplasia of the muscular wall of the pylorus. This results in narrowing of the pyloric canal and causes gastric outlet obstruction. There is commonly seen in first born males and between 3 and 12 weeks postnatally. Vomiting is typically non-bilious and projectile in nature. Hypokalaemic hypochloraemic metabolic alkalosis is seen in this condition. Severe cases develop paradoxical aciduria due to the retention of sodium and water by the kidneys in exchange of hydrogen ions.
- HPS may be associated with Turner syndrome, trisomy 18 and tracheo-oesophageal fistula.

RADIOLOGICAL FEATURES OF HPS

Upper gastrointestinal (GI) series (barium meal/ fluoroscopy)	• String sign = a small streak of barium passing through a narrowed and elongated pyloric canal (most specific) • Shoulder sign = hypertrophied muscular layer causing an impression on the distended gastric antrum and appearing as a shoulder • Caterpillar sign = peristaltic wavy contour of the stomach wall, just proximal to the pylorus • Mushroom sign = mushroom-like indentation on the duodenal cap • Beak sign = beak-like configuration of the pyloric entrance • Tit sign = indentation over distal antrum by the pyloric canal

Ultrasound	• Elongated and hypertrophied pyloric muscular wall
	  ◦ Pyloric muscle wall thickness >3 mm
	  ◦ Pyloric length > 15–17 mm
	  ◦ Pyloric transverse diameter > 13 mm
	• Target sign on cross-sectional view
	• Antral nipple sign = redundant pyloric mucosa protruding into the stomach antrum
	• Cervix sign = hypertrophied pylorus indenting into the fluid-filled stomach antrum

- Initially, the patient is managed medically with the aim to correct the electrolyte imbalance. Eventually, surgical treatment with pyloromyotomy is performed for definitive treatment.
- Differentials include pylorospasm and other causes of upper GI obstruction such as duodenal stenosis/web and midgut volvulus.

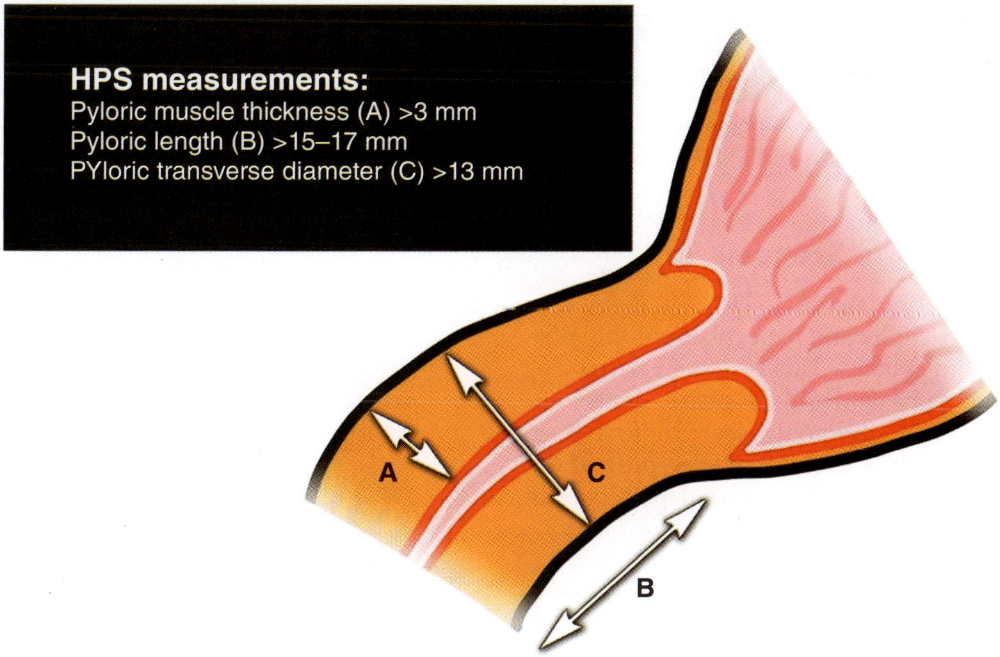

Adapted from Amini, B., Yap, J., Kearns, C., et al. Pyloric stenosis. Radiopaedia website. Updated on 7 January 2024. https://doi.org./10.53347/rID-1941

OSCE

35

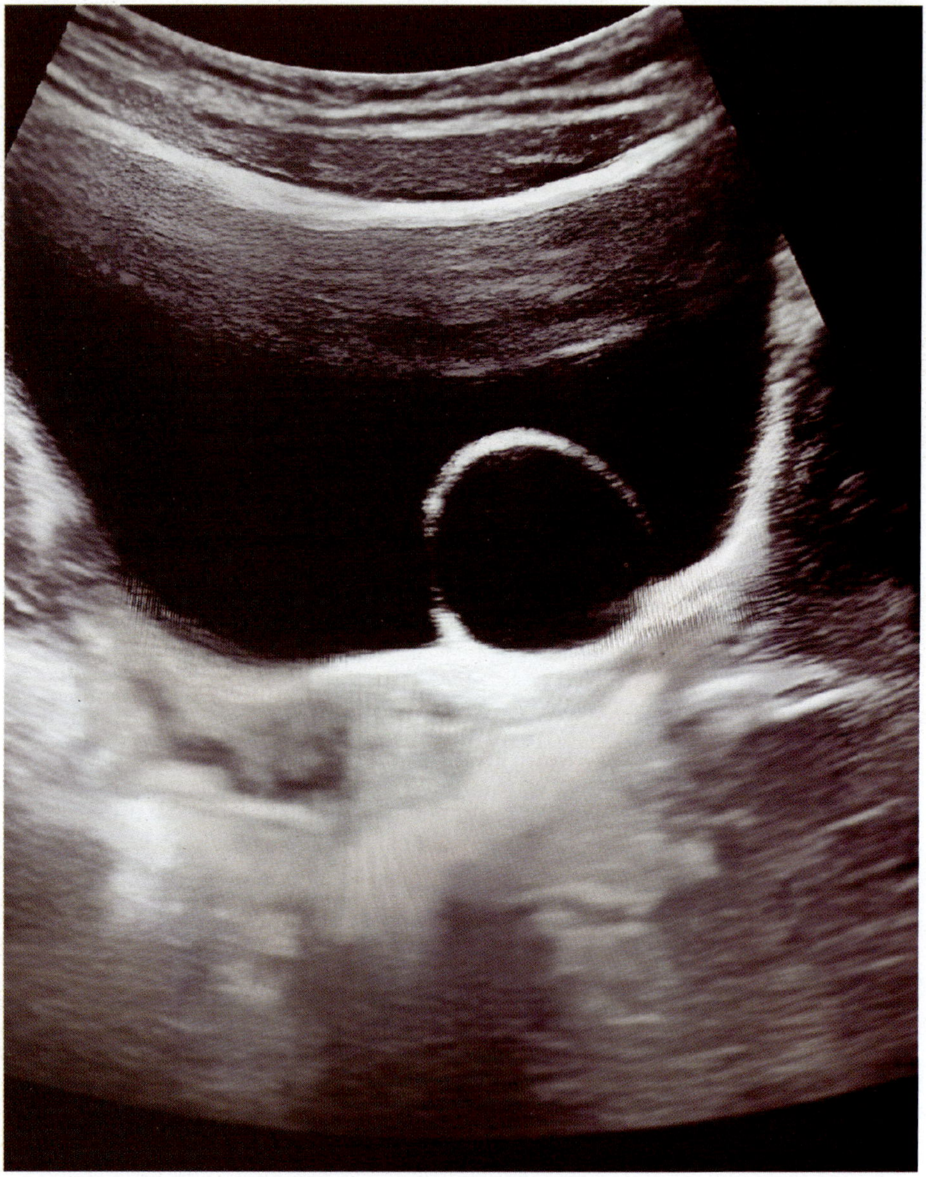

Clinical details: History withheld.

1. **Describe your findings in the provided image.**
2. **What is the most appropriate diagnosis?**
3. **What is the characteristic sign seen on intravenous pyelography (IVP) in this condition?**
4. **What is the Weigert–Meyer rule in duplicated renal collecting system?**

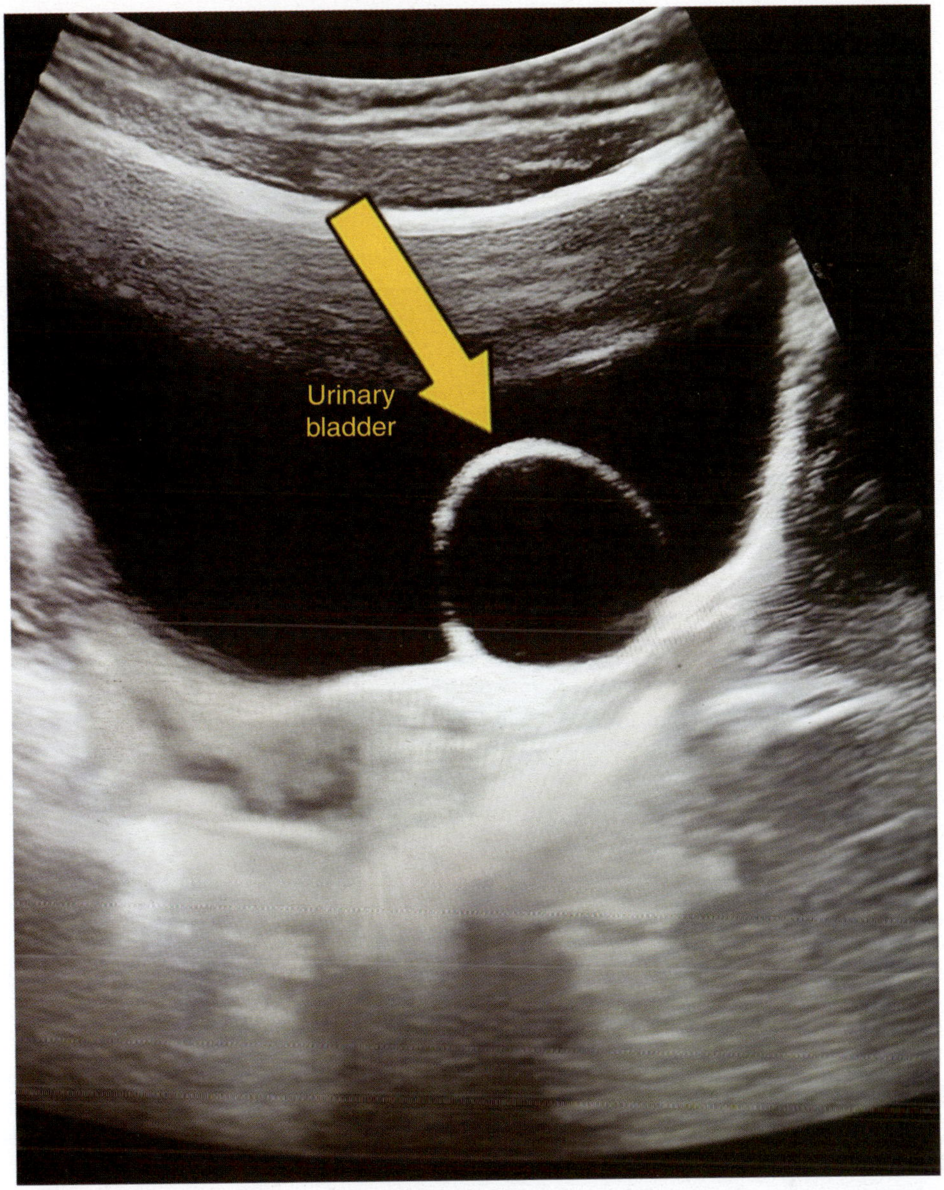

Ultrasound of the urinary bladder in the young male patient demonstrates a rounded cystic structure (*yellow arrow*) within the urinary bladder at the left vesicoureteric junction, consistent with a ureterocele.

Ureterocele

- A ureterocele is a focal congenital bulbous dilatation of the intravesical ureter. It maybe of two types: intravesical (occurring at the vesicoureteric junction) or extravesical (occurring ectopically near the bladder neck or urethra). The extravesical type is usually associated with a duplicated collecting system (duplex kidney).

Radiological Features

- On ultrasound, it appears as a cystic dilatation of the intravesical ureter at the vesicoureteric junction.
- On intravenous pyelography (IVP), the classic 'cobra-head' appearance may be seen, which refers to the cystic dilatation of the distal ureter and surrounded by a thin lucent rim, resembling the head of a cobra.
- An important differential is a pseudoureterocele which refers to obstruction of an otherwise normal intramural ureter, resembling a ureterocele.
- **Weigert–Meyer rule:** In a duplex collecting system or duplex kidney, the upper pole moiety inserts ectopically inferomedially into the bladder. The upper pole moiety is also prone to obstruction and is often associated with a ureterocele. The lower pole moiety is more likely to be associated with reflux.

OSCE

36

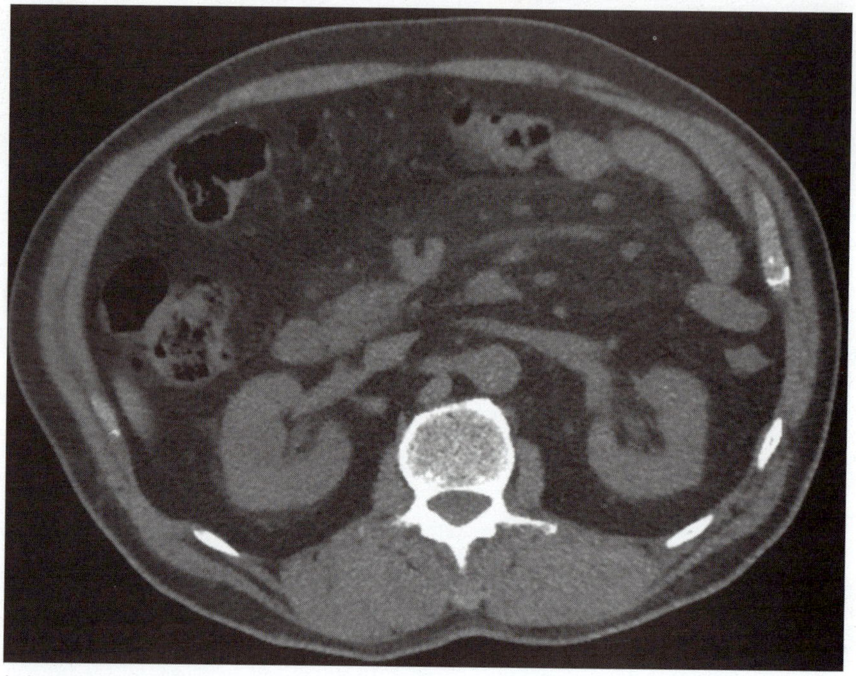

Clinical details: A middle-aged patient presented with fever and abdominal pain for 3 days.

1. **Describe the findings in the given image. What is the most appropriate diagnosis?**
2. **What is the most common malignancy associated with this pathology?**
3. **What is the ideal management plan?**
4. **What criteria is used on computed tomography (CT) to diagnose this condition?**
5. **What is the role of nuclear medicine in this condition?**

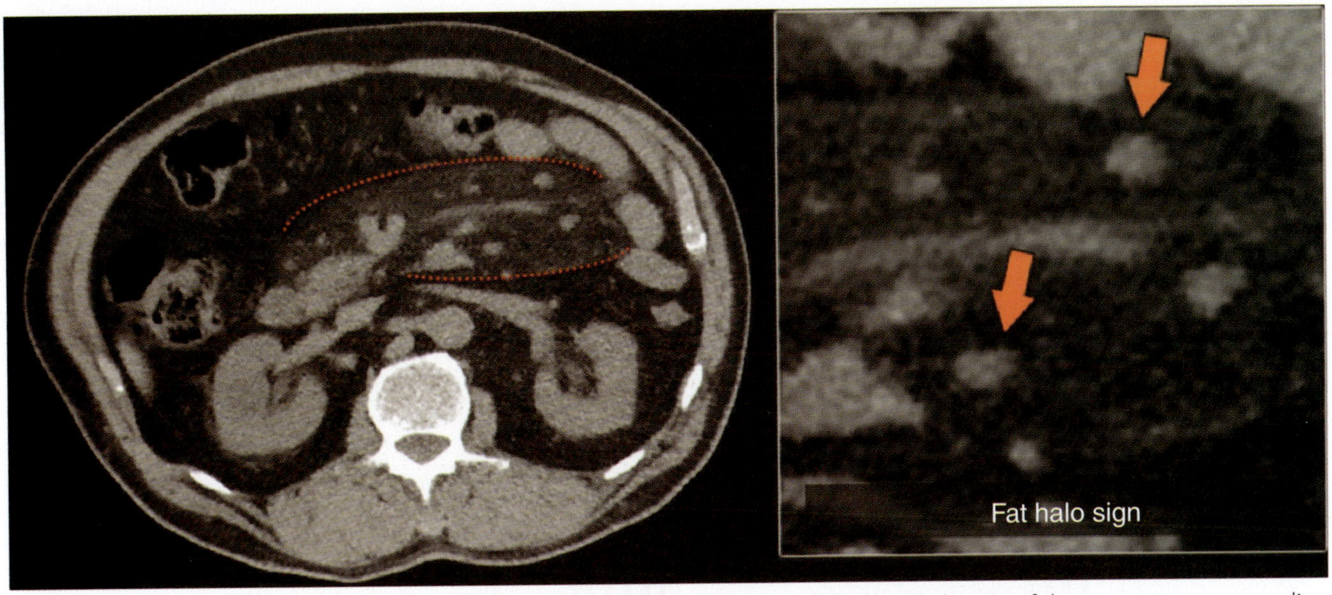

Axial NCCT abdomen image demonstrates a relatively well-demarcated area of increased density of the mesentery surrounding the mesenteric vessels ('misty mesentery'). Note the 'fat halo/fat ring sign' around the mesenteric vessels.

Mesenteric Panniculitis (Sclerosing Mesenteritis)

- Mesenteric panniculitis or sclerosing mesenteritis is a rare non-neoplastic idiopathic condition in which there is a characteristic inflammation of the mesenteric adipose tissue, usually affecting middle-aged to elderly adults with a median age of 65 years. It can cause abdominal pain, nausea, vomiting, diarrhoea, weight loss and fever.
- Various associated conditions have been reported, including malignancies such as systemic lymphoma (with up to a 10% risk), lung cancer, melanoma, colon cancer, renal cancer, myeloma and gastric carcinoma. Recent abdominal surgery is also linked, along with systemic inflammatory conditions like retroperitoneal fibrosis, sclerosing cholangitis, Riedel thyroiditis and orbital pseudotumor.

Radiological Features

- Computed tomography (CT) features include a well-demarcated or ill-defined mass like lesion involving the mesenteric fat ('misty mesentery'). The fat ring sign, or fat halo sign, is characterized by the preserved 'halo' of fat surrounding mesenteric vessels. This feature proves valuable in distinguishing mesenteric panniculitis from other mesenteric conditions like lymphoma, carcinoid tumour or carcinomatosis, where the fat ring sign is not present. The term 'misty mesentery' was coined by Mindelzun et al. in 1996.

THE COULIER CRITERIA, DESIGNED FOR CT DIAGNOSIS OF SCLEROSING MESENTERITIS, INCLUDE FIVE KEY SIGNS

1. **Well-defined mass effect:** Presence of distinct mass effect on neighbouring structures.
2. **Inhomogeneous higher attenuation:** Mesenteric fat showing higher attenuation compared to adjacent meso-colonic fat.
3. **Soft tissue nodes:** The presence of small soft tissue nodes within the lesion.
4. **Fat halo sign**
5. **Hyperdense pseudocapsule:** It may be surrounded by a hyperdense pseudocapsule.

Differentials: When encountering a 'misty mesentery' on CT, it is imperative for the radiologist to rule out alternative aetiologies for a localized increase in mesenteric fat density. Conditions such as oedema, haemorrhage, lymphoedema, inflammation (due to appendicitis, colitis and diverticulitis) and neoplastic involvement should be carefully considered before contemplating a diagnosis of mesenteric panniculitis.

Role of nuclear medicine: FDG PET-CT serves as a valuable tool for distinguishing between mesenteric panniculitis from malignant mesenteric involvement:

Mesenteric Panniculitis	Malignant Mesenteric Involvement
• Typically, not FDG-avid on PET-CT.	• Typically shows FDG avidity on PET-CT.

- Treatment for mesenteric panniculitis primarily involves supportive care, given the typically self-limiting nature of the condition. Surgical intervention is usually not done, as complete resection of mesenteric panniculitis is not feasible.
- It is important to note that in up to 15% of cases, there may be eventual development of local lymphoma.

OSCE

37

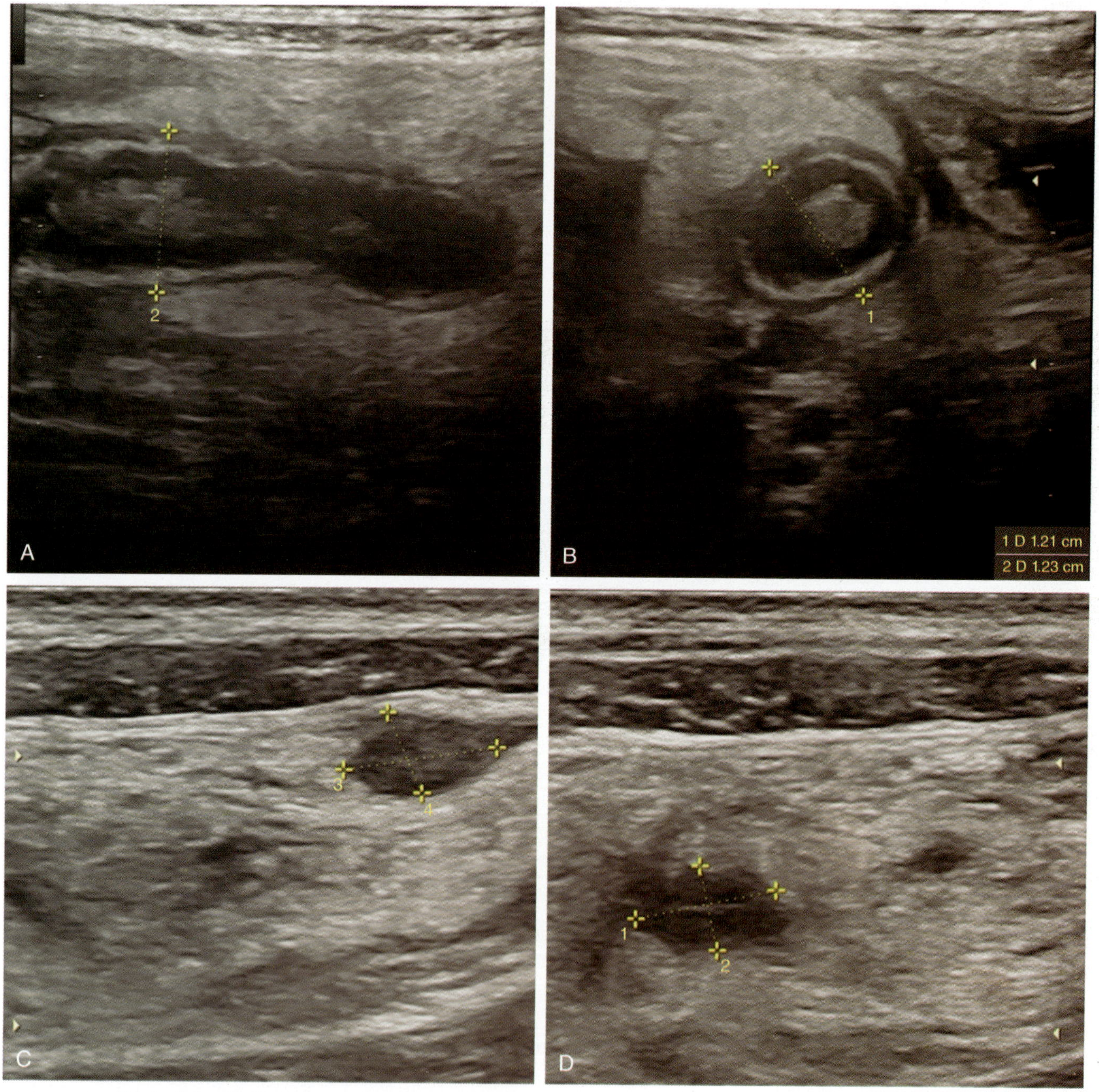

Clinical details: A young male presented with severe acute pain abdomen in the right iliac fossa.

1. **Describe the findings and the most appropriate diagnosis.**
2. **Can appendicitis occur in a post-appendicectomy status?**
3. **Which is the most sensitive modality to diagnosis appendicitis?**
4. **What is Amyand hernia?**

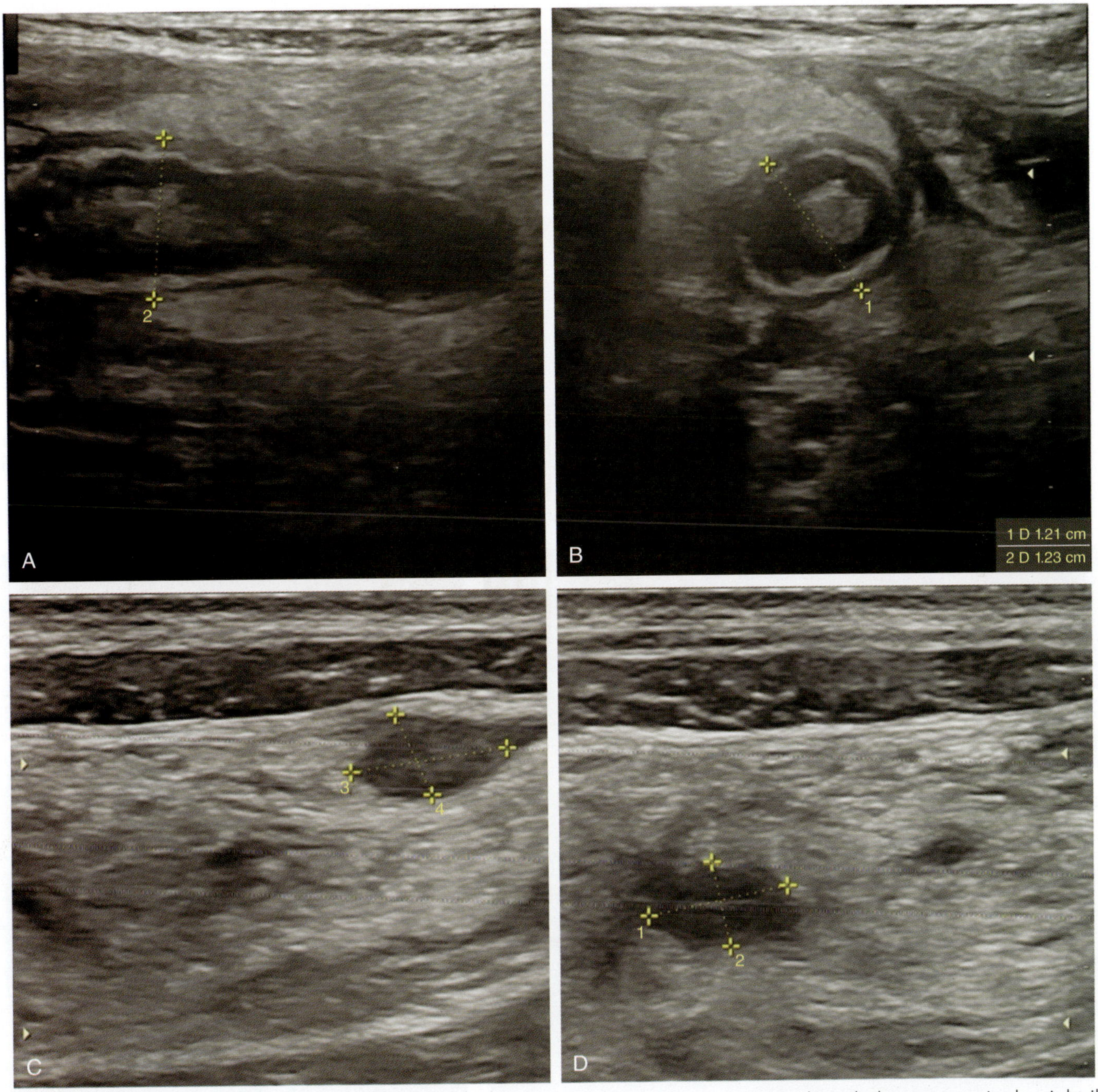

(A and B) Ultrasound of the right iliac fossa shows a non-compressible, blind ending, aperistaltic tubular structure in the right iliac fossa and measuring up to 12 mm in diameter. It was seen to arise from the base of the caecum. There is significant periappendiceal hyperechoic inflamed fat. (C and D) Periappendiceal reactive lymphadenopathy was observed. No periappendiceal fluid or other signs of perforation. No appendicolith.

Acute Appendicitis

Appendicitis is referred to acute inflammation of the appendix, frequently leading to abdominal surgery in young patients. It is one of the most common causes of acute abdomen. Among imaging methods, computed tomography (CT) stands out as the most sensitive diagnostic tool for detecting appendicitis. It may be caused by an appendicolith, faecolith, lymphoid hyperplasia, foreign bodies or tumours causing obstruction.

Even after an appendectomy, stump appendicitis remains a possible occurrence.

Radiological Features

USG:

- Ultrasound typically reveals the acute appendicitis as an aperistaltic, blind-ending, non-compressible tubular structure with a diameter >6 mm, often with the presence of an appendicolith (~10% of cases) casting an acoustic shadow.

- Additional findings:
  - Periappendiceal fat inflammation
  - Periappendiceal reactive lymphadenopathy
  - Periappendiceal fluid collection may be seen
  - Hyperaemia/increased vascularity of the appendiceal wall
- A study demonstrated that employing a dynamic ultrasound technique with a three-step patient positioning protocol enhances appendix detection. Initially examining patients in the supine position, followed by the left posterior oblique position (45-degree LPO), and then a 'second-look' supine position, resulted in increased detection rates.

Supine position → Left posterior oblique position (45-degree LPO) → 'Second look' supine position

CT:

- Increased appendiceal diameter (≥8–9 mm) with thickened wall (>3 mm)
- Caecal apex thickening, known as 'caecal bar' or 'arrowhead sign'
- Periappendiceal fat stranding and reactive lymphadenopathy
- Presence of extraluminal fluid, phlegmon or abscess
- Appendicolith

Complications of acute appendicitis include perforation with or without appendiceal abscess, portal venous infective thrombophlebitis and liver abscess.

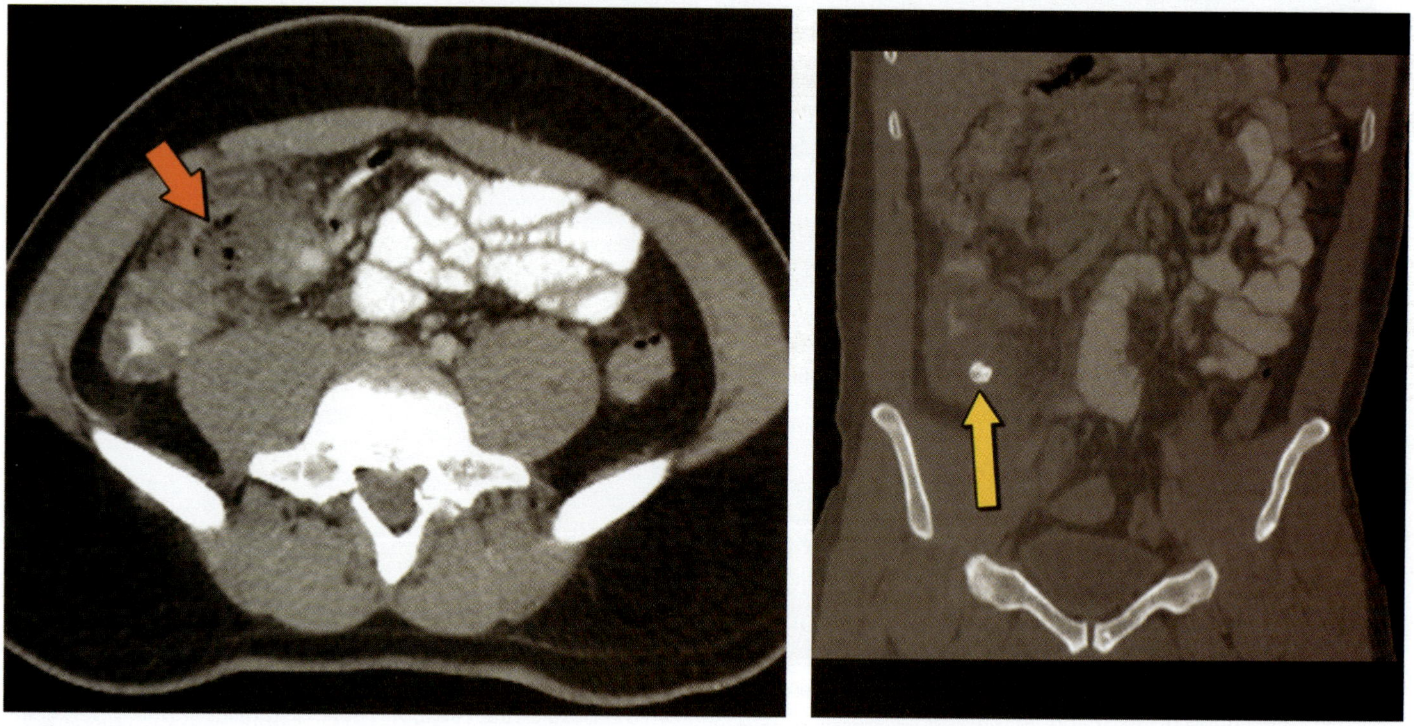

Axial and coronal computed tomography (CT) abdomen shows a common complication of acute appendicitis – appendicular abscess due to perforated appendix. Ill-defined heterogenous fluid collection is observed in the right iliac fossa with locules of air (*red arrow*) and the presence of an appendicolith (*yellow arrow*). Note the thickened caecal base.

Amyand hernia is a type of inguinal hernia which involves the presence of the appendix within the hernial sac. A femoral hernia that includes the appendix is referred to as a De Garengeot hernia.

OSCE

38

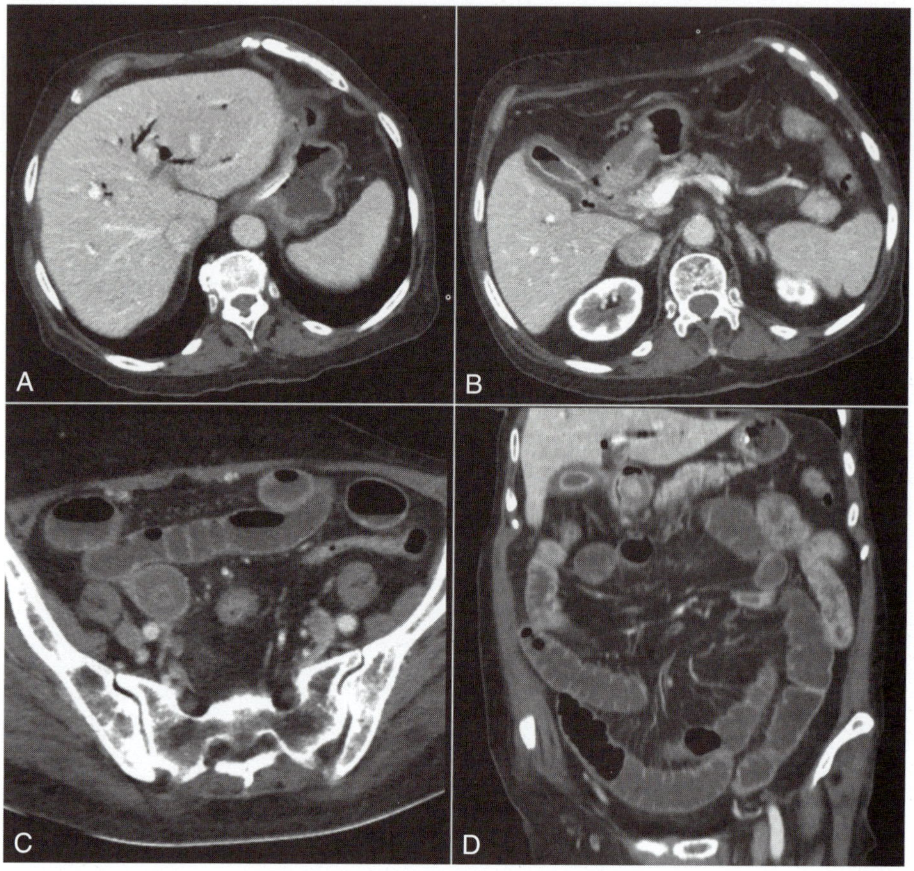

Clinical details: History withheld.

1. **Describe the findings in the provided images.**
2. **What is the most appropriate diagnosis?**
3. **What is the classic triad seen here?**
4. **What is 'Bouveret syndrome'?**

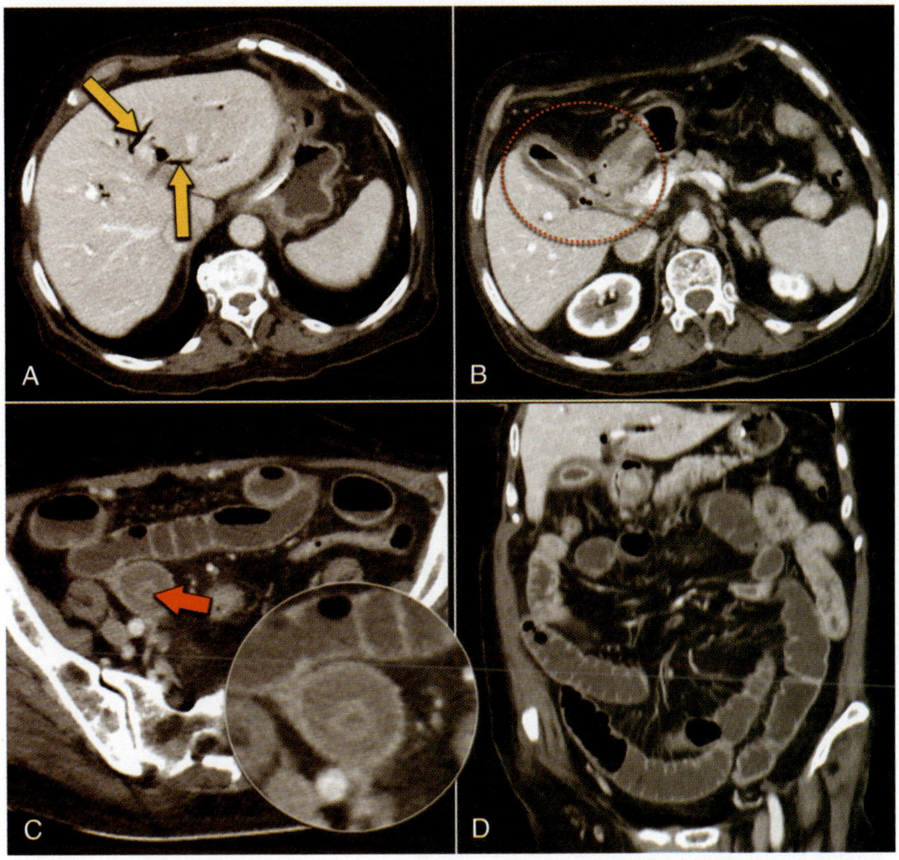

Axial and coronal post-contrast computed tomography (CT) abdomen images demonstrate: (A) gas within the biliary tree or pneumobilia (*yellow arrows*), (B) gas within the gallbladder with close communication of the gallbladder neck with the adjacent duodenum with formation of a cholecystenteric fistula and (C and D) ectopic gallstone (*red arrow*) in distal small bowel with dilated obstructed bowel loops.

Gallstone Ileus

- Gallstone ileus refers to a mechanical obstruction in the gastrointestinal tract caused by impaction of gallstones. This aetiology accounts for less than 1% of cases of intestinal obstruction.
- Gallstone ileus often follows chronic or recurrent cholecystitis, where inflammation leads to adhesion formation. This leads to erosion through the gallbladder wall, forming a fistula with the adjacent gastrointestinal tract, usually the duodenum, due to its close proximity. This gallstone becomes ectopic and may get impacted distally (typically at the ileocecal junction or terminal ileum) leading to intestinal obstruction. The term 'ileus' is a misnomer in this context, as the obstruction is a true mechanical obstruction rather than a functional ileus.

Radiological Features

- Classically, abdominal radiographs and computed tomography (CT) reveal the triad of findings known as Rigler triad, which includes:

RIGLER TRIAD (GALLSTONE ILEUS)

1. Small bowel obstruction
2. Pneumobilia
3. Ectopic gallstone, commonly in right iliac fossa

- One must document the site of fistulization in the reports. Care must be taken to look for free air (pneumoperitoneum), mural gas or portal venous gas.
- The definitive treatment for gallstone ileus involves surgery, specifically the removal of the stone through enterolithotomy. Additionally, the fistula is repaired and a cholecystectomy is performed.

Mirizzi Syndrome	Bouveret Syndrome
Extrinsic compression of an extrahepatic biliary duct due to calculus in the cystic duct or gallbladder.	Gastric outlet obstruction resulting from a gallstone impacted in the pylorus or proximal duodenum, representing a very proximal form of gallstone ileus.

PART

F

Musculoskeletal System

OSCE

39

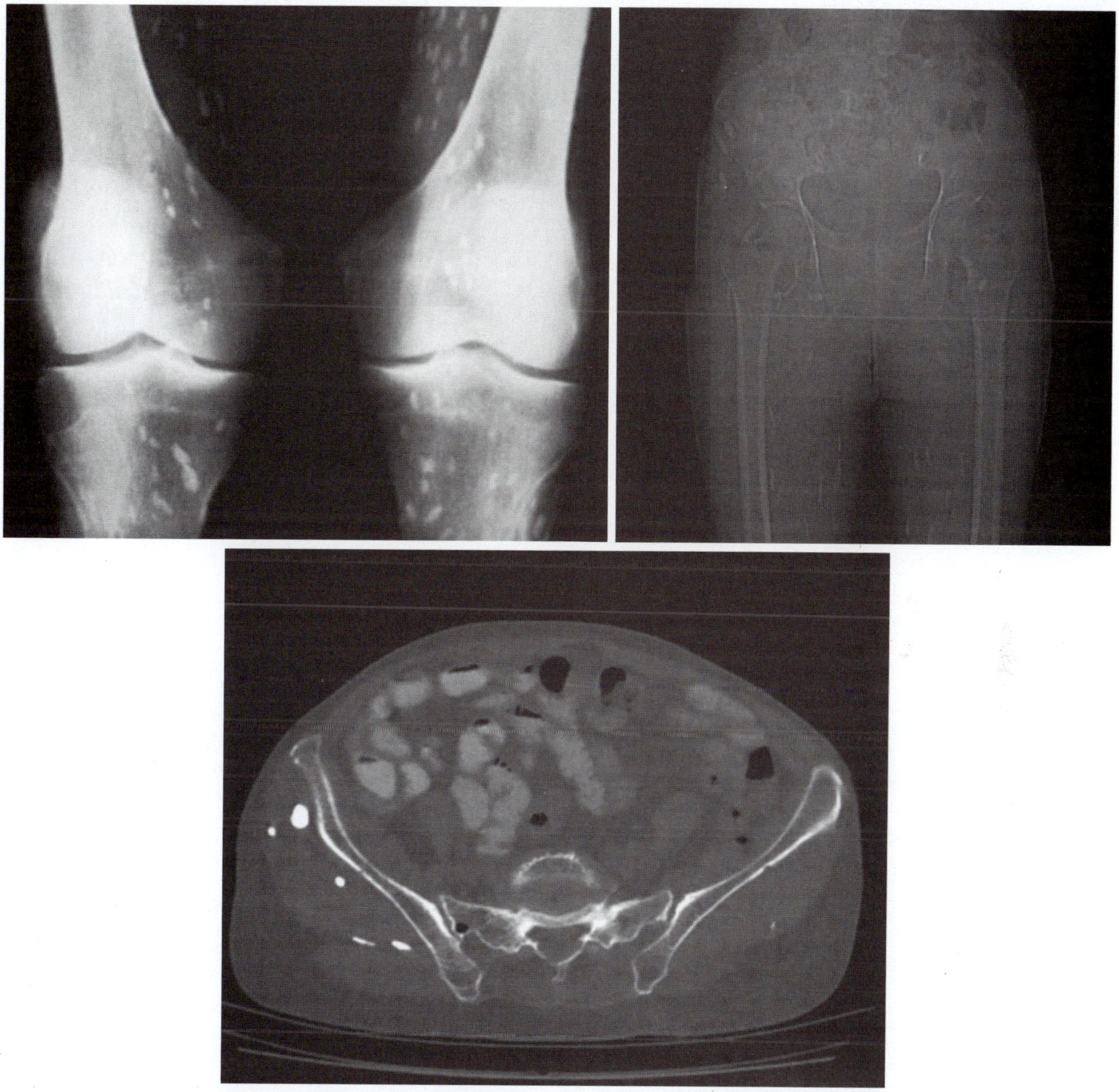

Clinical details: A 36-year-old-male with multiple subcutaneous nodules.

1. **What is the most appropriate diagnosis?**
2. **How is it caused?**
3. **What is the characteristic sign seen here?**
4. **What should be the next line of imaging?**

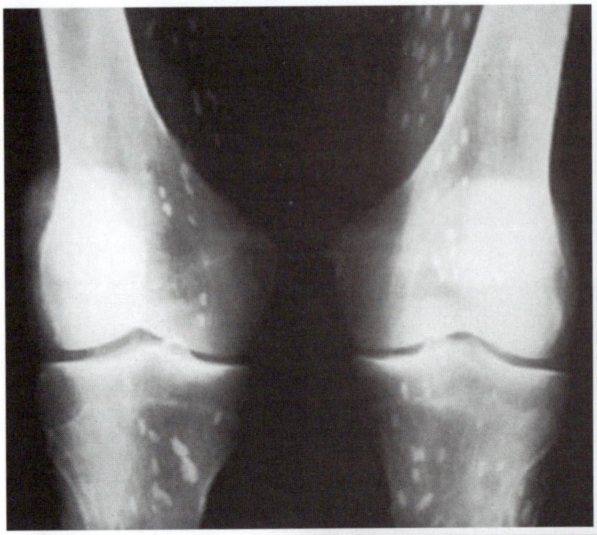

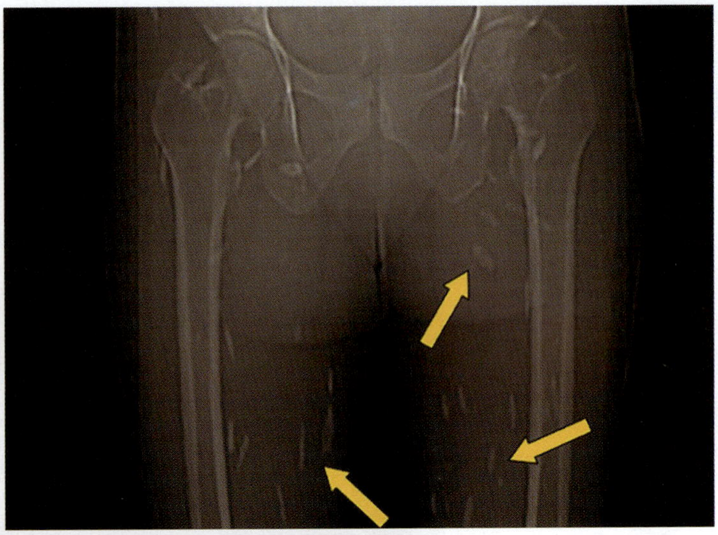

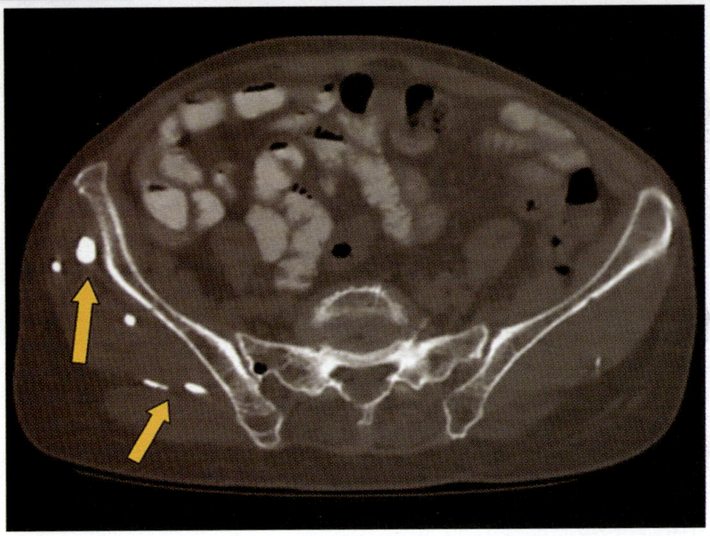

Frontal knee radiograph, computed tomography (CT) scout image and axial NCCT pelvis reveal multiple oblong calcific densities in the skeletal muscles around knees, thighs and pelvis (rice-grain or cigar-shaped calcifications) – myocysticercosis.

Myocysticercosis

- Cysticercosis is a parasitic infection caused by the tapeworm *Taenia solium*. It occurs via faeco-oral transmission. Intake of undercooked pork is a known aetiological factor.
- Muscular involvement is characterized by the presence of solitary or multiple specks of calcification, giving the 'rice-grain calcification' or 'cigar-shaped calcification' appearance on imaging. Imaging of the brain should be the next line of imaging.
- Central nervous system (CNS) manifestation of cysticercosis is known as neurocysticercosis (NCC) and is a common differential of multiple ring-enhancing lesions in the brain.

(Refer to OSCE 83: Neurocysticercosis)

OSCE

40

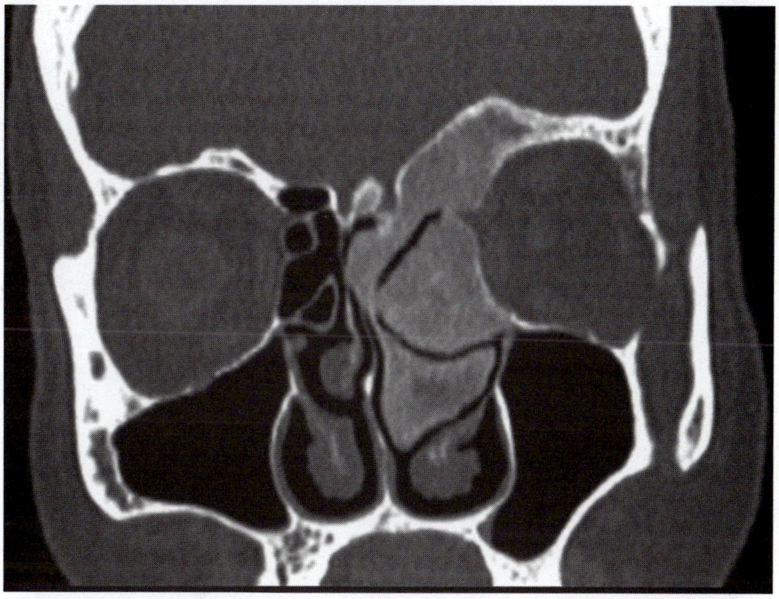

Clinical details: A 30-year-old presented with gradually developing facial asymmetry.

1. **What is the most appropriate diagnosis?**
2. **What is McCune–Albright syndrome?**
3. **Give one differential diagnosis.**
4. **What syndrome would it be if the patient had intramuscular myxomas?**

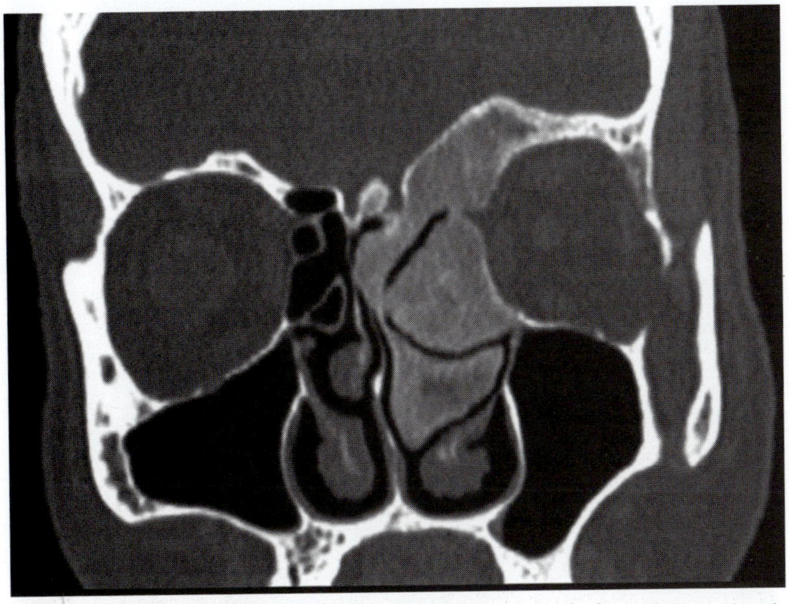

Coronal NCCT PNS shows asymmetric expansion of the bony cortex with ground glass attenuation involving the bony walls of left ethmoid sinus, left cribriform plate, left middle nasal turbinate – craniofacial fibrous dysplasia.

Craniofacial Fibrous Dysplasia

- Craniofacial fibrous dysplasia is a type of fibrous dysplasia involving the cranium and facial bones. It usually affects the younger age group. The cortex is usually intact with an expanded ground glass appearance.
- Fibrous dysplasia may be monostotic or polyostotic.
- McCune–Albright syndrome comprises of:
  - 'Café au lait' spots
  - Precocious puberty
  - Polyostotic fibrous dysplasia.
- Paget's disease is the main differential and is more common in elderly. Paget's involves the inner table, while fibrous dysplasia spares it.

OSCE

41

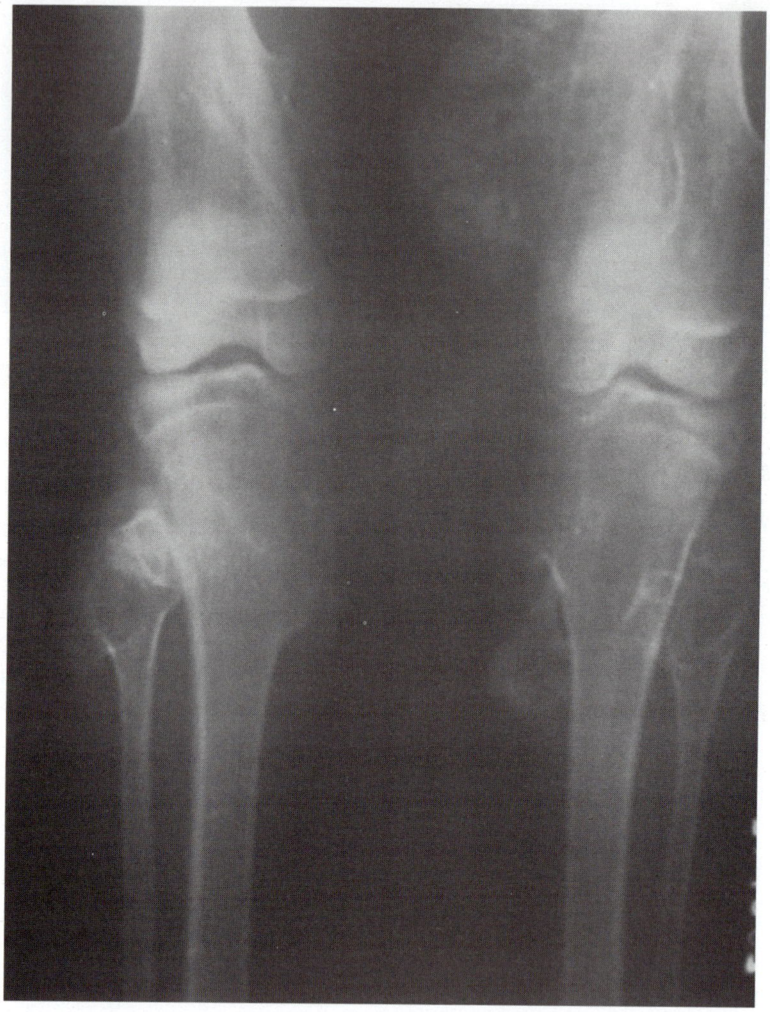

Clinical details: A 20-year-old male with multiple bony swellings around the knee joint.

1. **What is the most appropriate diagnosis?**
2. **What is the inheritance pattern?**
3. **Name any two complications other than malignant transformation.**
4. **Enumerate any two features to suggest sarcomatous transformation.**

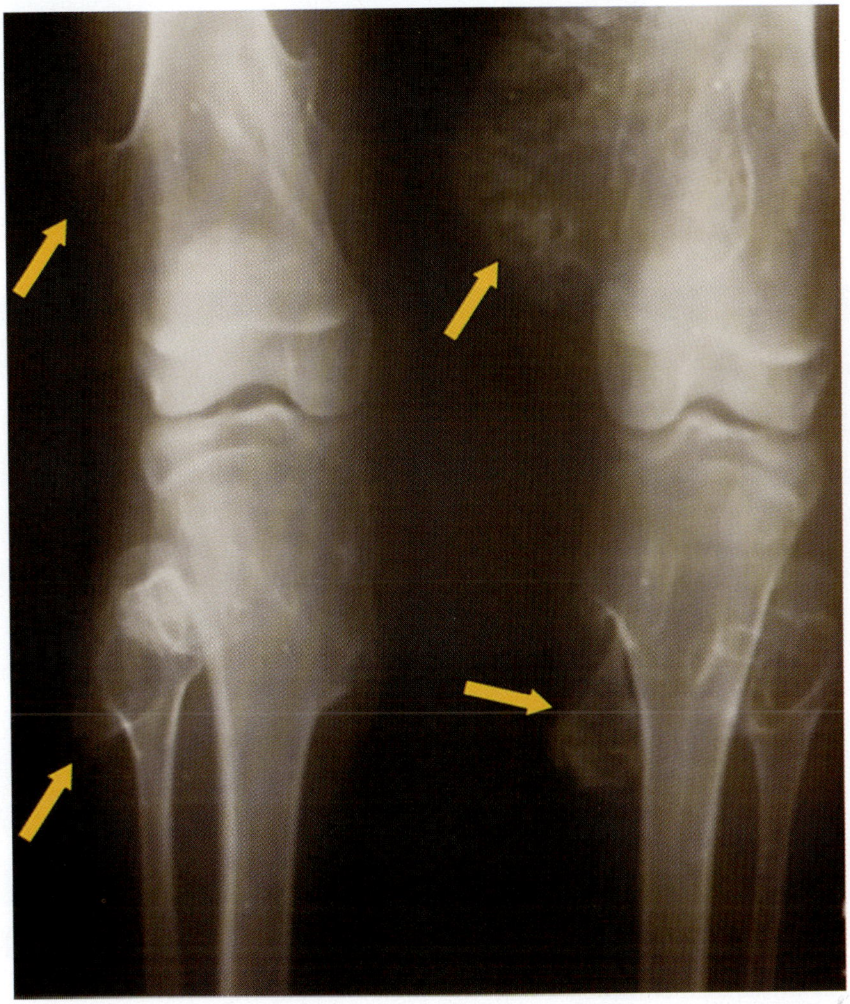

Frontal radiographs of bilateral knee joints in a skeletally mature patient shows few bony outgrowths (osteochondromas) around the knee joints. These point away from the joint. Findings are consistent with diaphyseal aclasia (hereditary multiple exostosis)

Diaphyseal Aclasia (Hereditary Multiple Exostosis)

- Diaphyseal aclasia (hereditary multiple exostosis [HME]) is characterized by multiple osteochondromas and is inherited in an autosomal dominant inheritance pattern. Patient may be asymptomatic or present with obvious bony deformities. Complications include fractures, vascular or neural impingement, and malignant (sarcomatous) transformation (~3%–5% in HME).

- Features suggesting sarcomatous transformation in an osteochondroma can be memorized by the mnemonic GLAD PAST.

G: Growth in the osteochondroma after skeletal maturation

L: Any new Lucency

A: Any scintigraphy activity

D: Destruction of cortex

P: Pain after skeletal maturation

A: and

S: associated Soft-tissue mass lesion

T: Thickening of cartilage cap more than 1.5 cm

OSCE

42

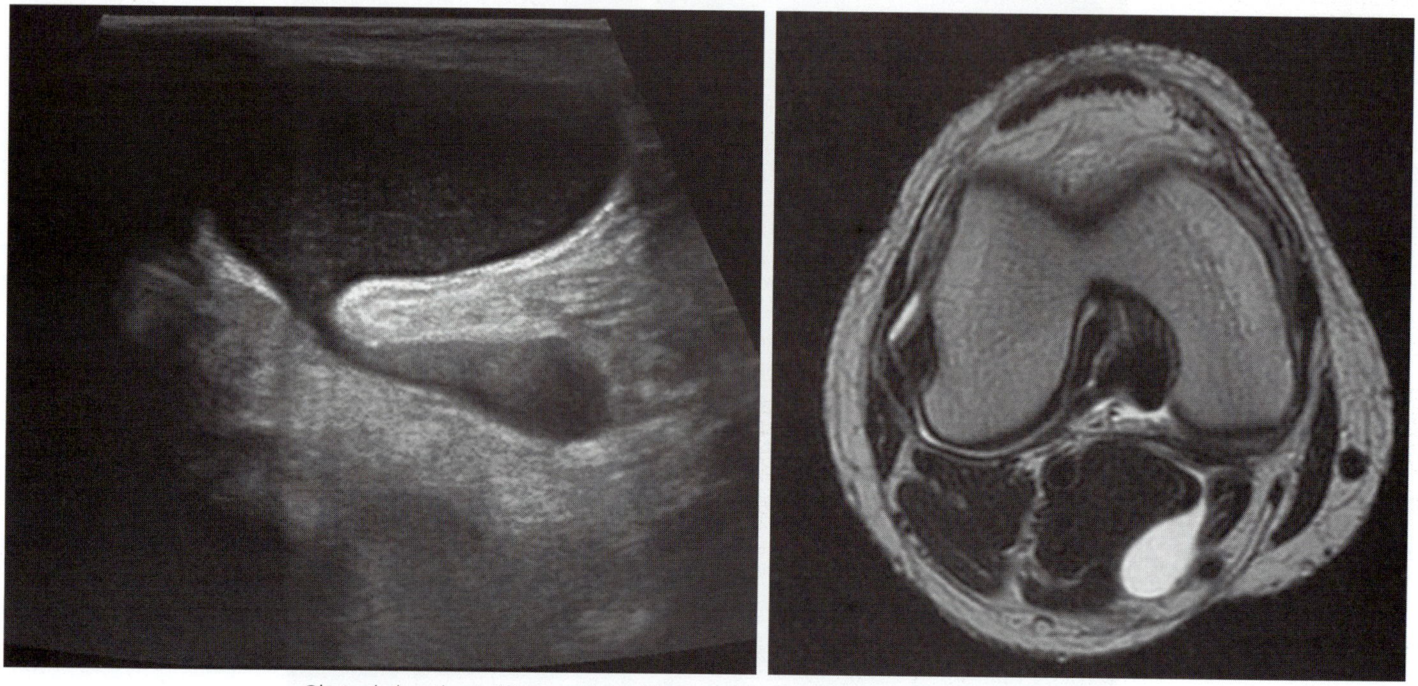

Clinical details: A 35-year-old athlete with boggy swelling behind the knee.

1. **Provided imaging of two different patients with the same entity. Identify the imaging modalities.**
2. **What is the most appropriate diagnosis?**
3. **Which radiological sign do you see in the ultrasound image?**
4. **Between which two muscles does this entity arise from?**

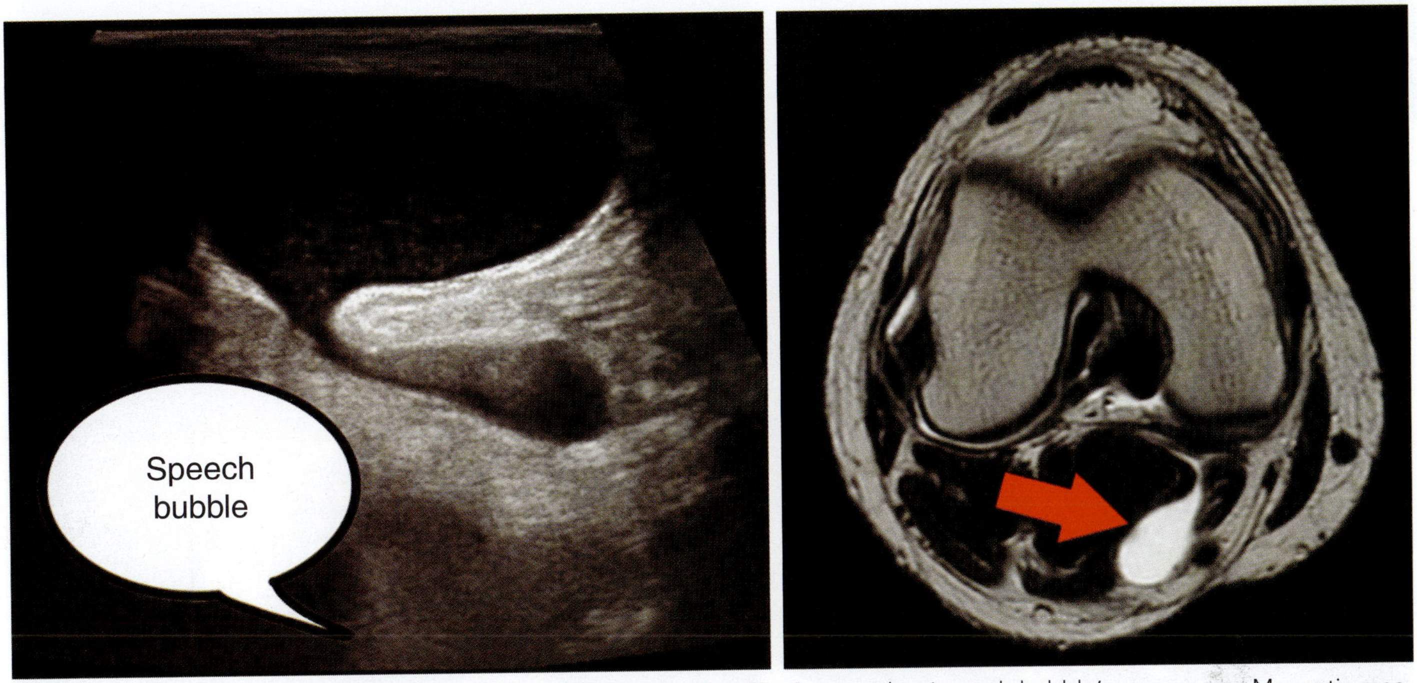

(Baker cyst) Ultrasonography (USG) of popliteal fossa shows a fluid-filled cyst with a 'speech bubble' appearance. Magnetic resonance imaging (MRI) of the knee joint in another case demonstrates a T2 hyperintense lesion within the popliteal fossa (*red arrow*). It shows a thin 'neck' extending between the semi-membranous and medial head of gastrocnemius.

Baker Cyst

- Baker cyst is a commonly occurring popliteal cyst. It is usually encountered incidentally during ultrasonography (USG)/magnetic resonance imaging (MRI) for alternate reasons.
- It can be associated with degenerative knee and rheumatoid arthritis.

RADIOLOGICAL FEATURES

- On ultrasound, it is seen in the medial popliteal fossa as an anechoic fluid-filled cystic between the semi-membranous and the medial head of the gastrocnemius. The thin 'neck' gives it as 'speech bubble' like appearance. On MRI, it shows high signal intensity on T2WI and low signal intensity on T1WI. No post-contrast enhancement is seen.

OSCE

43

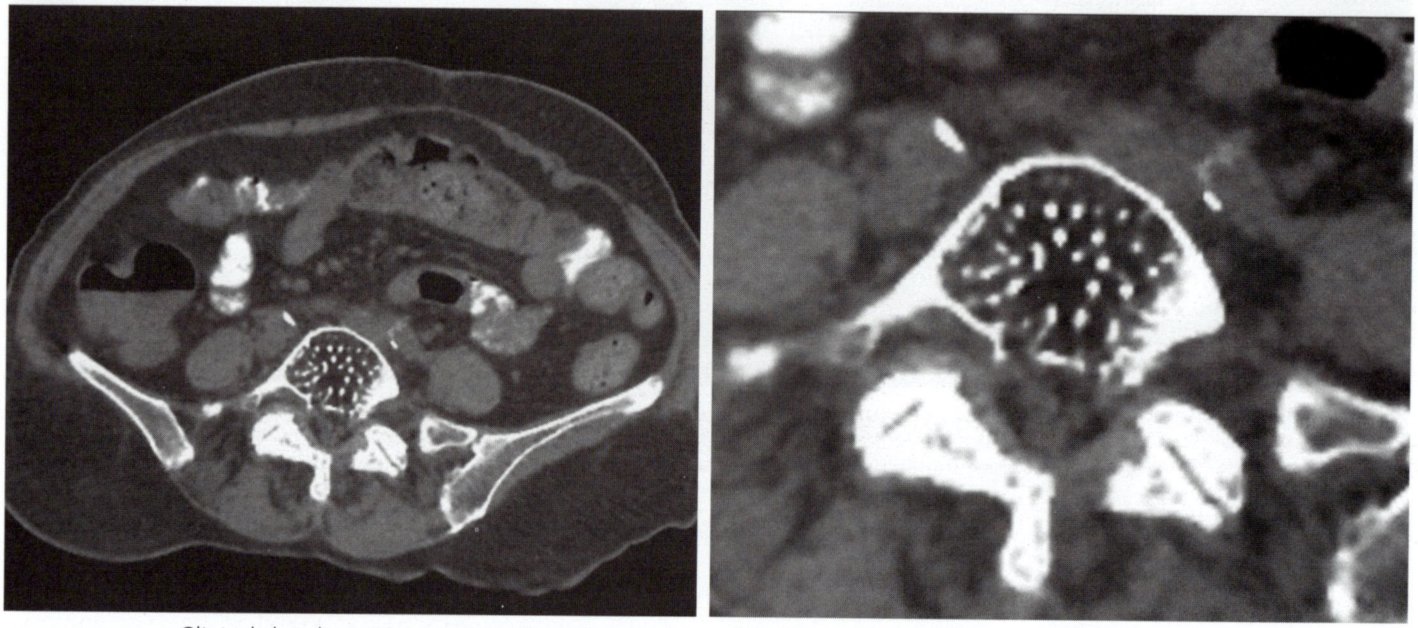

Clinical details: A 50-year-old male with an incidental finding on computed tomography (CT) scan.

1. **What is the diagnosis?**
2. **Which characteristic radiological sign is seen here?**
3. **Name the sign that would be seen on the sagittal image.**
4. **What is the expected signal intensity on T1 and T2 magnetic resonance imaging (MRI) images?**

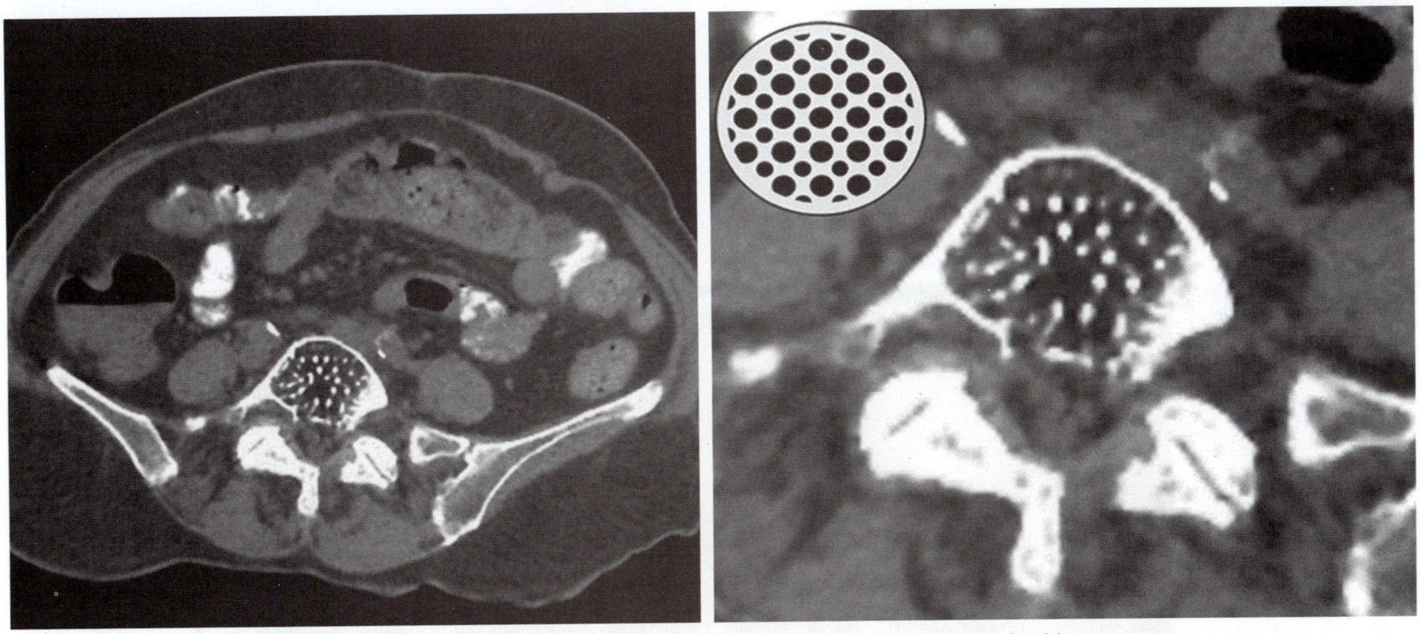

Axial NCCT abdomen shows the typical 'polka-dot' appearance of a vertebral haemangioma.

Vertebral Haemangioma

- Vertebral haemangioma (VH) is usually an incidental finding on imaging. On axial computed tomography (CT), the characteristic polka-dot appearance has been described which is due to the thickened trabeculae seen on cross section. On sagittal images, it is known as the 'corduroy cloth' appearance.
- VH usually shows high signal intensity on both T1- and T2-weighted magnetic resonance imaging (MRI) images owing to their lipid content. Post-contrast enhancement is seen.

Lipid-poor haemangiomas or atypical haemangiomas may exhibit T1 isosignal, T2 hypersignal, and lack suppression on STIR due to their small lipid content.

Another type is aggressive vertebral haemangioma, a rare form characterized by significant vertebral expansion, extra-osseous component with epidural extension, and potential complications such as compression fractures, spinal cord, or nerve root compression.

OSCE

44

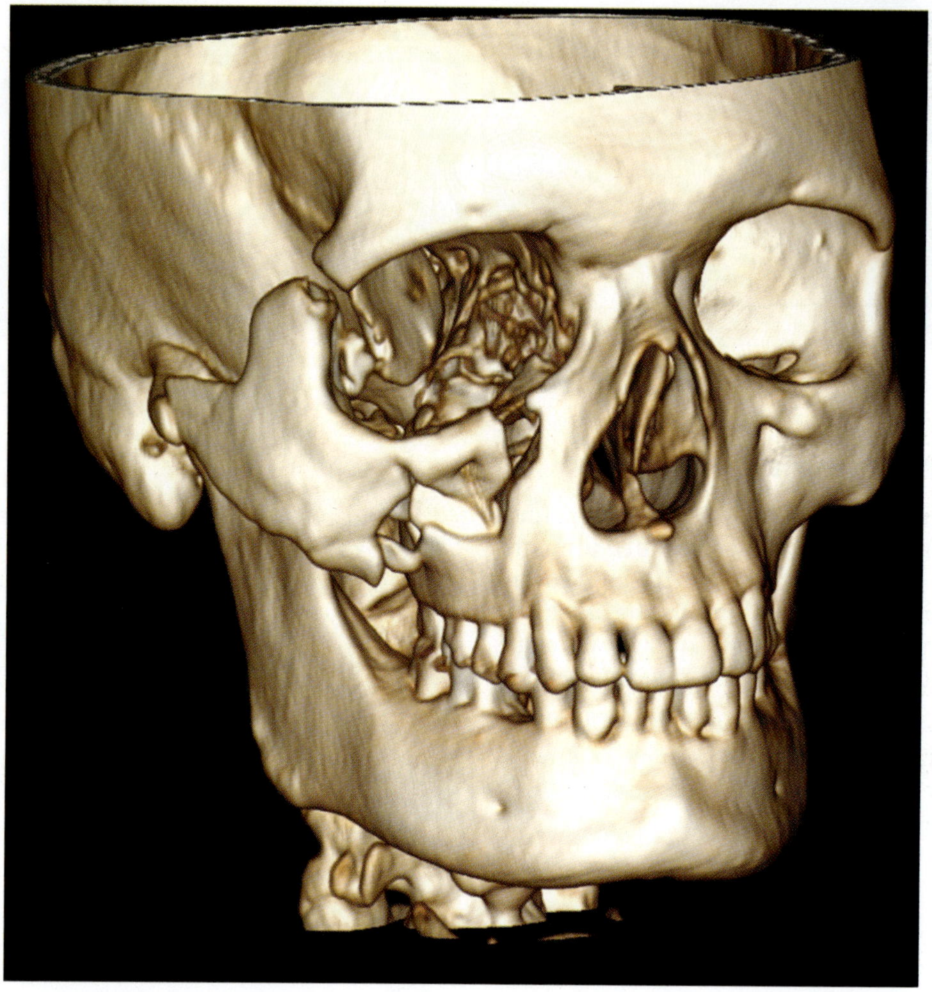

Clinical details: A young male with facial injury due to motor vehicle accident.

1. **Describe your findings.**
2. **What is the appropriate diagnosis?**
3. **Which nerve may get compromised?**
4. **Which is the most common type of facial fracture?**

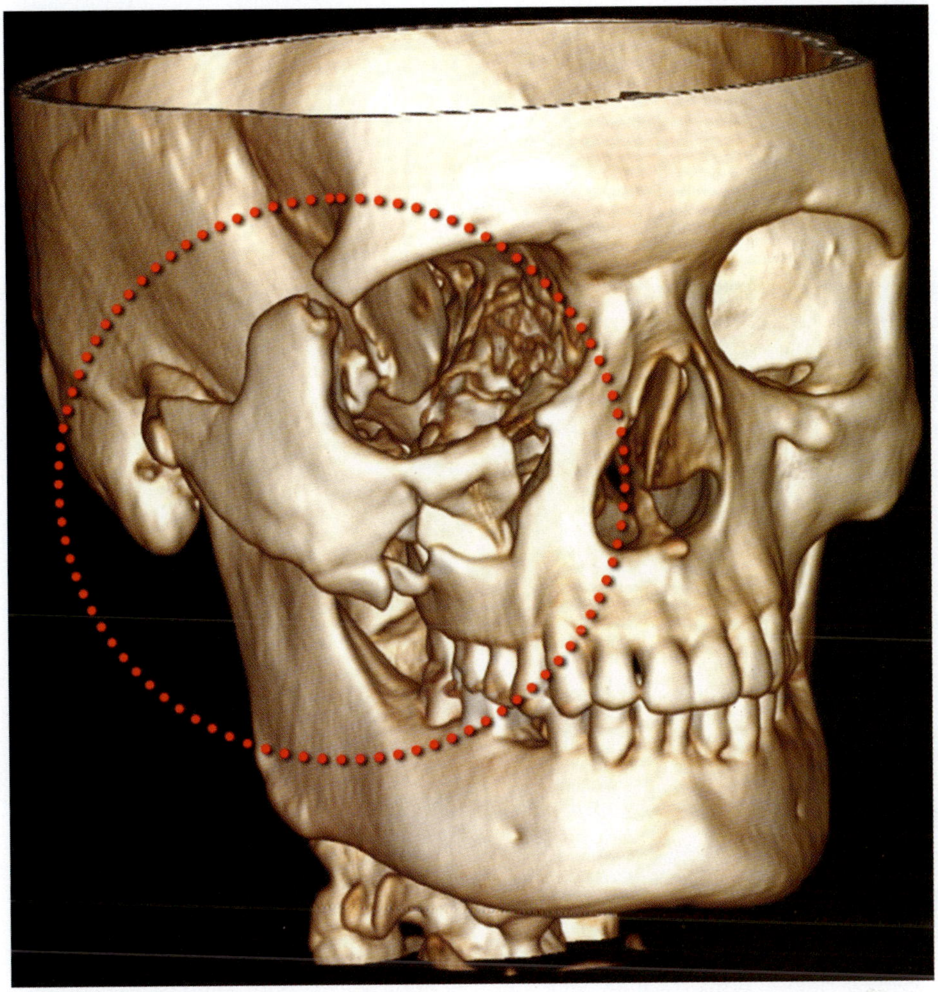

VRT (Volume Rendering Technique) (3D) image demonstrates a right zygomaticomaxillary complex fracture, also known as the tripod fracture – involving the zygomatic arch, lateral orbital wall, inferior orbital wall and lateral wall of the maxillary sinus.

Tripod Fracture

- Tripod fracture or zygomaticomaxillary complex fracture is usually caused by a direct impact to the malar eminence of the cheek. It is the second most common facial fracture after nasal bone fractures.
- Fracture lines involving the tripod fracture are zygomatic arch, lateral orbital wall, inferior orbital wall and lateral wall of the maxillary sinus.
- Tripod fracture may involve the infraorbital foramen and cause compromise of the infraorbital nerve.

OSCE

45

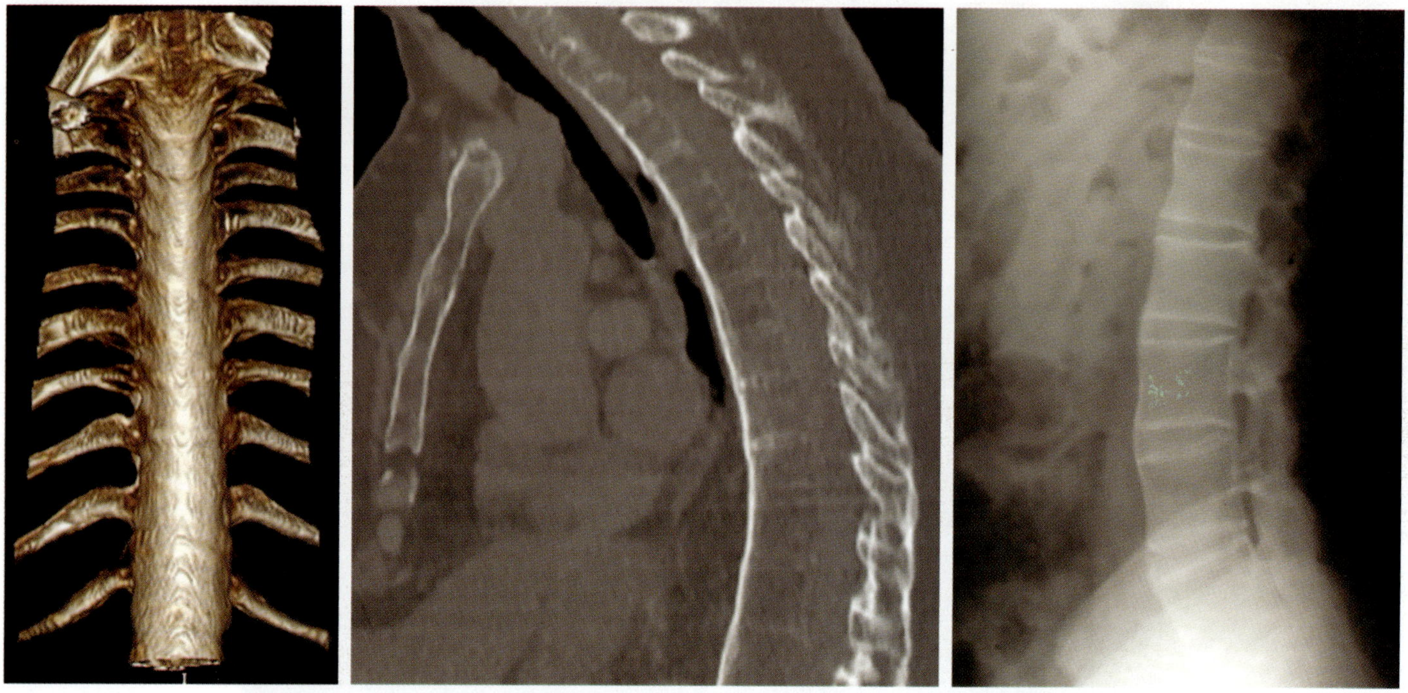

Clinical details: A male patient with a history of backache after lifting heavy weight.

1. **Describe your findings in the provided images.**
2. **What is the most appropriate diagnosis?**
3. **What is the characteristic radiological sign seen here?**
4. **What is usually the first manifestation of this pathology?**

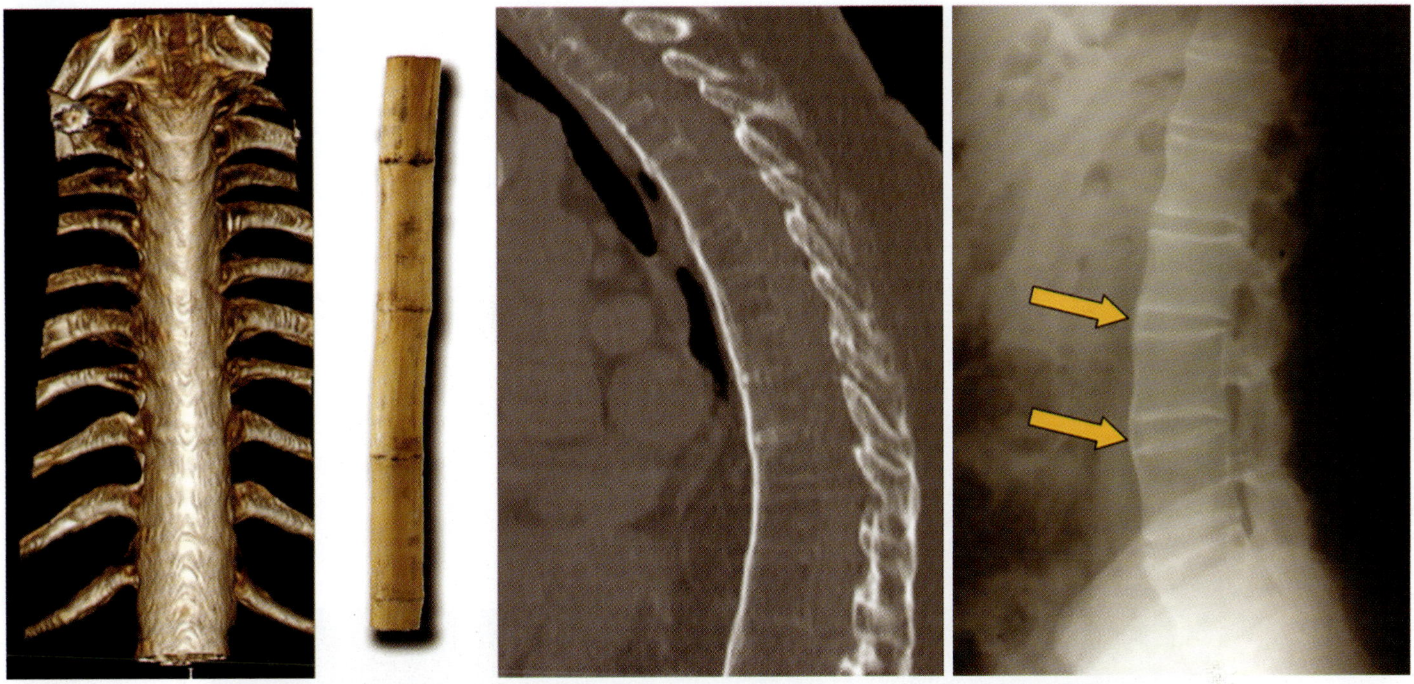

VRT (Volume Rendering Technique) (3D) and sagittal computed tomography (CT) dorsal spine (bone window) and X-ray dorsolumbar spine: Extensive syndesmophyte formation and vertebral body 'squaring' in the entire dorsal spine leading to diffuse ankylosis with the characteristic 'bamboo spine' appearance in ankylosing spondylitis.

Ankylosing Spondylitis

- Also known as Bechterew disease, ankylosing spondylitis is an autoimmune seronegative spondyloarthropathy (rheumatoid factor negative). It causes fusion of the sacroiliac joints and the spine. Sacroiliitis is usually the first manifestation of ankylosing spondylitis and is bilateral and symmetrical. HLA-B27 gene is associated with ankylosing spondylitis in majority of cases.

RADIOLOGICAL FEATURES

- Extensive ankylosis of the spine leads to the characteristic 'bamboo spine' appearance. Other important skeletal manifestations of ankylosing spondylitis include Romanus lesion, Andersson lesion, shiny corner sign, vertebral body squaring, dagger spine appearance and 'trolley track' sign.

IMPORTANT SKELETAL MANIFESTATIONS OF ANKYLOSING SPONDYLITIS

Romanus lesion	Erosions or inflammatory changes at the corners of the vertebra
Shiny corner sign	Superior endplate sclerosis (shiny corners)
Dagger sign (frontal X-ray)	Posterior interspinous ligament ossification – midline vertical opaque line
Trolley track sign (frontal X-ray)	Central vertical opaque line (ossified supraspinous and interspinous ligaments) + two parallel vertical lines (ossified apophyseal joint capsules)
Bamboo sign	Extensive ankylosis of the spine
Andersson lesion	Central abnormal discovertebral hemispherical signal affecting adjacent endplates of vertebral bodies

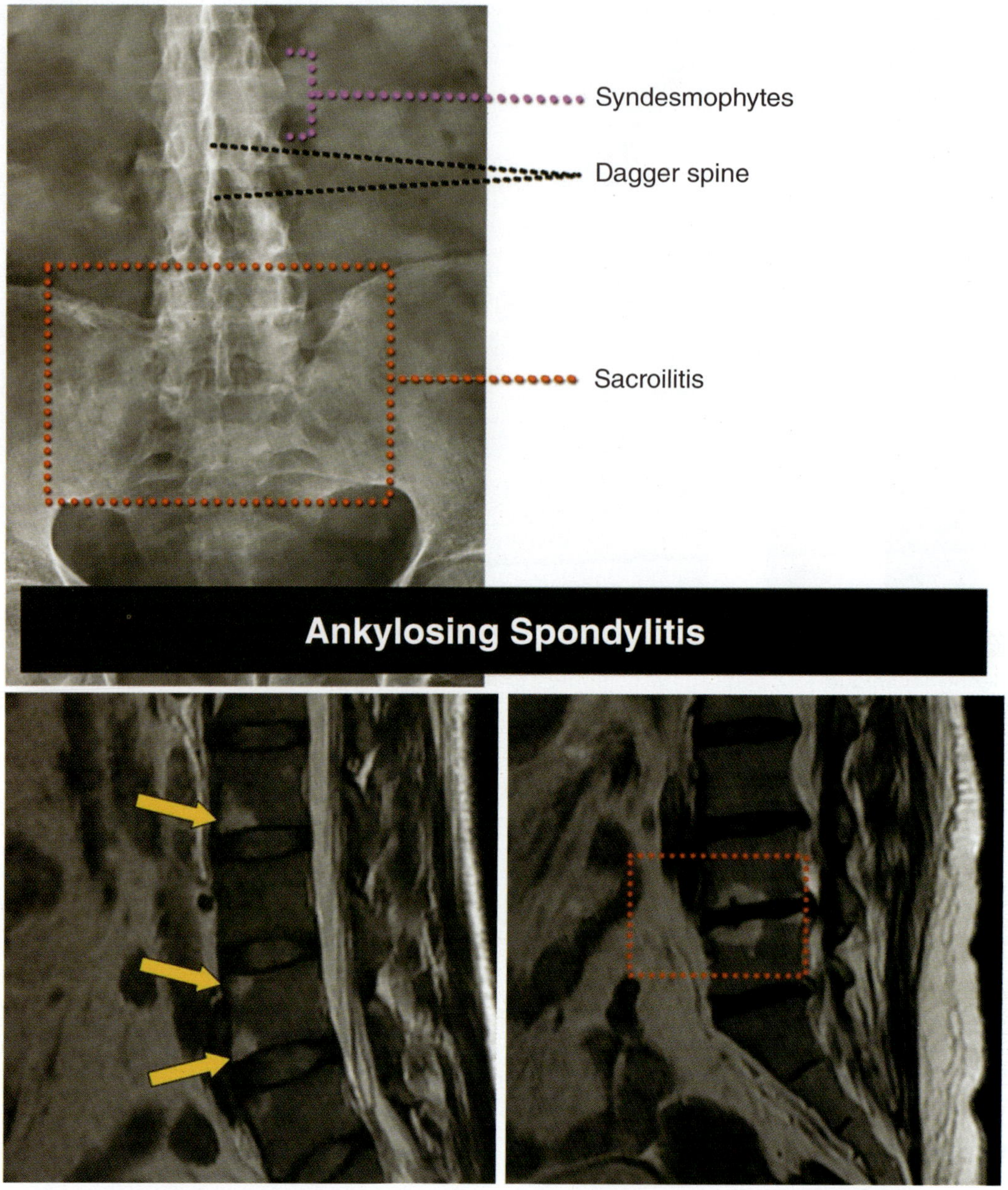

Romanus lesions **Andersson lesions**

OSCE

46

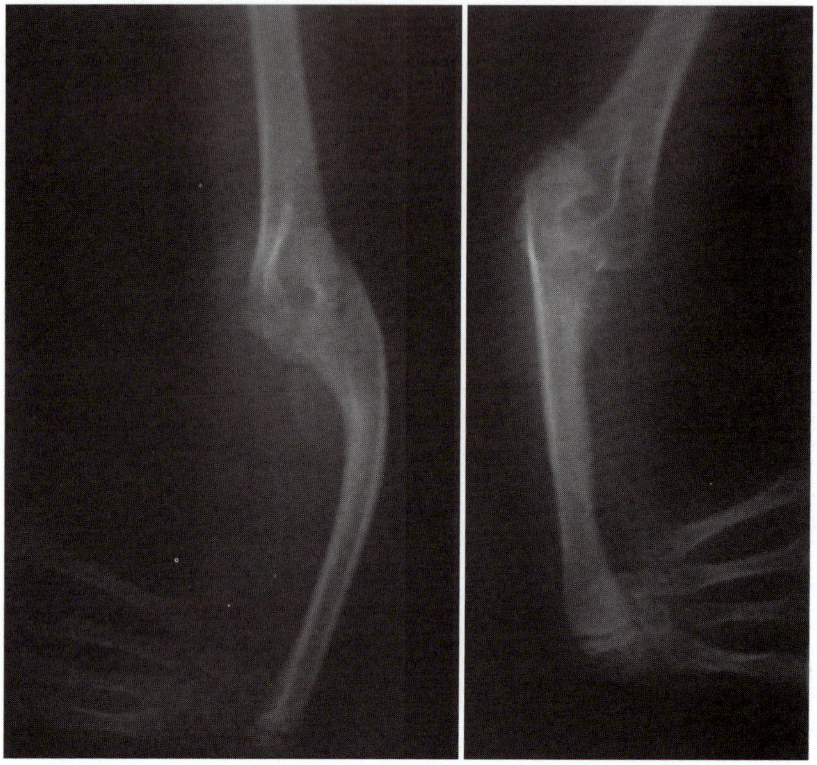

Clinical details: A young boy with congenital anomaly involving both forearms.

1. **Describe your findings.**
2. **What is the probable diagnosis?**
3. **Name two syndromes associated with this.**
4. **Which imaging modality can diagnose this entity at the earliest?**

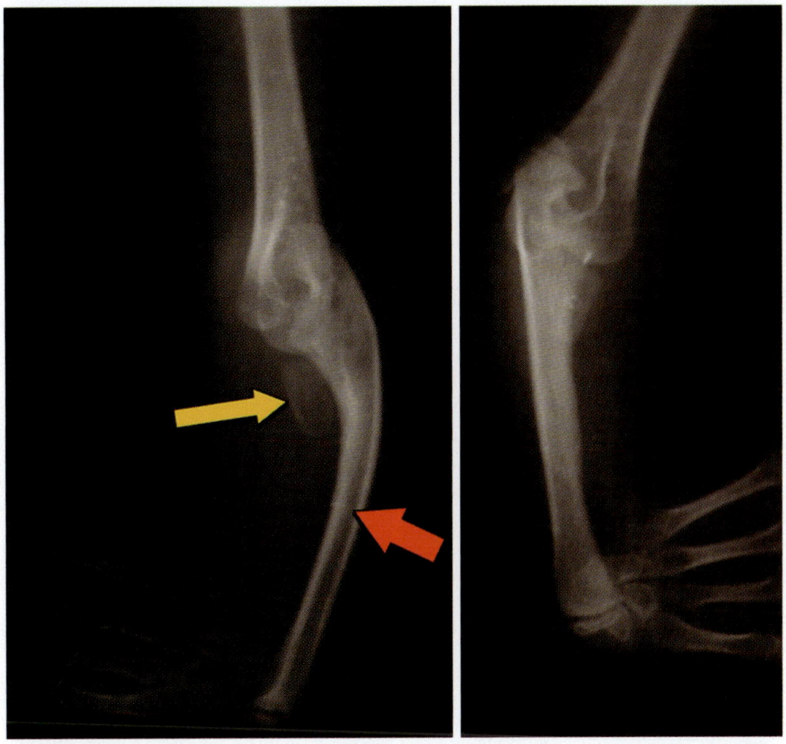

Radiographs of the forearm show a severely hypoplastic radius bone (*yellow arrow*) with bowing of ulna (*red arrow*). Hand is rotated with the absence of thumb.

Radial Ray Anomaly

- Radial ray anomaly belongs to a spectrum of upper limb abnormalities characterized by the aplasia/hypoplasia of radius, thumb or carpal bones.
- Foetal ultrasonography can detect the absence of radius bone in the prenatal period.

- Radial ray anomaly is associated with various syndromes:
  1. Holt–Oram syndrome
  2. Fanconi anaemia
  3. TAR syndrome (thrombocytopenia absent radius)
  4. VACTERL
  5. Amniotic band syndrome

OSCE 47

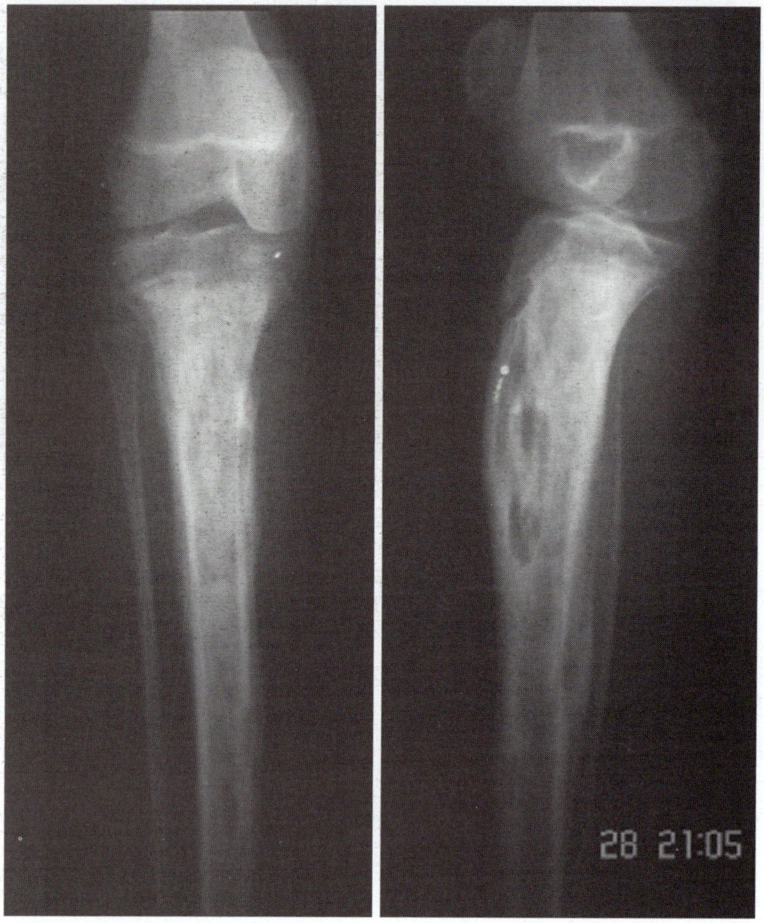

Clinical details: A 35-year-old male with chronic discharging sinus over right leg.

1. **Describe your findings.**
2. **What is the most appropriate diagnosis?**
3. **What are the differentials for this lesion?**
4. **Name another investigation/s that you would recommended.**

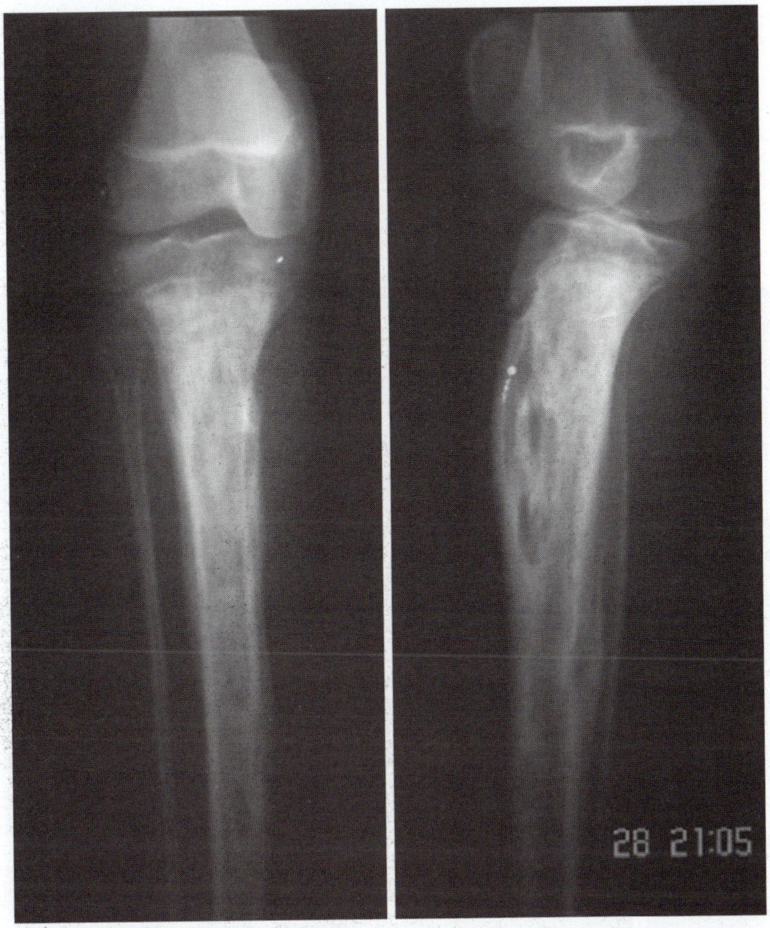

Frontal and lateral radiographs of right knee and upper leg show multiple ovoid, osteolytic lesions involving the metadiaphyseal region at the medial aspect of proximal left tibia. It shows thick sclerotic borders, a narrow zone of transition and lamellated type of periosteal reaction. An irregular thickening of the cortex is noted at the medial aspect of tibia with irregular and distorted trabecular pattern as compared to that of normal bone. A discrete sclerotic focus is seen within one of these lytic areas likely suggestive of sequestrum. A subtle lucent gap is seen in the cortex of a bone at medial end at the proximal end likely suggestive of cloaca. No obvious soft tissue component is seen.

Chronic Osteomyelitis

- Osteomyelitis is of three distinctive clinical and radiological types: acute, subacute and chronic osteomyelitis. Acute <2 weeks, subacute 2–6 weeks and chronic >6 weeks.
- Three routes of infection: Haematogenous, by contiguity, or direct implantation through a penetrating wound/foreign body.
- Common sites are the fast-growing and large metaphysis around the knee joint, wrist joint and proximal humerus.
- Chronic osteomyelitis may be indolent for a long time and then reactivate due to continuous low-grade infection.

RADIOLOGICAL FEATURES

- Radiographs are usually the first investigation. The earliest imaging feature is soft tissue swelling. Other features such as bone destruction and periosteal reaction are seen 10–21 days after onset.
- Bone scintigraphy may also assist in localizing osteomyelitis and distinguishing it from cellulitis. MRI and computed tomography (CT) provide complementary and detailed evaluation of osseous and soft tissue changes. Magnetic resonance imaging (MRI) is considered the gold standard for osteomyelitis evaluation. Ultrasound application for soft tissues evaluation and abscess drainage guidance has encouraging reports.
- Possible complications comprise septic arthritis, pathologic fracture, growth disturbances and rarely squamous cell carcinoma decades after chronic osteomyelitis with longstanding sinus tract drainage. Early diagnosis and prolonged antibiotic therapy are vital to eradicate osteomyelitis and prevent sequelae.

OSCE

48

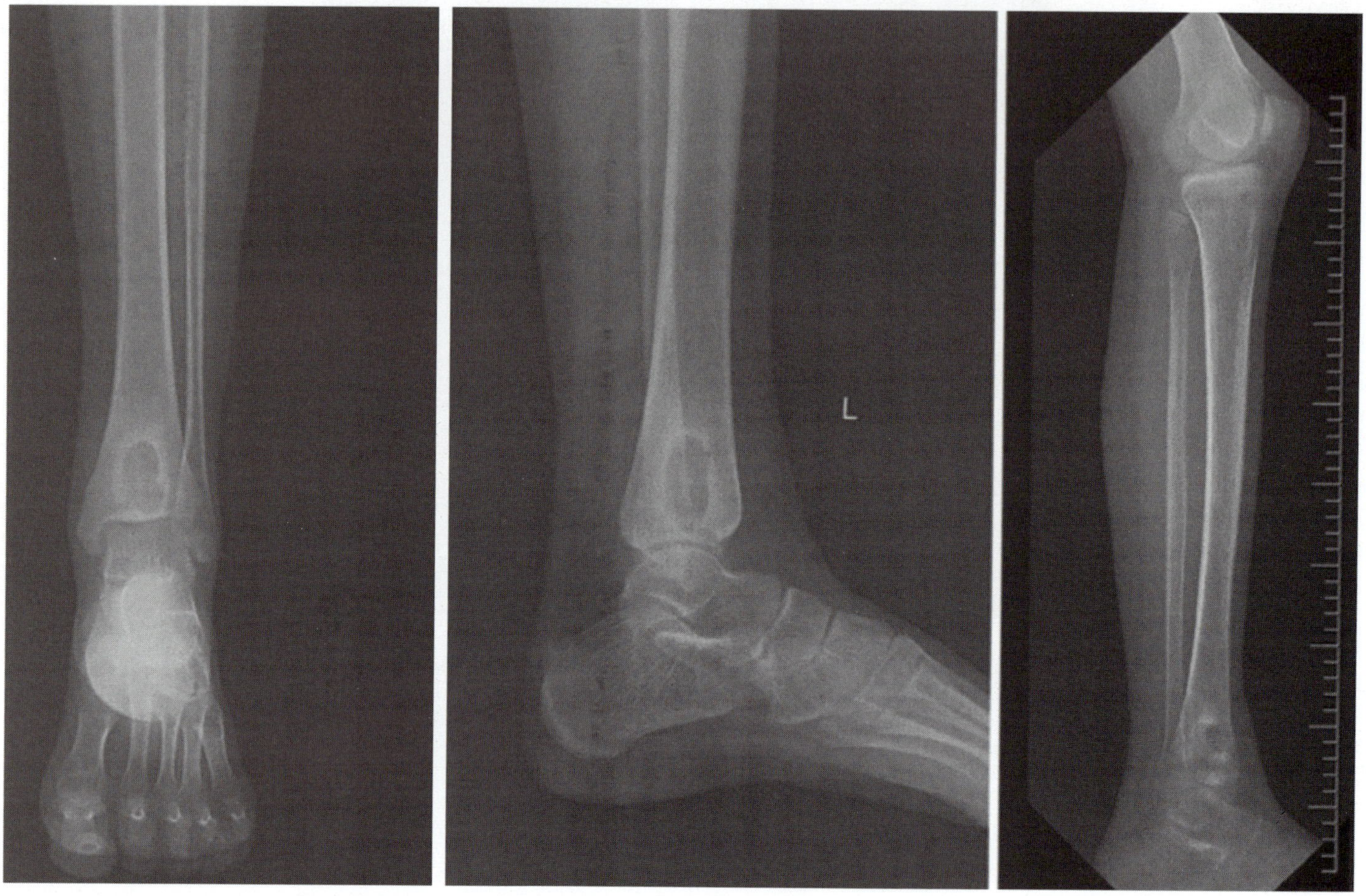

Clinical details: Chronic localized pain with history of night pains.

1. **Describe your findings.**
2. **What is the most appropriate diagnosis?**
3. **What are the differentials for this lesion?**
4. **What another investigation/s would be recommended?**

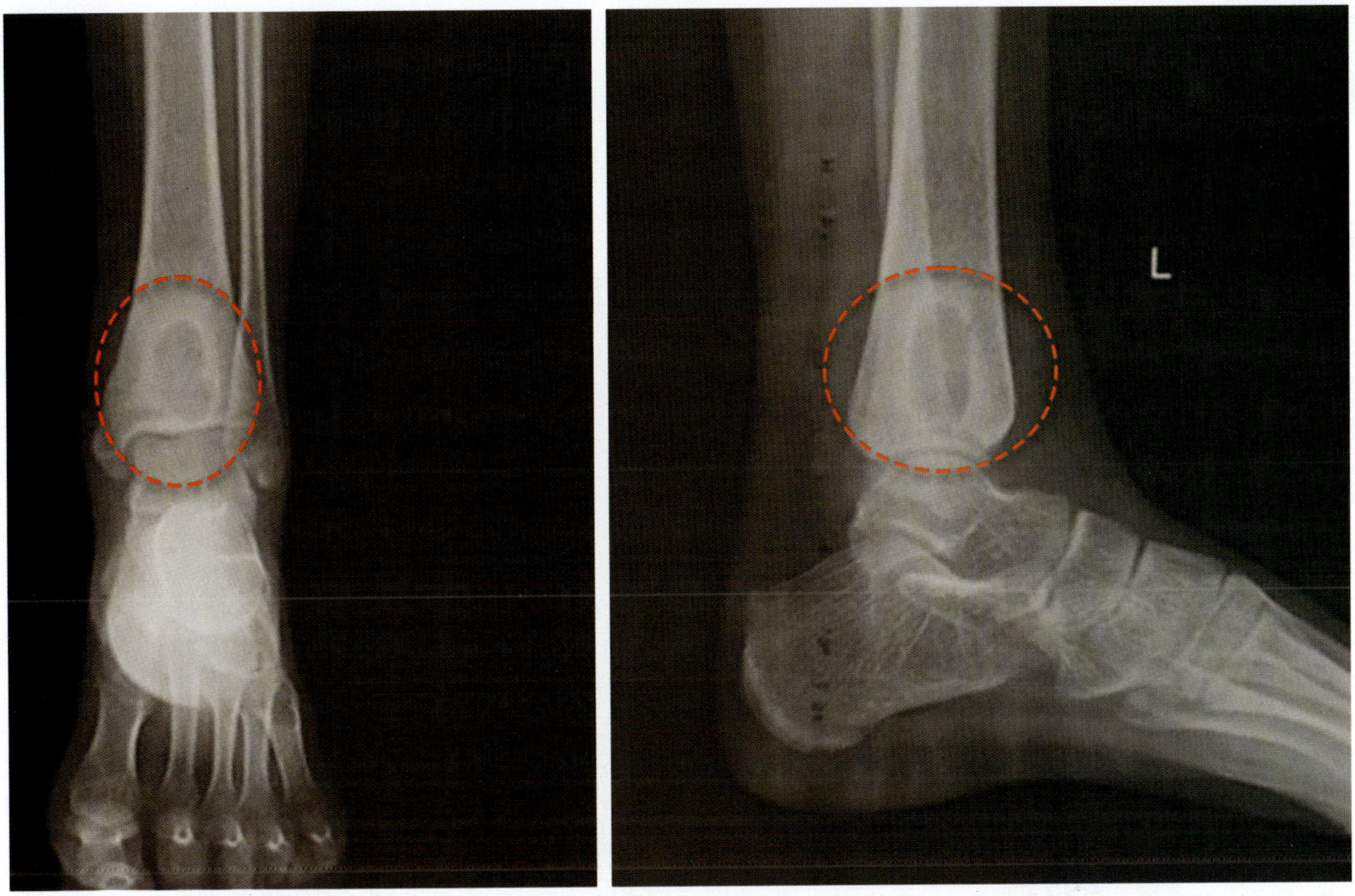

Radiographs showed a well-defined, flame-shaped lucency in the distal tibial metaphysis surrounded by considerable sclerosis. No evidence of bony expansion/fracture.

Brodie's Abscess

- Brodie's abscess is a complication of subacute osteomyelitis.

RADIOLOGICAL FEATURES

- On radiographs, it is seen as a well-defined metaphyseal central lucency with surrounding zone of reactive sclerosis.
- A channel/tract connecting this lucency to the physis is commonly seen. Cortical extension results in periostitis and involvement of extra-osseous soft tissues.
- Technetium-99m methylene diphosphonate (MDP) scintigraphy demonstrates intense uptake of tracer on flow, diffusion and delayed images and is particularly useful in excluding other areas of clinically occult infection.
- Computed tomography (CT) defines the margins of the abscess cavity and the extent of soft tissue involvement more clearly. It is highly sensitive in identifying sequestrum. Rarely fat-fluid levels/gas may also be demonstrated within the abscess.
- On magnetic resonance imaging (MRI), Brodie's abscesses appear as well-defined intra-osseous regions of low-to-intermediate signal intensity on T1-weighted images and of high signal intensity on T2-weighted images. A rim of low signal intensity due to sclerotic bone is seen. They are surrounded by extensive changes in the bone marrow which may extend into the extra-osseous soft tissues. Sequestrum is a dead bone, appears as areas of low signal on all sequences and does not enhance.
- The differential diagnosis of Brodie's abscess includes bone neoplasms including, particularly when small and cortically located, osteoid osteomas.

OSCE

49

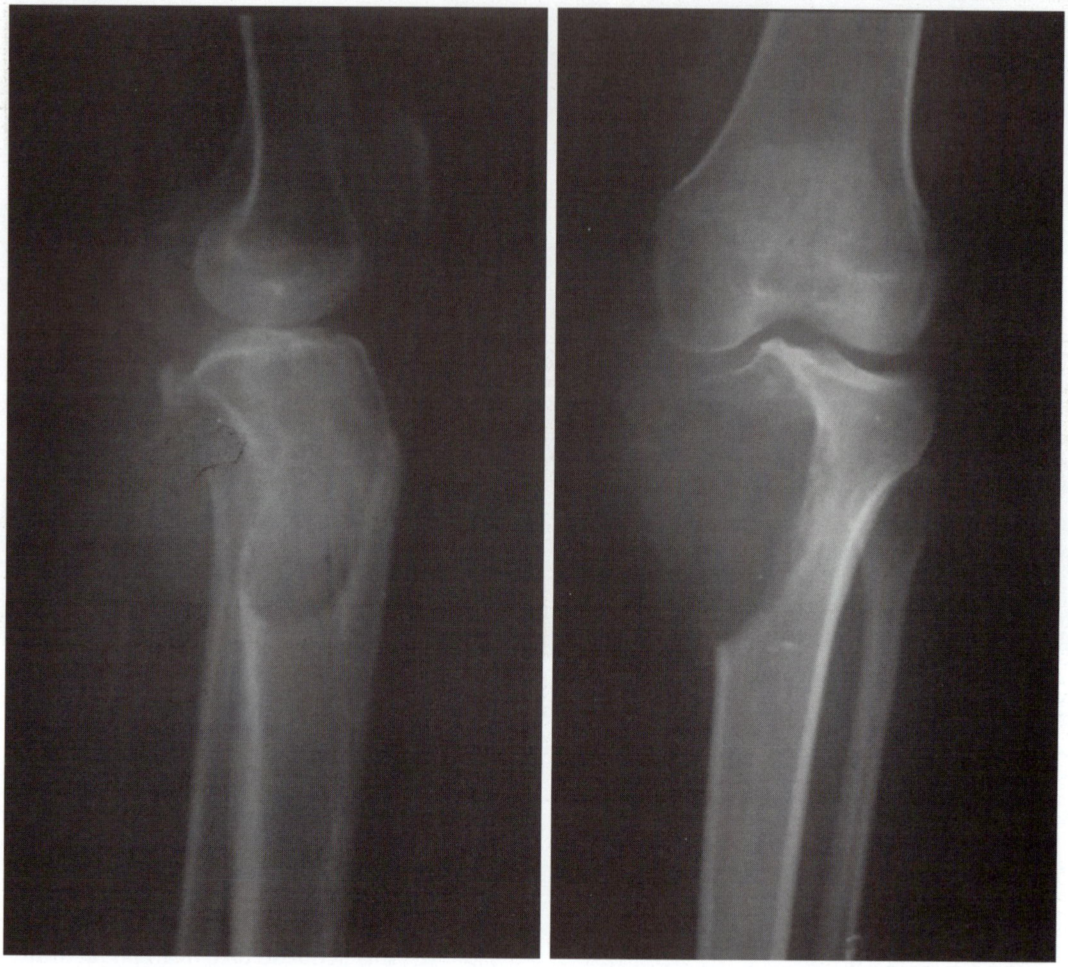

Clinical details: A 36-year-old male with pain and swelling over left knee.

1. **Describe your findings.**
2. **What is the most appropriate diagnosis?**
3. **What are the differentials for this lesion?**
4. **What another investigation/s would be recommended?**

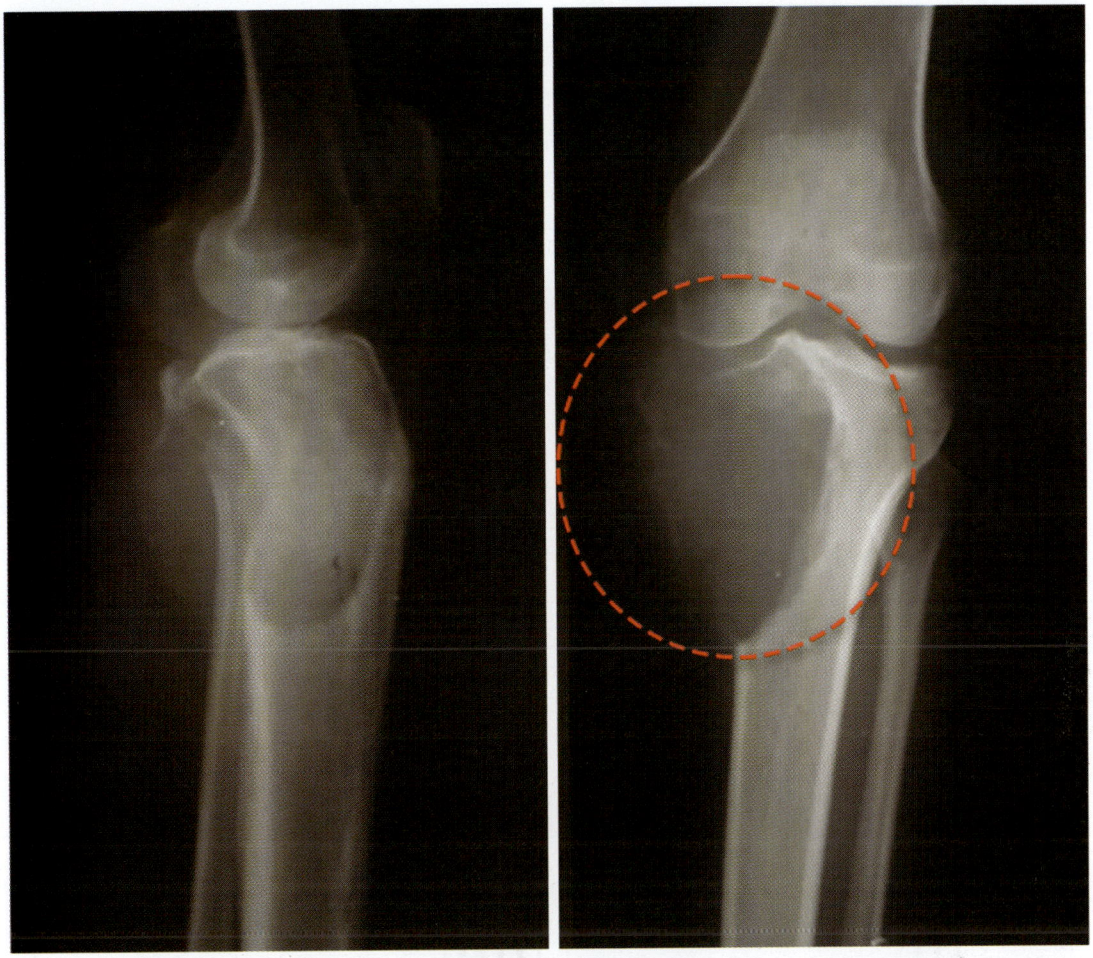

Frontal and lateral radiographs of left knee in a mature skeleton show a well-defined, eccentric, osteolytic lesion is seen in the subarticular region of the left tibia. It shows narrow zone of transition without obvious sclerosis/periosteal reaction or pathological fracture.

Giant Cell Tumour

- Giant cell tumours (GCTs) are locally aggressive bone neoplasms, typically occurring at the epiphysis of long bones in skeletally mature patients of 20 to 40 years. GCT account for 5% of the bone tumours with a slight female predilection.
- Most frequent sites include distal femur, proximal tibia and distal radius.
- Although they tend towards the benign end of the spectrum, there is a tendency to recur locally and may undergo sarcomatous transformation or metastasize to the lungs in 1%–9% of cases. They usually present with pain and swelling of the affected area or post-traumatic pathological fracture.

RADIOLOGICAL FEATURES

- It usually presents as a lytic epiphyseal expansile lesion, extending to the subchondral bone without surrounding sclerosis. Septations vary from fine striations to coarse trabeculation.
- The Campanacci system of grading maybe used to characterize plain radiographs.

Campanacci System Grade	Description
I	No cortical disruption and have a well-defined sclerotic medullary margin
II	Bone insufflation, with cortical thinning, and a well-defined non-sclerotic medullary margin
III	Unclear/indistinct margins, cortical disruption and soft tissue extension

- Magnetic resonance imaging (MRI) can be used for pre-operative local evaluation and to assess the extraosseous component. GCT usually shows a low to intermediate signal on T1-weighted (best to appreciate the intramedullary component) and T2-weighted images (fluid levels), and low signal due to haemosiderin deposition with significant enhancement of the solid component after contrast.
- The usual treatment is curettage with or without bone graft and cement.

OSCE 50

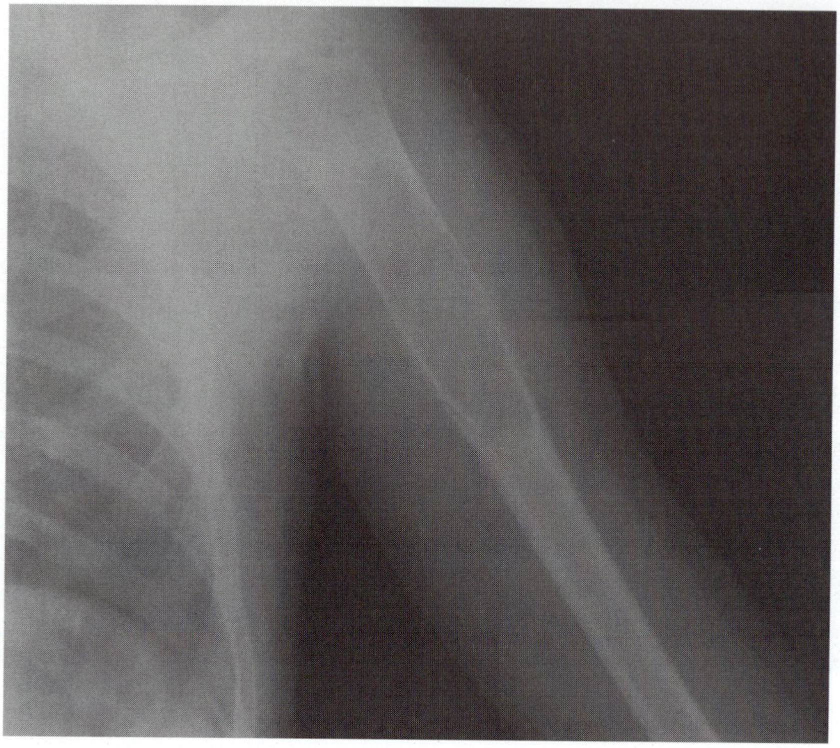

Clinical details: Young boy with pain and swelling over left proximal arm.

1. **Describe your findings in the above radiograph.**
2. **What is the most likely diagnosis?**
3. **What is the most common location for this pathology?**
4. **What is the 'fallen fragment sign'?**

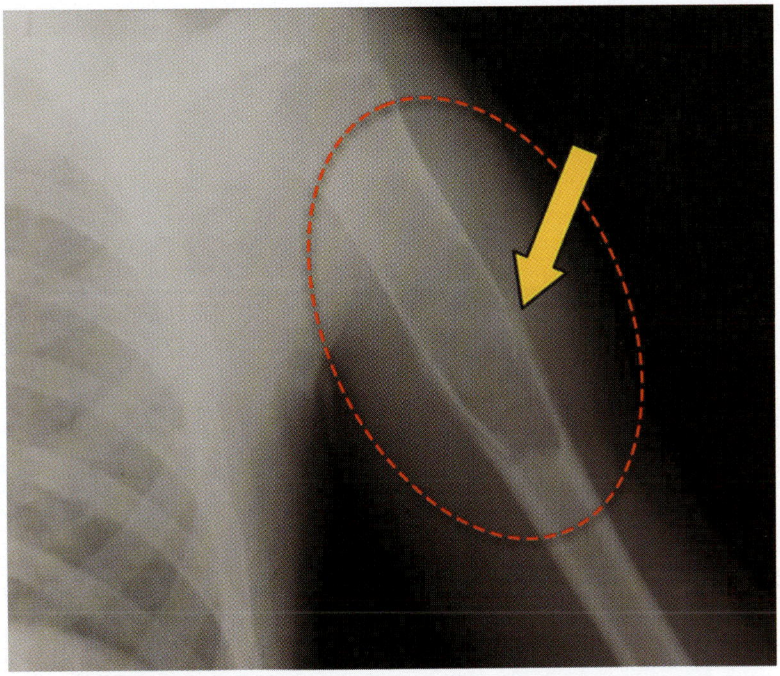

Radiograph of the left humerus of a 10-year-old boy shows a well-defined, intramedullary expansile lytic lesion with a narrow zone of transition and a thin sclerotic rim in the metadiaphysis. Associated pathological fracture (*yellow arrow*).

Simple Bone Cyst (Unicameral Bone Cyst)

- Simple bone cysts (SBCs) or unicameral bone cysts (UBCs) are benign bony lesions that are most frequently encountered in children and normally do not cause any symptoms.
- UBCs are typically seen in the first and second decades (young age group) and are more frequently seen in males.
- Men are more likely to have them than women (M:F 2–3:1).

RADIOLOGICAL FEATURES

- SBC is characterized radiologically as a centrally located well-defined intramedullary geographic expansile lytic lesion with a narrow zone of transition and a thin sclerotic rim.
- Magnetic resonance imaging (MRI) features include a low T1 signal, a high T2 signal and peripheral enhancement post-contrast. Fluid-fluid levels can be seen if fibrous septations are present.
- 'Fallen fragment sign' is defined by the presence of a bone fracture fragment within a cystic bone lesion. It can be seen in pathological fracture associated with SBC, eosinophilic granuloma or aneurysmal bone cyst.
- Differential includes aneurysmal bone cyst (eccentric location).

OSCE

51

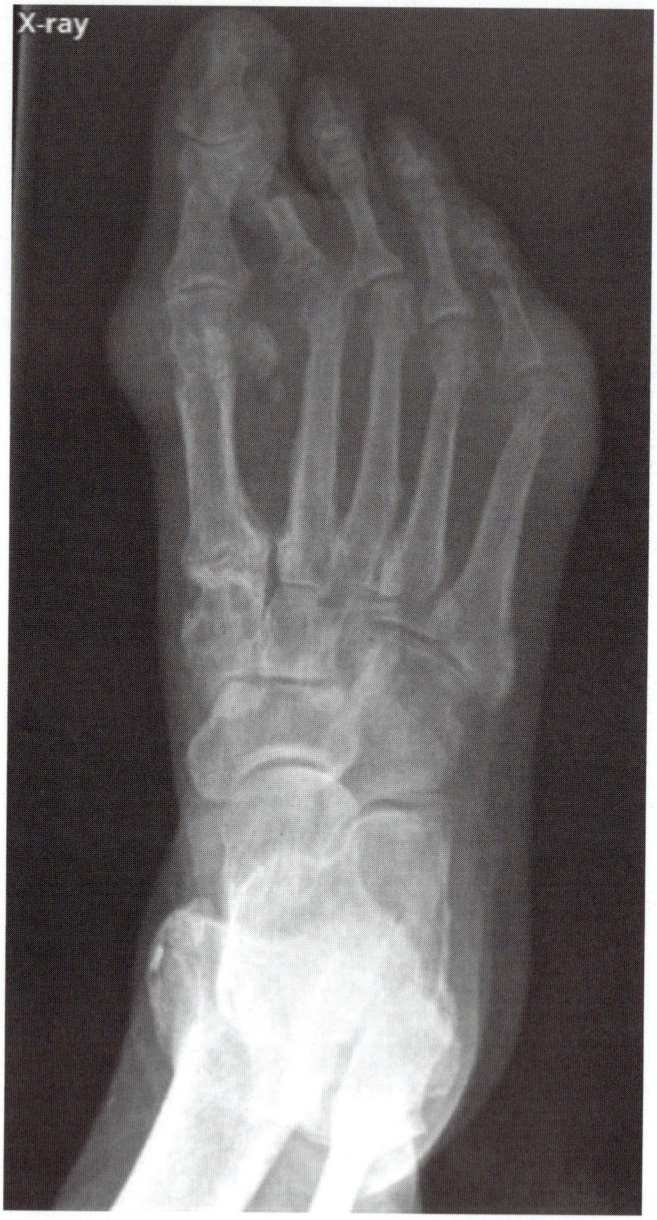

Clinical details: Middle aged man with polyarthralgia.

1. **Describe your findings.**
2. **What is the most appropriate diagnosis?**
3. **What is the underlying cause?**
4. **What are the differentials for this lesion?**

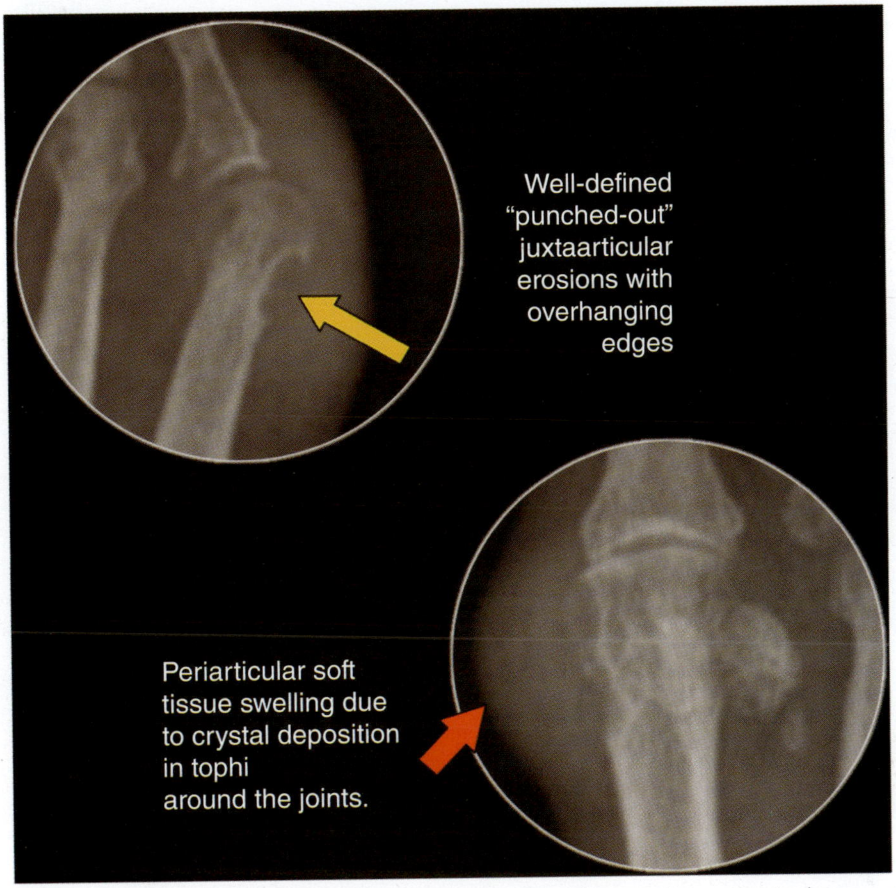

Zoomed images of the frontal radiograph of forefoot show soft tissue swelling with juxta-articular punched-out erosions at the metatarsophalangeal joints. The joint space is maintained.

Gouty Arthropathy (Crystal Arthropathy)

- Gout is a systemic metabolic disorder which occurs due to deposition of monosodium urate crystals in and around joints. It is characterized by hyperuricaemia which may be due to either an increase in production or a decrease in excretion of uric acid.
- It usually occurs in adults; age >40 years. Males are affected more than females.

LOCATION

- First metatarsophalangeal (MTP) joint most common
- Hands, wrists, elbows and knees

Characteristic radiographic findings of chronic tophaceous gout include following:

Erosions:

- Marginal = bare area
- Periarticular = metaphysis/diaphysis
- Intraosseous = well-defined, oval-shaped radiolucencies intramedullary
- Well-defined 'punched-out' erosions
- Overhanging edges
- Sclerotic margins
- Preserved joint space
- Normal mineralization

Tophi:

- Periarticular soft tissue swelling due to crystal deposition in tophi around the joints
- Hyperdense due to the crystals, tophi can calcify
- Juxta-articular
- Olecranon and prepatellar bursitis
- T1 WI: Intermediate signal intensity (SI) (isointense relative to muscles)
- T2 WI: Intermediate to low SI
- Post-contrast: Homogeneous and intense enhancement

OSCE

52

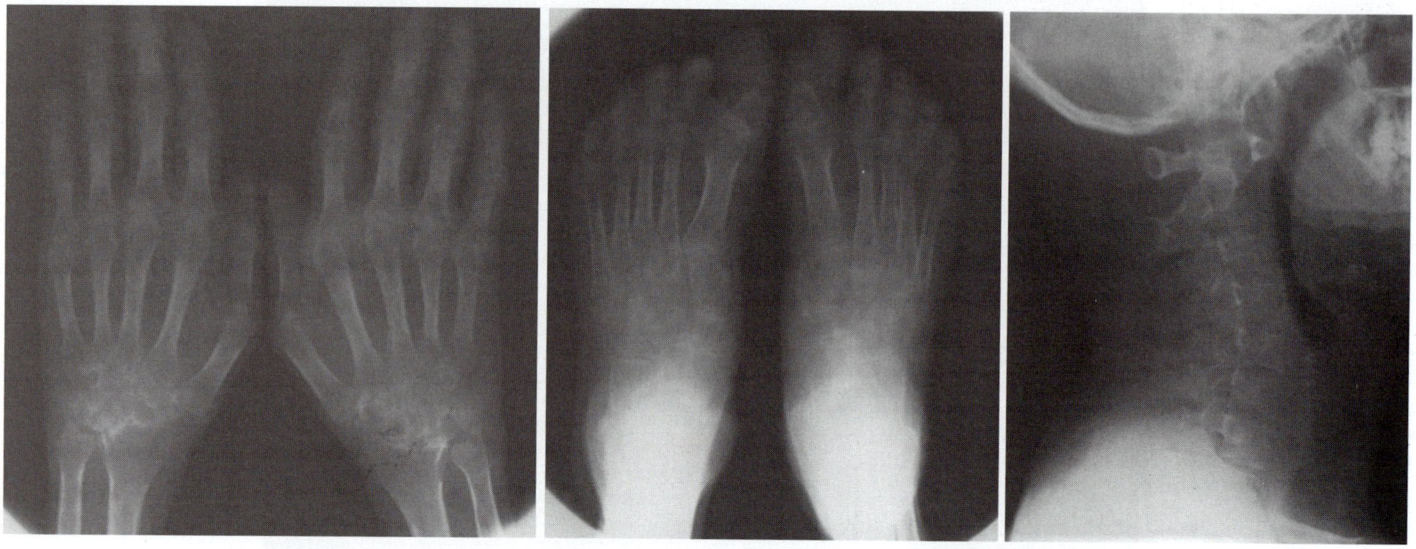

Clinical details: A 45-year-old lady with polyarthralgia.

1. **Describe your findings in the above radiographs.**
2. **What is the unified diagnosis?**
3. **Name two characteristic deformities seen in wrist radiographs in this pathology.**
4. **Give two appropriate differential diagnosis.**

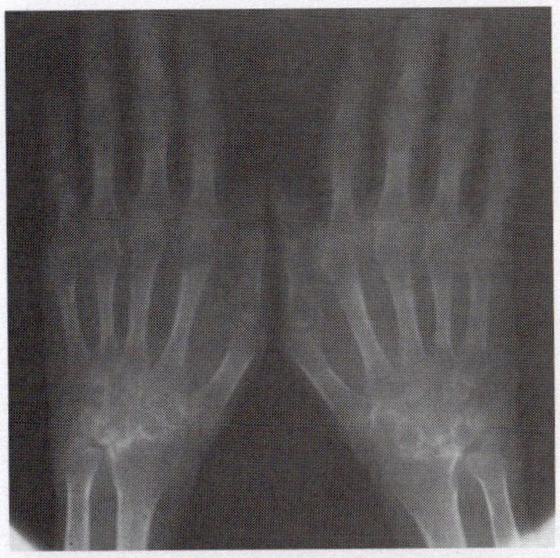

Radiograph both hands:
- Diffuse osteopenia in carpals
- Periarticular osteopenia in all metacarpophalangeal (MCP) joints
- Erosions involving articular surfaces of radius and ulna in both hands
- Reduced Intercarpal (IC) joint space in both hands
- Ulnar deviation of digits (more in right hand)

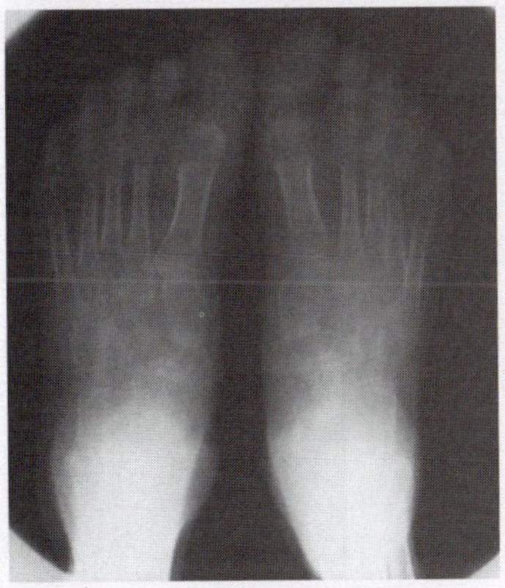

Radiograph both feet:
- Diffuse osteopenia
- Erosions in distal interphalangeal (DIP) joints of great toe in both feet
- Tibial subluxation of all metatarsophalangeal (MTP) joints in bilateral feet
- Loss of intertarsal joint spaces

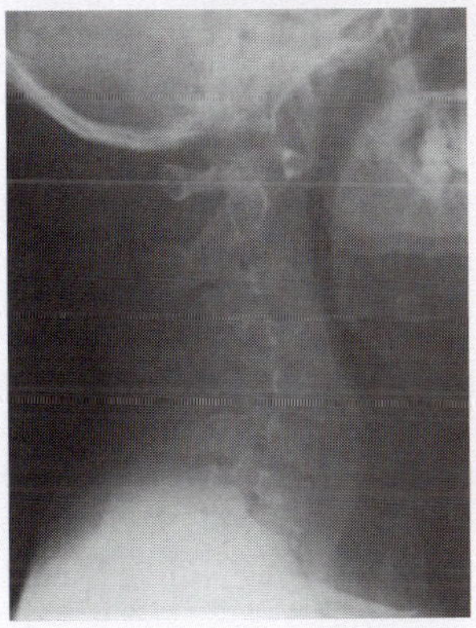

Radiograph cervical spine
- Atlantoaxial distance (AAD) >3 mm on a flexion radiograph

Rheumatoid Arthritis (Musculoskeletal Manifestations)

Rheumatoid arthritis (RA) is an autoimmune disorder characterized by chronic inflammation of the synovial tissue, leading to the progressive destruction of cartilage, bone and other joint structures. It is caused by the complex interplay of genetic, environmental and immunologic factors.

Common radiographic manifestations of RA:

- Periarticular osteopenic changes
- Uniform loss of joint space
- Marginal erosions
- Subchondral cyst formation
- Subluxations

Hand involvement:

- Symmetrical arthritis
- Typically, the hands are affected before the feet
- Primarily involves the MCP joints, proximal interphalangeal (PIP) joints and carpal bones
- Boutonnière deformity: Characterized by flexion at the PIP joint and extension at the DIP joint
- Swan neck deformity: Characterized by extension at the PIP joint and flexion at the DIP joint
- ‘Telescoping’ of fingers: Phalanges are dislocated, leading to subsequent shortening

Feet involvement:

- Initially involves the MTP joints (preference for fourth and fifth MTP joints)
- Erosions occur on the bare areas of the metatarsal heads
- Joint subluxations as disease progresses
- Bony ankylosis can develop with chronic disease

Cervical spine:

- Dens erosion
- Atlantoaxial subluxation with atlantoaxial distance more than 3 mm
- Uncovertebral, facet joint and spinous process erosions

Differentials include following:

1. Osteoarthritis:
   - PIP and DIP joints and thumb carpometacarpal joint are involved; MCP joints are spared
   - Subchondral sclerosis, osteophytes
   - Loss of joint space
   - Absence of erosive changes/ankylosis
2. Erosive osteoarthritis:
   - 'Gull-wing' type central erosions
3. Psoriatic arthritis:
   - Interphalangeal predominance
   - Erosive changes with proliferation of bone
   - Osteoporosis is not seen

OSCE

53

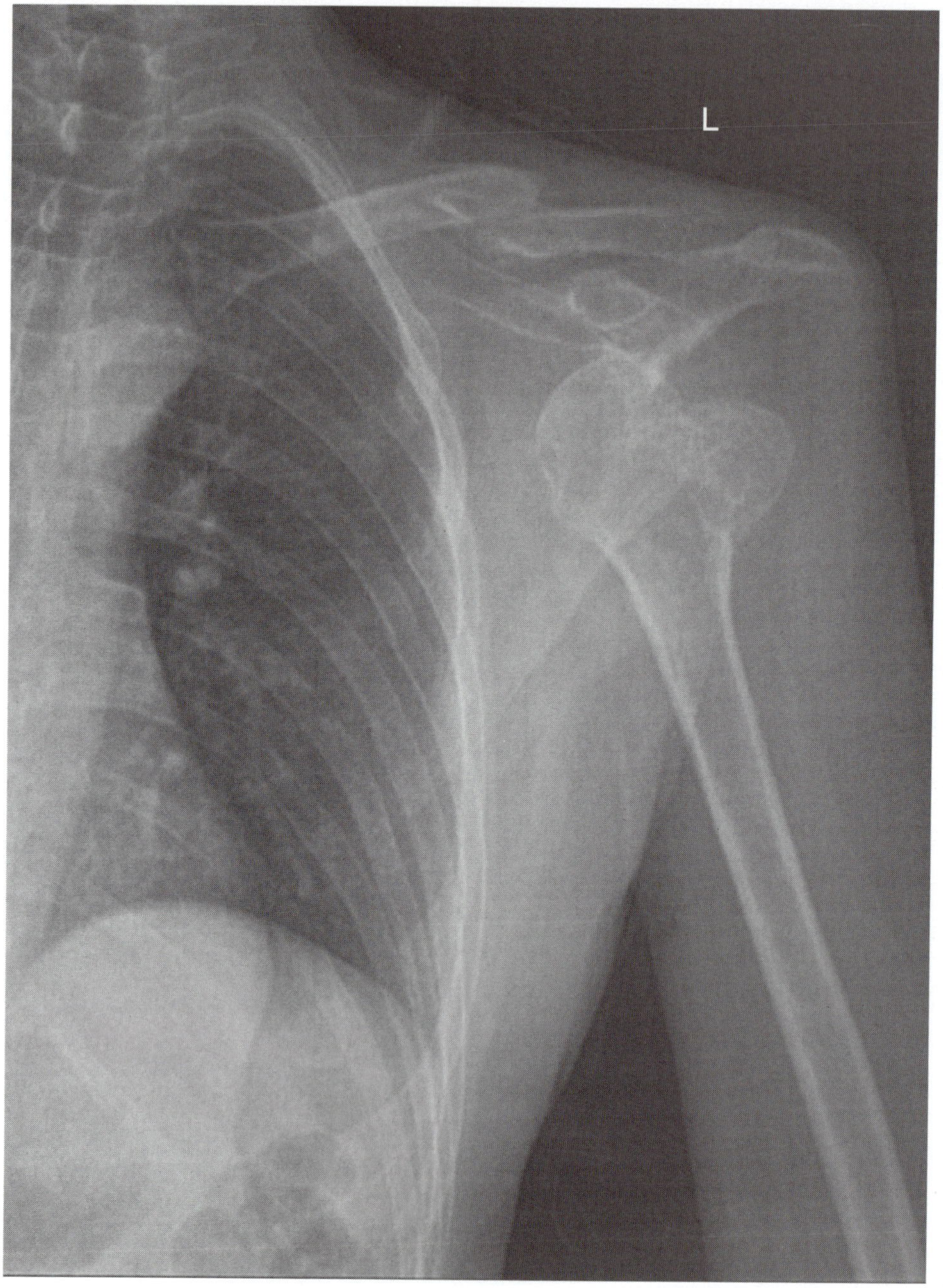

Clinical details: Adult male with a history of shoulder trauma.

1. **What is the most appropriate diagnosis?**
2. **Describe your findings.**
3. **What other view would you recommended?**
4. **How much is the radiation dose for this view?**

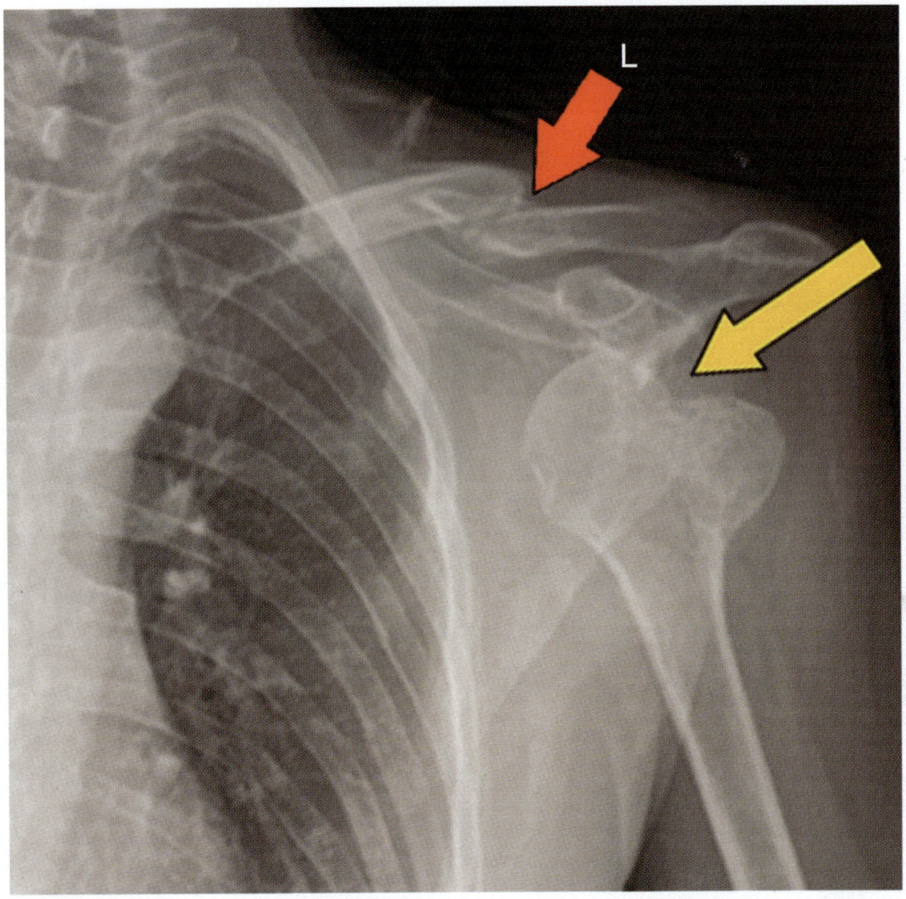

Frontal radiograph of left shoulder joint and proximal humerus shows presence of a wedge-shaped defect (*yellow arrow*) in the posterolateral aspect of the humeral head with fracture of the anteroinferior aspect of the glenoid. Also noted is displaced fracture of the middle third of the left clavicle (*red arrow*).

Recurrent Dislocation of Shoulder With Hill–Sachs Defect

- The glenohumeral joint is the most common site of subluxation or dislocation in the human body. Anterior dislocations, constituting 97% of cases, are particularly prevalent, with approximately 40% of them being recurrent.
- Complications include Hill–Sachs and bony Bankart lesions, avulsion fractures of the greater tuberosity (10%–15%), and injuries to the rotator cuff and brachial plexus (7%–45%).

RADIOLOGICAL FEATURES

- Hill–Sachs defect is a compression fracture of the posterolateral aspect of the humeral head. Its prevalence is 25% in acute dislocations and rises to 75% in cases of recurrent dislocations. This defect occurs during the dislocation event when the humeral head impacts the anteroinferior margin of the glenoid. Notably, its size tends to be more substantial in shoulders dislocated for extended durations and in instances of recurrent dislocations. Optimal visualization of the Hill–Sachs lesion is achieved through the anteroposterior projection of the shoulder with internal rotation of the arm.
- A bony Bankart lesion refers to a fracture occurring at the anterior aspect of the inferior glenoid rim, a less frequent occurrence. This pathology is clearly visible on the anteroposterior (AP) view with the arm positioned neutrally.
- Occasionally, supplementary views like the Abduction and external rotation (ABER) view and shoulder Y view may be necessary for a comprehensive assessment.
- Employing additional imaging modalities such as computed tomography (CT) arthrography, magnetic resonance (MR) and MR arthrography may be essential to effectively reveal abnormalities in the labrum and capsule.
- The radiation dosage associated with the shoulder AP view is measured at **0.01 mSv**.

OSCE

54

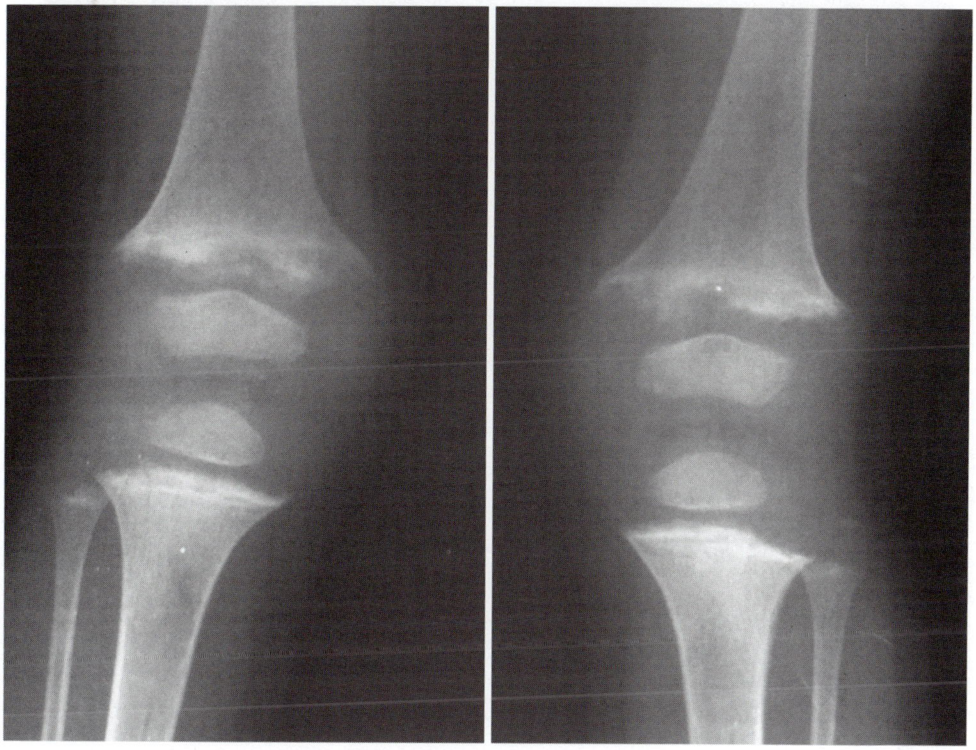

Clinical details: Young boy with lethargy bone pain and bleeding gums.

1. **What is the most appropriate diagnosis?**
2. **What is the underlying cause?**
3. **What are the classical radiological signs seen here?**
4. **Explain two causes of 'lucent metaphyseal bands' in a radiograph.**

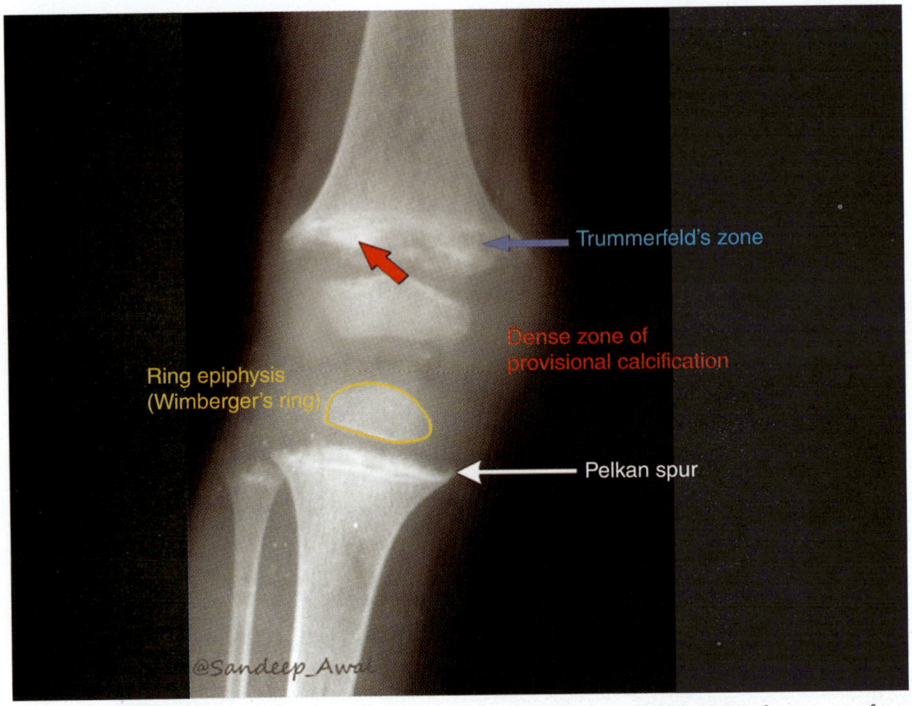

Frontal radiograph of a paediatric knee joint showing some of the classic features of scurvy.

Scurvy

- Scurvy is caused by the deficiency of vitamin C in children, commonly arising from insufficient dietary intake of the vitamin.
- **Radiographic features** are osteopenia, thinning of the cortex, subperiosteal haemorrhage and the following classic radiological signs listed:

White line of Frenkel	Dense zone of provisional calcification (*red arrow*)
Trummerfeld's zone	Lucent zone beneath the Frenkel line (*blue arrow*)
Wimberger's ring	Ring-shaped thin calcification surrounding the epiphyses
Pelkan spur	Beak-like prominence of the metaphyseal corners (*white arrow*)

- Differential diagnosis for 'lucent metaphyseal bands' includes scurvy, neuroblastoma metastasis, leukaemia and lymphoma.

OSCE

55

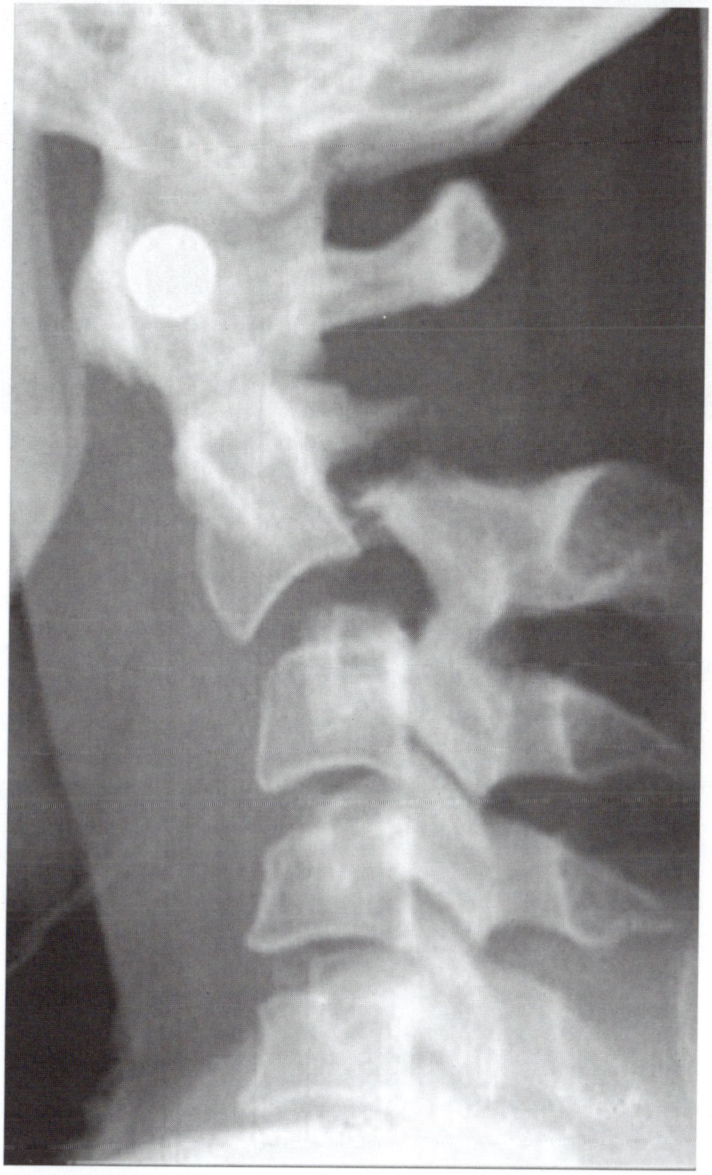

Clinical details: An adult male met with a motor vehicle accident.

1. **What is this fracture known as?**
2. **Define Jefferson fracture.**
3. **What is Clay-Shoveler's fracture?**
4. **How many types of odontoid fractures are there?**

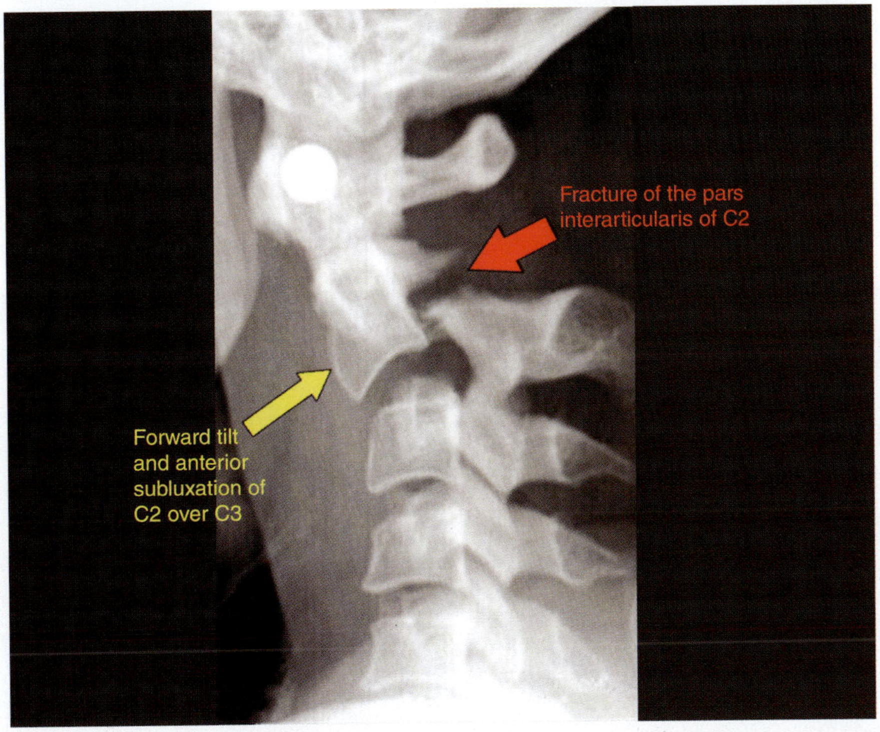

Lateral cervical spine radiograph, the case of Hangman fracture: Fracture through the pedicles of C2 vertebra. There is forward tilt and anterior subluxation of C2 over C3.

Cervical Spine Fractures

Jefferson fracture:	A burst fracture of the first cervical vertebra (C1) caused by axial compression. It is a **stable** injury.
Hangman's fracture:	A fracture of the second cervical vertebra (C2) caused by hyperextension injury, resulting in a bilateral fracture of the pars interarticularis.
Odontoid fracture:	A fracture of the dens or odontoid process of the second cervical vertebra (C2), which can be classified into three types: type I (**stable**), a fracture of the tip of the dens; type II (**unstable**), a fracture at the base of the dens; and type III (**unstable**), a fracture extending into the C2 vertebral body.
Clay-shoveler's fracture:	A fracture of the spinous process of a lower cervical or upper thoracic vertebra (C6–T1) caused rotation of the upper trunk with a fixed cervical spine. It is a **stable** injury.
Chance fracture:	Transverse fracture through the posterior elements of a vertebra, usually in the thoracolumbar region, usually due to a seat belt injury.

OSCE 56

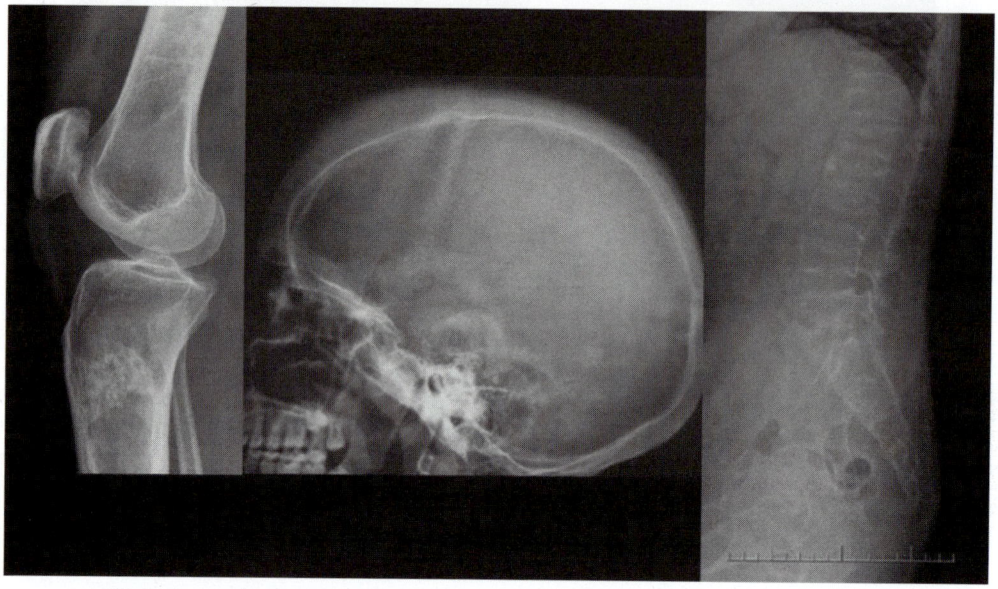

Clinical details: A young boy with anaemia and acute onset loss of vision.

1. **What is the most appropriate diagnosis?**
2. **Enumerate the systems involved and some of the systemic manifestations?**
3. **What is the inheritance pattern?**
4. **Enumerate a few complications?**

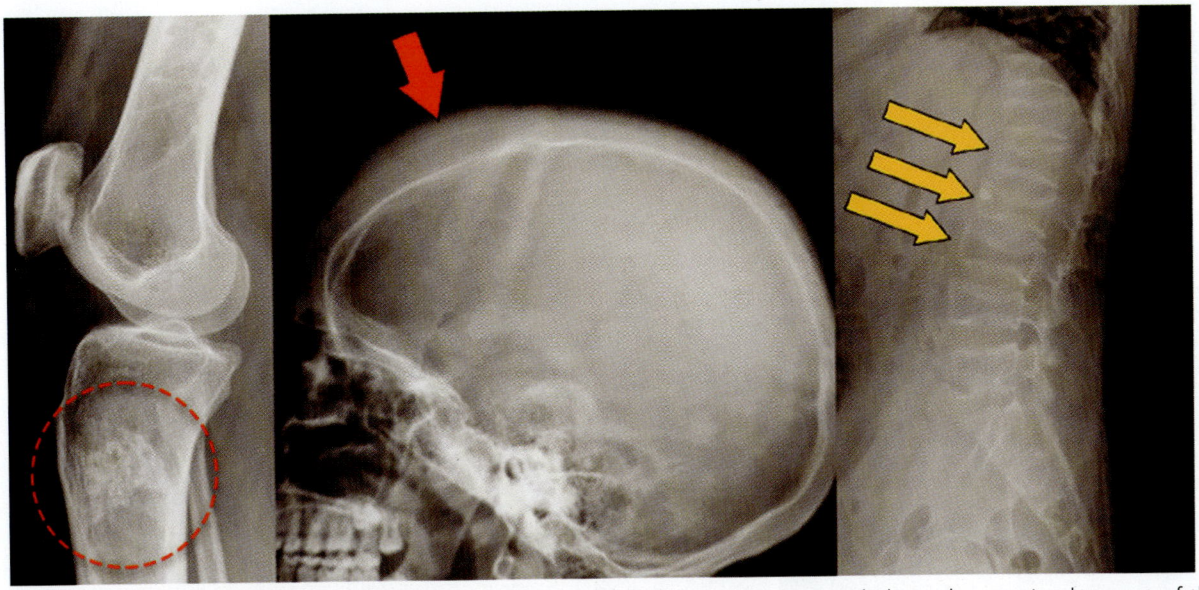

Radiograph of knee: There are abnormal, serpiginous, medullary radiodensities observed along the proximal aspect of the tibia in keeping with bone infarcts. Lateral radiograph of the skull: There is widening of the diploic space of the calvarium, hair on end appearance (*red arrow*) of diploic space due to thickening of trabeculae. Lateral radiograph of spine: There are central endplate depressions of multiple lumbar vertebrae (*yellow arrows*) – H-shaped or Lincoln log vertebrae.

Sickle Cell Disease

- Sickle cell disease (SCD) is an autosomal recessive (AR) disorder which leads to haemoglobinopathy and causes haemolytic anaemia. There is mutation involving the beta chain of haemoglobin. SCD commonly involves the skeletal system, pulmonary system, cardiovascular system, abdominal system and cerebral system.
- Skeletal system: The commonest manifestations include
  - (a) Bone infarcts most commonly of proximal long bones and vertebral bodies
  - (b) Characteristic endplate infarction
  - (c) Dactylitis or hand-foot syndrome
  - (d) Osteomyelitis caused by *Salmonella* or *Staphylococcus aureus*.
- Pulmonary system: The commonest manifestations include
  - (a) Pneumonia
  - (b) Acute chest syndrome due to sepsis or pulmonary fat embolism
  - (c) Long-term pulmonary fibrosis.
- Cardiovascular system: The commonest manifestations include
  - (a) Increased cardiac output resulting in cardiomegaly
  - (b) Ventricular dysfunction.
- Abdominal system: The commonest manifestations include
  - (a) Splenomegaly in early childhood
  - (b) Auto-splenectomy
  - (c) Haemosiderosis due to repeated blood transfusions
  - (d) Portal hypertension
  - (e) Liver abscesses
  - (f) Cholelithiasis
  - (g) Nephrotic syndrome
  - (h) Papillary necrosis
  - (i) Renal vein thrombosis
  - (j) Bowel ischaemia.
- Cerebral system: The commonest manifestations include
  - (a) Cognitive impairment
  - (b) Cerebral infarction
  - (c) Cerebral aneurysms and their complications and Moyamoya disease.
- Patients are at increased risk of renal medullary carcinoma.
- Diagnostic test is haemoglobin electrophoresis.
- Bone marrow transplant and supportive management are the main stay of management with normal life expectancy.

OSCE

57

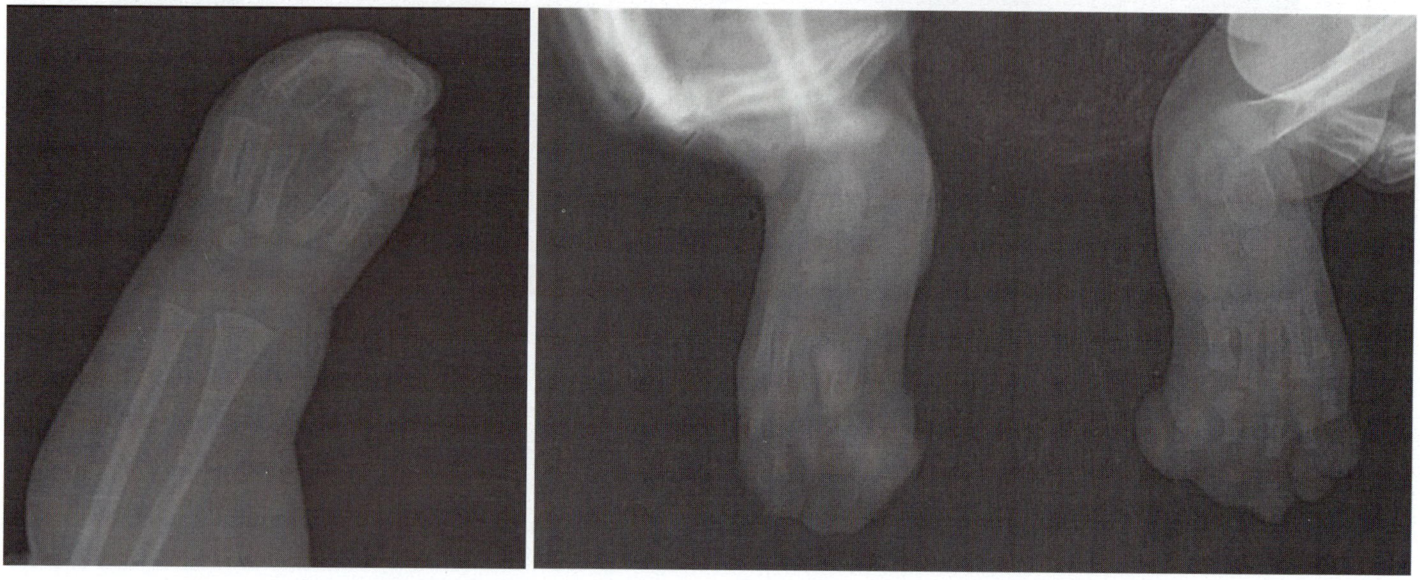

Clinical details: A toddler with a tower-shaped head with prominent forehead.

1. **What is the most appropriate diagnosis?**
2. **What is the inheritance pattern?**
3. **Enumerate the associations?**
4. **Is there any risk factor?**

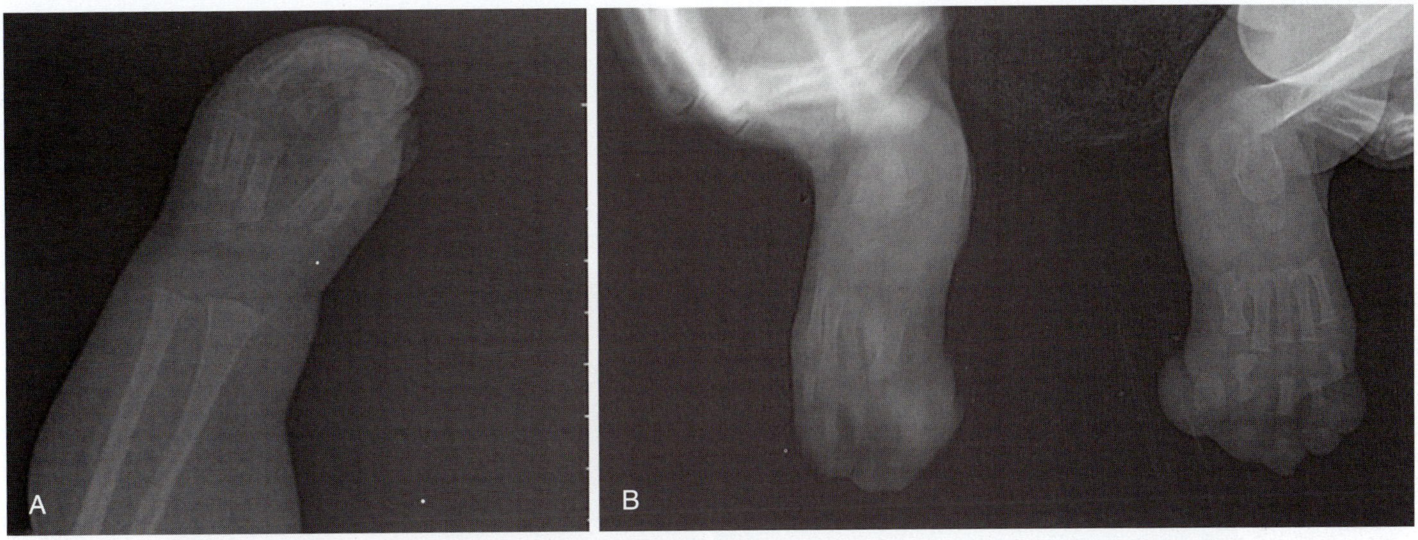

(A) Radiograph of the hand demonstrates syndactyly with fusion of multiple phalanges. (B) A radiograph of the demonstrated polydactyly and syndactyly with fusion of multiple phalanges.

Apert Syndrome

- Apert syndrome is also known as type I acrocephalosyndactyly which is a rare autosomal dominant malformation.
- Mutation of fibroblast growth factor receptor ($FGFR_2$) gene, a fibroblast growth factor.
- Triad = brachycephaly, syndactyly and maxillary hypoplasia.
- Associated with symphalangism (fusion of interphalangeal joints). Webbed fingers and toes are also a feature.
- There are central nervous system anomalies such as multisuture craniosynostosis most commonly involving the coronal suture causing a brachycephalic skull.
- Complex cyanotic heart diseases are the congenital cardiac anomaly associated with Apert syndrome.
- A known risk factor is increased paternal age.
- Additional abnormalities include cloverleaf skull, hypertelorism, exophthalmos, intellectual disability and prominent forehead.

OSCE

58

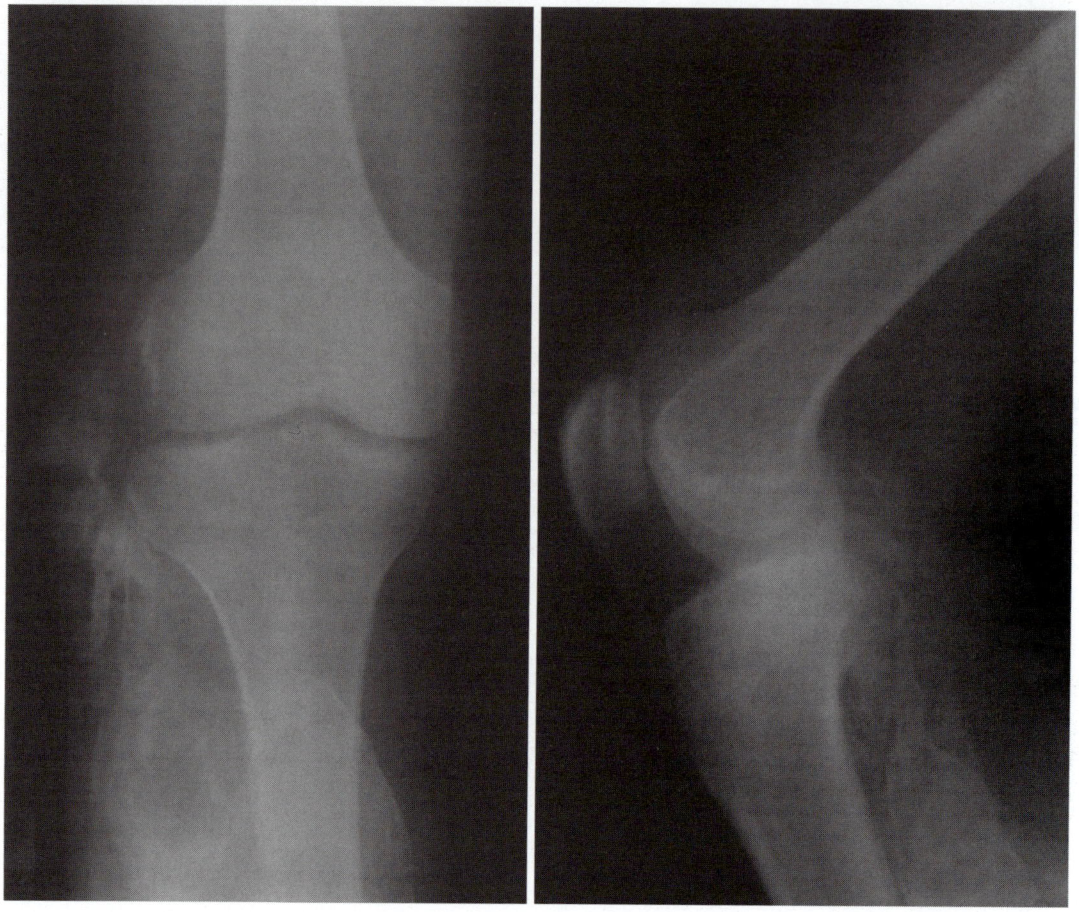

Clinical details: An adult male with a history of musculoskeletal trauma.

1. **Describe your findings.**
2. **What is a common trigger for this pathology to occur?**
3. **In what pattern does the calcification begin?**
4. **Name a genetic cause.**

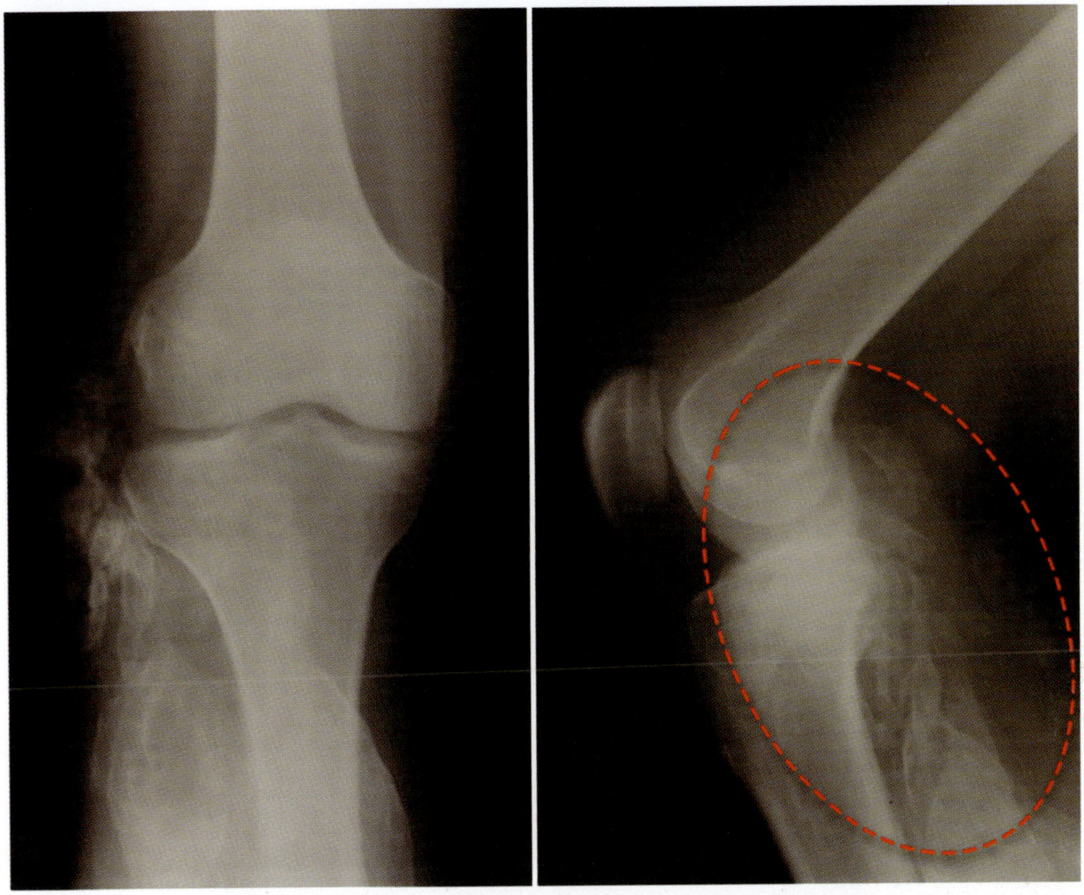

Heterotopic ossification: Ossification surrounding the knee joint in an adult male patient with a history of traumatic injury few months ago.

Heterotopic Ossification

Heterotopic ossification (HO) is the formation of bone tissue in soft tissue where bone should not be present. It is a well-known complication of trauma, central nervous system injury, burns and orthopaedic procedures. In some rare cases, a genetic condition called fibrodysplasia ossificans progressiva (FOP) can lead to HO.

RADIOLOGICAL FEATURES

Plain radiographs:

- Soft tissue mass without calcification is seen in early stages of HO which may be missed during initial imaging.
- Calcification usually begins peripherally and evolves centrally.
- Lesions can be poorly organized without a recognizable pattern.
- Mature cortical bone is formed in untreated cases.

Computed tomography (CT):

- CT can identify mineralization earlier than plain radiographs and has a good overall specificity for HO.
- Early-stage HO is seen as a low-attenuation soft tissue mass with indistinct surrounding soft tissue planes that may show contrast enhancement.
- Mineralization is seen as a zonal pattern with peripheral calcification.
- A central fatty marrow component can occasionally be seen in mineralized lesions.
- Mature cortical bone is seen at the periphery of the lesion.

Magnetic resonance imaging (MRI):

- MRI can provide detailed soft tissue contrast and is useful in the early detection of HO before mineralization occurs.
- T1-weighted imaging can show the soft tissue mass with surrounding oedema and inflammation.
- T2-weighted imaging can show peripheral calcification and a central fatty marrow component.

OSCE

59

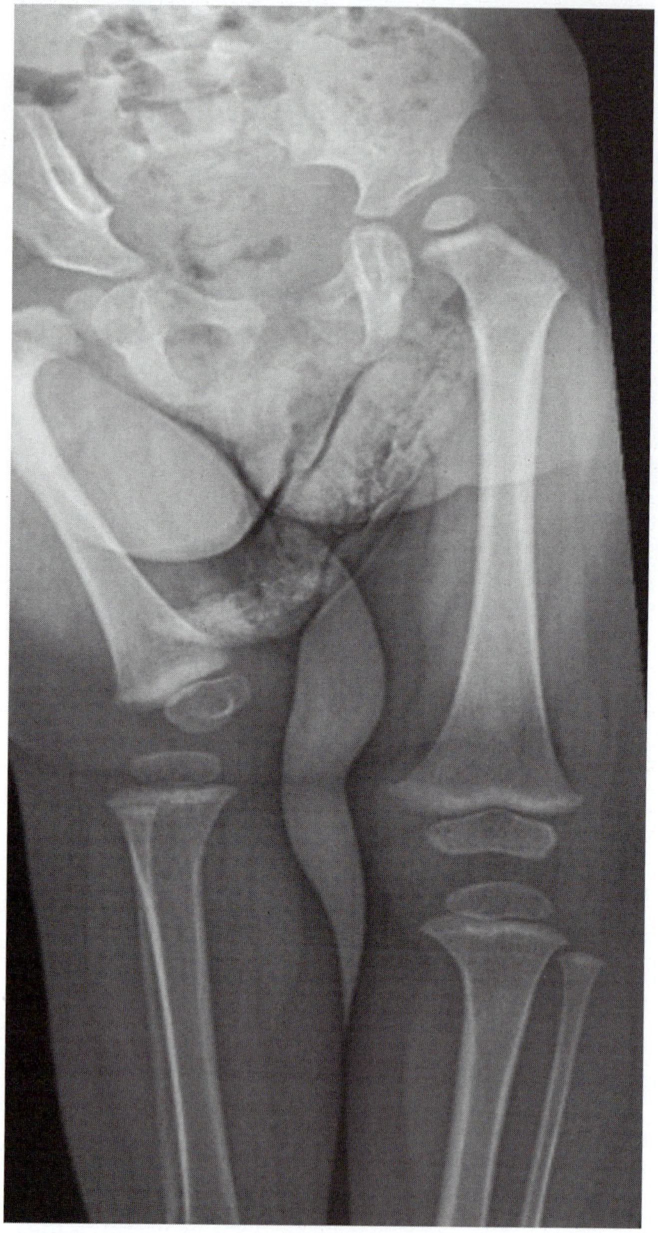

Clinical details: Congenital abnormality of lower limb.

1. **Describe your findings.**
2. **What is the most appropriate diagnosis?**
3. **Name the most widely used classification.**
4. **Enumerate two other anomalies associated with this disease.**

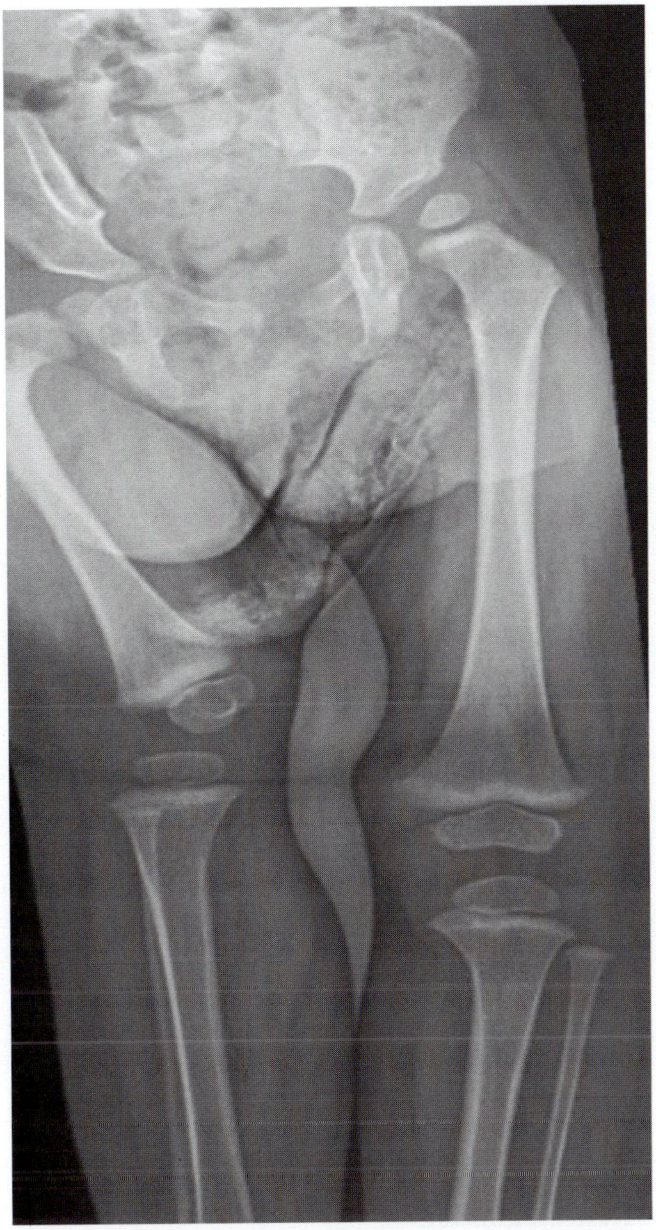

Small-sized right femoral head and neck showing an abnormal orientation and an acute angle with the femoral shaft is noted. There is a marked shortening of right femoral shaft. Acetabulum appears dysplastic and widened.

Proximal Focal Femoral Deficiency

- Proximal focal femoral deficiency (PFFD) is a rare congenital limb anomaly characterized by a partial or complete absence of the proximal femur.
- PFFD is usually unilateral (~85% of cases), affecting the right side more commonly than the left. The severity of the defect can vary, with some cases involving complete absence of the femoral head, neck and trochanter, while others involve partial absence of the femoral head or neck.

RADIOLOGICAL FEATURES

- Shortening of the femur on the affected side
- Partial or complete absence of the femoral head, neck and/or trochanter
- Dysplastic acetabulum
- Absence of patella
- Fibular hemimelia
- Abnormal pelvic morphology
- Classification: There are several classification systems for PFFD, including the Aitken classification (widely used) and the Papadimitriou classification, which take into account the severity of the deformity and the presence or absence of associated anomalies.

OSCE

60

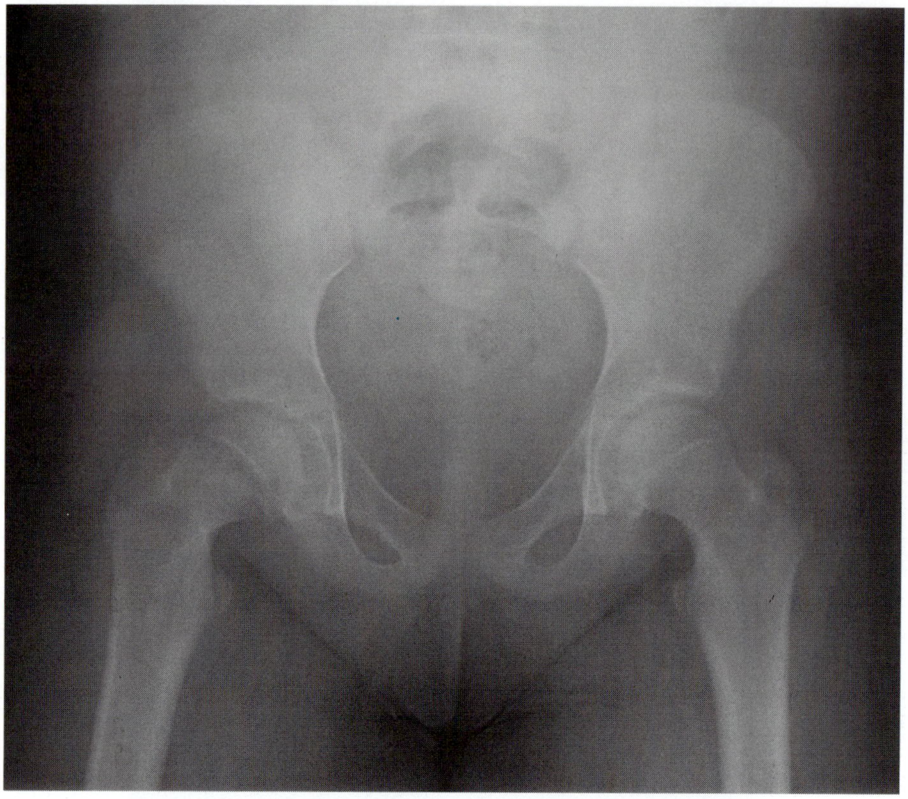

Clinical details: Overweight child with limping gait.

1. **Describe your findings.**
2. **What is the most appropriate diagnosis?**
3. **Which type of Salter–Harris injury is this?**
4. **Name one possible complication.**
5. **What is the line of Klein?**

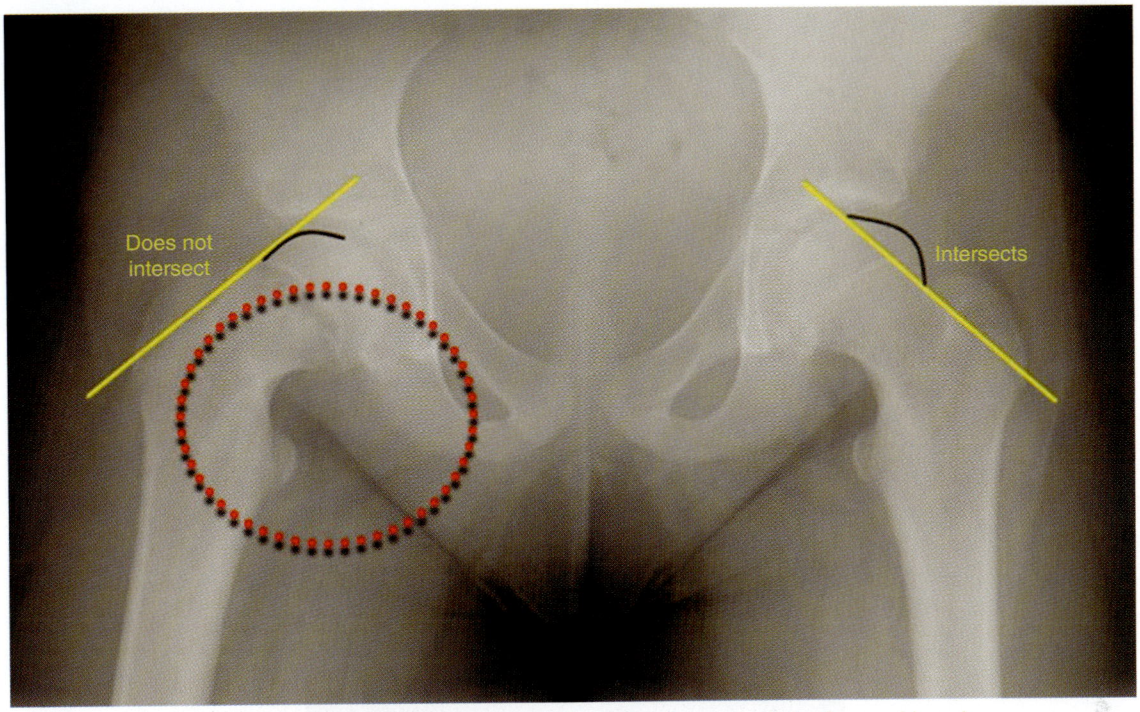

Klein line should normally intersect the lateral aspect of the femoral head.

Slipped Capital Femoral Epiphysis

Slipped capital femoral epiphysis (SCFE) is a common hip disorder affecting adolescents.

It occurs when the femoral growth plate at the hip joint weakens and separates from the femoral head, allowing the head to slip out of the socket. This results in pain, reduced range of motion and altered gait.

- Bilateral in 15%–40% of cases (roughly one-third of cases)
- Most commonly affects obese adolescents between the ages of 11 and 16 years
- More common in boys
- Salter–Harris type 1 epiphyseal plate injury of proximal femur
- Growth plate widening and irregularity, and femoral head slip/displacement (posteromedial).
- The severity of the slip is classified based on the amount of displacement of the femoral head.
- Anteroposterior (AP) and frog leg view radiographs are usually done to diagnose SCFE
- Treatment is done by surgical pinning and is aimed at preventing further slip and avoiding complications such as long-term osteoarthritis and avascular necrosis (AVN) of the femoral head.

Klein line is an important radiological tool used in the evaluation of SCFE. The Klein line is a line drawn along the superolateral aspect of the femoral neck on a frontal radiograph.

In a normal hip, the Klein line should intersect with the lateral portion of the femoral neck. In SCFE, the epiphysis slips posteriorly and inferiorly relative to the femoral neck, and as a result, the Klein line no longer intersects the lateral aspect of the femoral neck.

OSCE

61

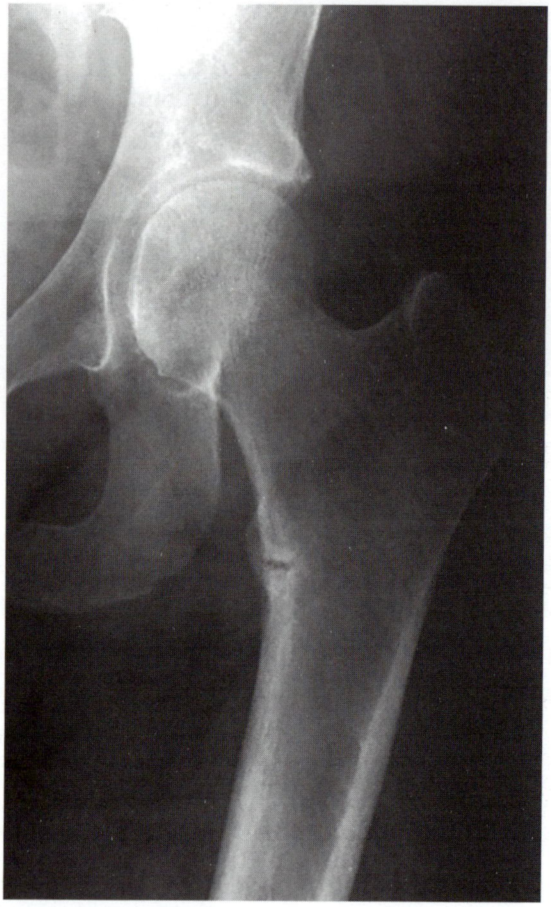

Clinical details: An adult male post-bariatric surgery.

1. **What is the most appropriate diagnosis?**
2. **What is the underlying aetiology?**
3. **What are Looser zones?**
4. **What is Milkman syndrome?**

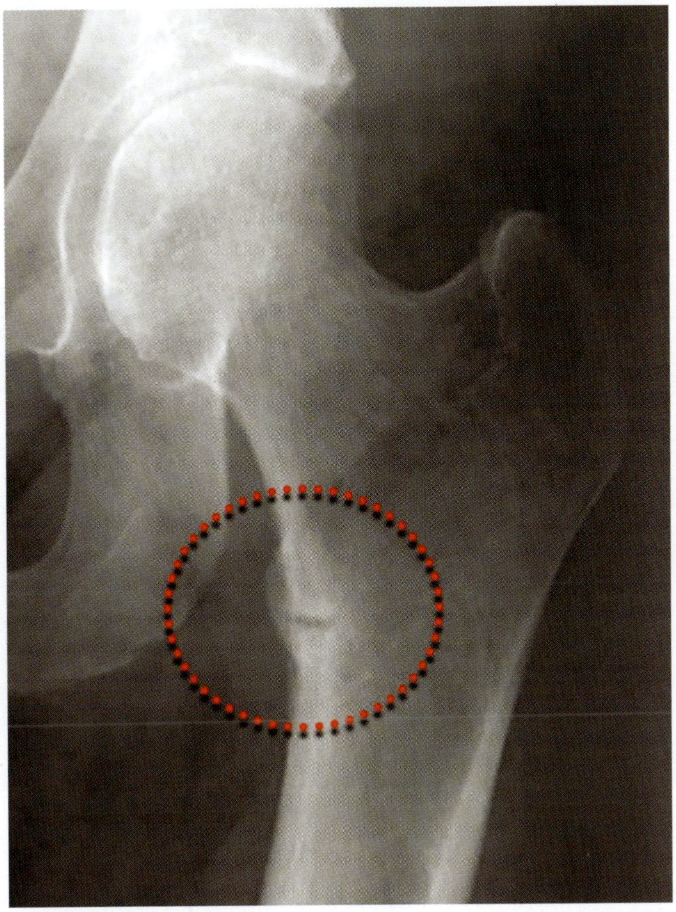

Frontal radiograph of left femur exhibits a focal lucency with surrounding sclerotic changes, along the inner margin of the left femur. The lucency is aligned perpendicular to the cortex and does not traverse the entire thickness of the femur bone. Features are in keeping with a Looser zone.

Osteomalacia

Osteomalacia is a metabolic bone disease characterized by impaired mineralization of bone matrix, resulting in bone softening and weakening. It is often caused by a deficiency of vitamin D, calcium or phosphorus, which are essential for bone mineralization.

Other causes include bariatric surgery, malabsorption (e.g. celiac disease and inflammatory bowel disease), chronic renal failure, renal tubular acidosis, chronic liver disease, etc.

RADIOLOGICAL FEATURES

- Diffuse osteopenia, decreased bone density and thinning of the cortices. These changes are most prominent in the weight-bearing bones of the lower extremities, such as the femoral neck and proximal tibia.
- Looser zones, also known as cortical infractions or pseudofractures or Milkman lines, are a characteristic radiologic finding in osteomalacia. These are transverse lucent lines with sclerotic margins, perpendicular to the cortex.
- **Milkman syndrome:** Osteomalacia with multiple Looser zones.
- Late: Protrusion acetabuli.

OSCE

62

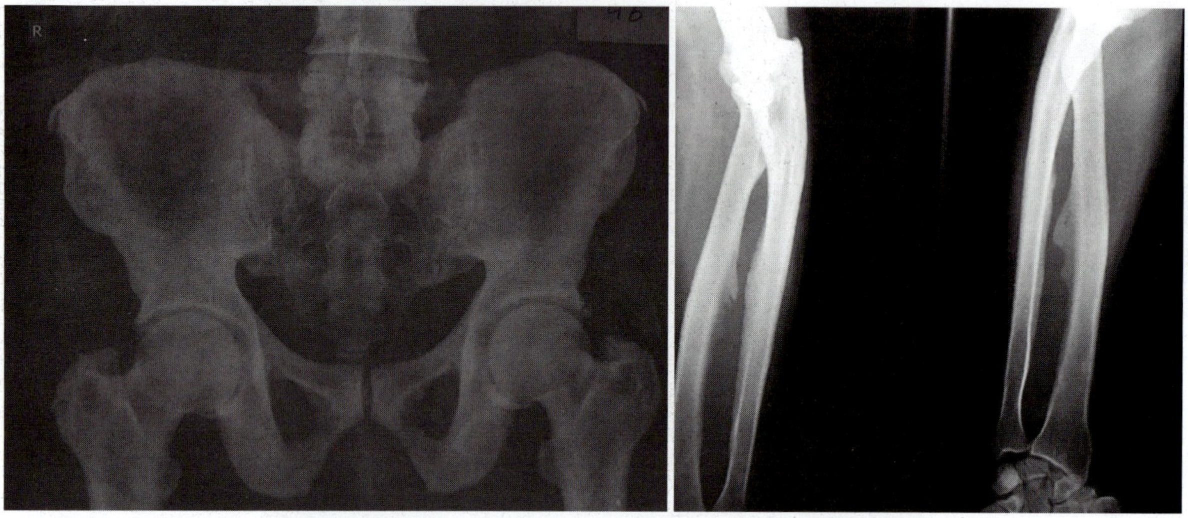

Clinical details: An adult male with mottled dental enamel.

1. **What are the findings and diagnosis?**
2. **What is the underlying aetiology?**
3. **What are the differentials?**
4. **What are the complications?**

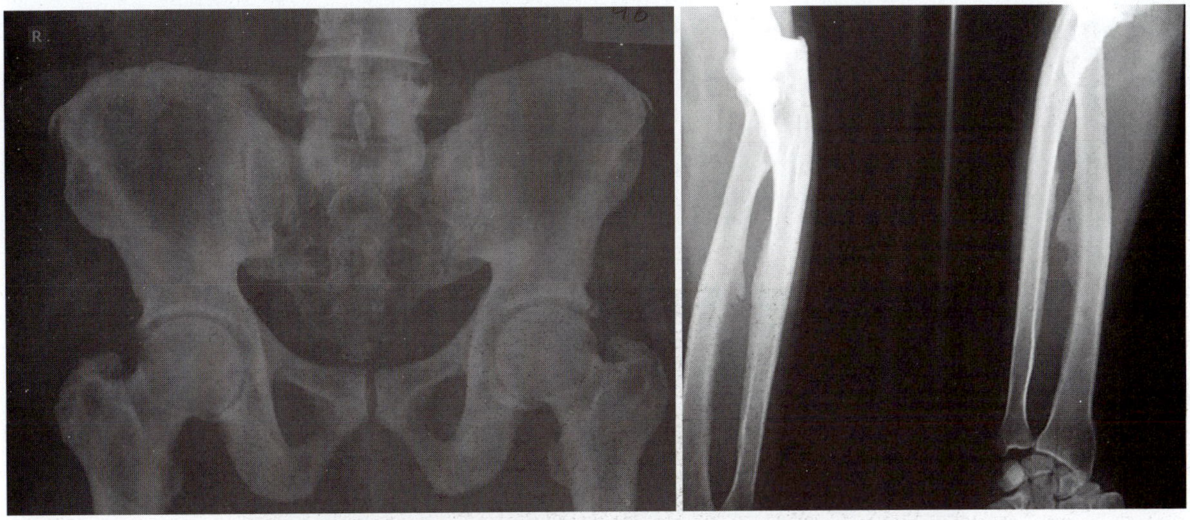

Radiograph pelvis anteroposterior (AP) view shows generalized increased bone density in the visualized bones. No focal lesions/periosteal reaction/calcified ligaments.

Radiograph forearm AP view shows generalized increased density with focal solid irregular periosteal reaction along the medial aspect of midshaft radius and solid smooth periosteal reaction along the lateral aspect of ulna. No focal lesions/soft tissue calcification.

Skeletal Fluorosis

Skeletal fluorosis is a metabolic bone disease caused by chronic ingestion of fluoride via contaminated water or food.

RADIOLOGICAL FEATURES

- Initial osteopenia
- Diffuse osteosclerosis
- Blurred trabeculae
- Periostitis
- Ossification of ligamentous attachments
- Sacrotuberous ligament calcification is considered a characteristic feature of fluorosis
- Vertebral osteophytosis and hyperostosis
- Sclerotic vertebral bodies with paraspinal ligament calcification
- Findings are more marked in axial skeleton than appendicular skeleton
- Complications include pathological fracture and neurological compression
- In India, it is endemic in Nalgonda region of Telangana.
- Differentials include renal osteodystrophy, osteoblastic metastasis, mastocytosis and myelofibrosis.

OSCE

63

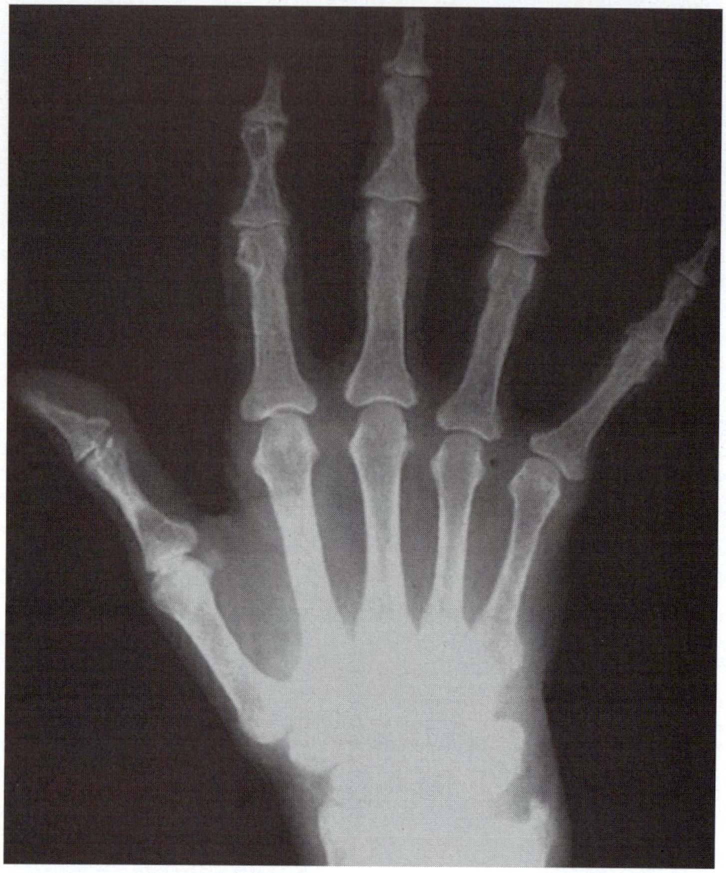

Clinical details: A 55-year-old lady with chronic renal failure.

1. **Describe your findings in the above radiograph.**
2. **What is the most appropriate diagnosis?**
3. **What causes tertiary hyperparathyroidism?**
4. **What is salt and pepper skull?**

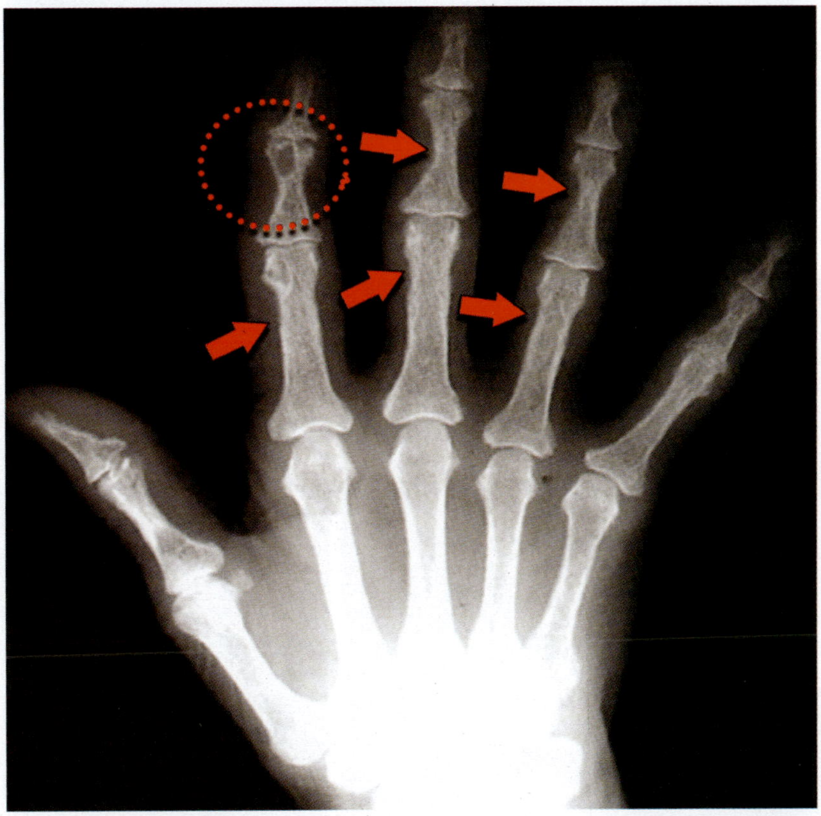

Frontal radiograph of hand in a mature skeleton:

1. Subperiosteal resorption (*red arrows*) of the radial aspect of the middle phalanges of the second, third and fourth fingers. Additionally, there is acro-osteolysis involving the second and third fingers.
2. Fairly well-circumscribed, osteolytic, non-expansile lesion (*red dotted circle*) in distal metaphysis of middle phalanx of right index finger. The lesion is eccentric in location and shows a narrow zone of transition. There is no obvious calcification of matrix or periosteal reaction. No fracture is noted although the lateral cortex appears thin. The lesion does not transgress the adjacent joint. Findings indicate benign pathology – likely Brown's tumour in a case of hyperparathyroidism.

Hyperparathyroidism

Primary hyperparathyroidism:

- Increased parathyroid hormone production
- Caused by parathyroid adenoma (most common), hyperplasia or carcinoma

Secondary hyperparathyroidism:

- Vitamin D deficiency, intestinal calcium malabsorption or chronic renal failure

Tertiary hyperparathyroidism:

- Caused by an autonomous adenoma within a hyperplastic parathyroid gland

MUSCULOSKELETAL FEATURES OF HYPERPARATHYROIDISM

- Subperiosteal bone resorption: Subperiosteal bone resorption, along the radial aspects of middle phalanges of the index and middle fingers of hand
- Salt and pepper skull: Bone resorption in the skull, resulting in a radiographic appearance that resembles the pattern of salt and pepper
- Brown tumours: These are expansile, well-defined lytic lesions with thinning of the adjacent cortex
- Acro-osteolysis
- Pathologic fractures
- Osteoporosis (mainly occurs in primary disease)
- Osteosclerosis (mainly are causing secondary disease)
- Floating teeth

OSCE

64

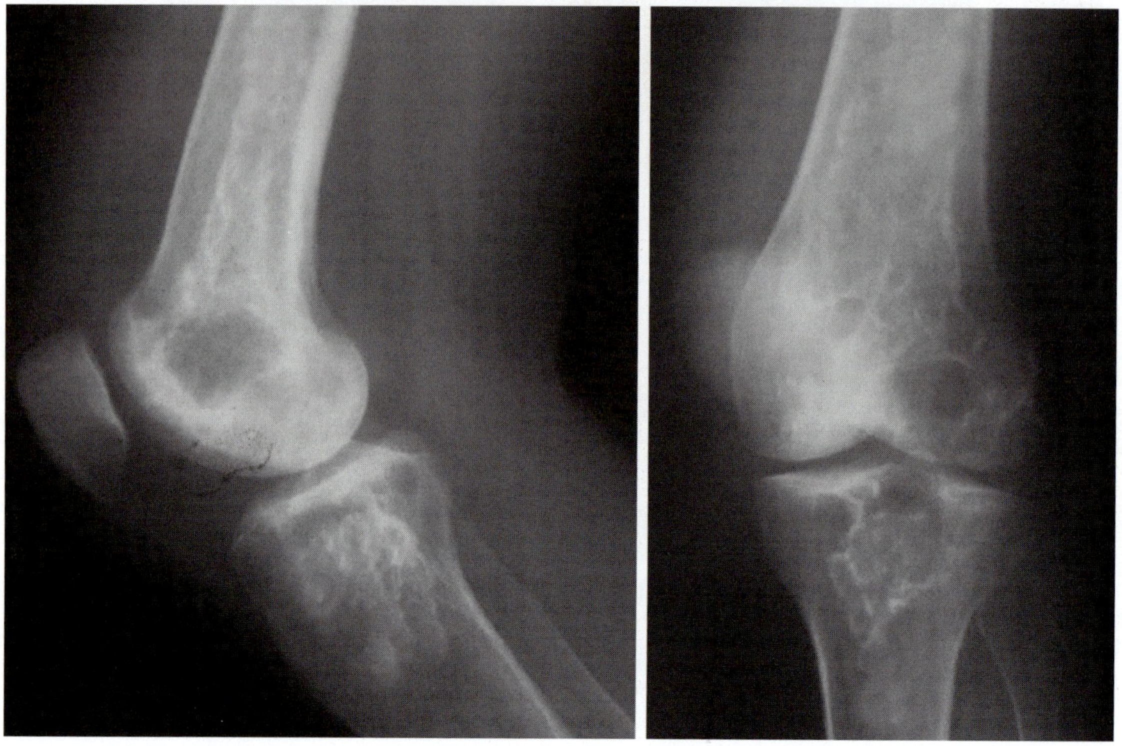

Clinical details: A known case of sickle cell disease with joint pains.

1. **What is the diagnosis?**
2. **Enumerate two causes.**
3. **What is 'double line sign'?**
4. **Name one differential diagnosis for this imaging appearance.**

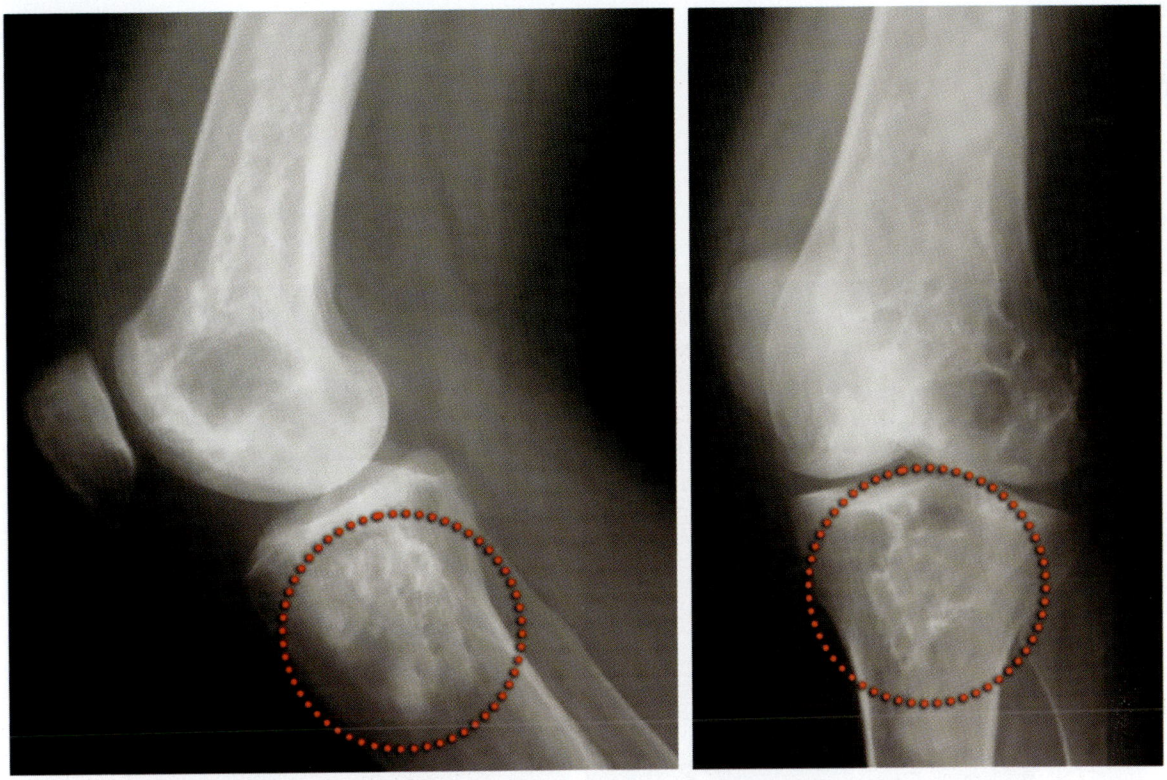

Lateral and anteroposterior (AP) radiographs of the knee joint demonstrate patchy areas of 'serpiginous' sclerosis in the metadiaphyseal region of proximal tibia and distal femur.

Bone Infarcts

Bone infarct or medullary infarct is characterized by osteonecrosis involving the medullary cavity of the metadiaphyseal region of a bone caused by ischaemia.

It can occur due to many pathologies which include following:

- Sickle cell anaemia
- Trauma
- Connective tissue disorders
- Radiotherapy
- Excessive corticosteroid use
- Pancreatitis
- Chronic alcoholism

RADIOLOGICAL FEATURES

- On radiograph, it is seen as sheet like serpiginous areas of sclerosis within the medullary cavity of a long bone.
- Magnetic resonance imaging (MRI) is more sensitive in the diagnosis of medullary bone infarcts. On MRI, bone infarcts are seen as irregular serpiginous areas of abnormal signal intensity within the medullary cavity. On T2-weighted imaging, bone infarcts show a hyperintense inner ring (granulation tissue) surrounded by a hypointense outer ring (sclerosis) – 'double line sign'.
- Differentials include following:
  - Enchondroma: Ring and arcs type of chondroid calcification
  - Healing non-ossifying fibroma
- Bone infarcts may rarely differentiate into a malignancy (malignant fibrous histiocytoma, osteosarcoma and fibrosarcoma)

The skeletal manifestations observed in sickle cell disease include following:

- Bone infarcts
- H-shaped vertebrae, tower vertebra
- Extramedullary haematopoiesis
- Skull changes: Expanded diploic space, thinning of the outer table and 'hair-on-end' appearance.
- Avascular necrosis (AVN) – hip joints and shoulder joints ('snow-capping')
- Dactylitis, also known as 'hand–foot' syndrome
- Osteomyelitis

OSCE

65

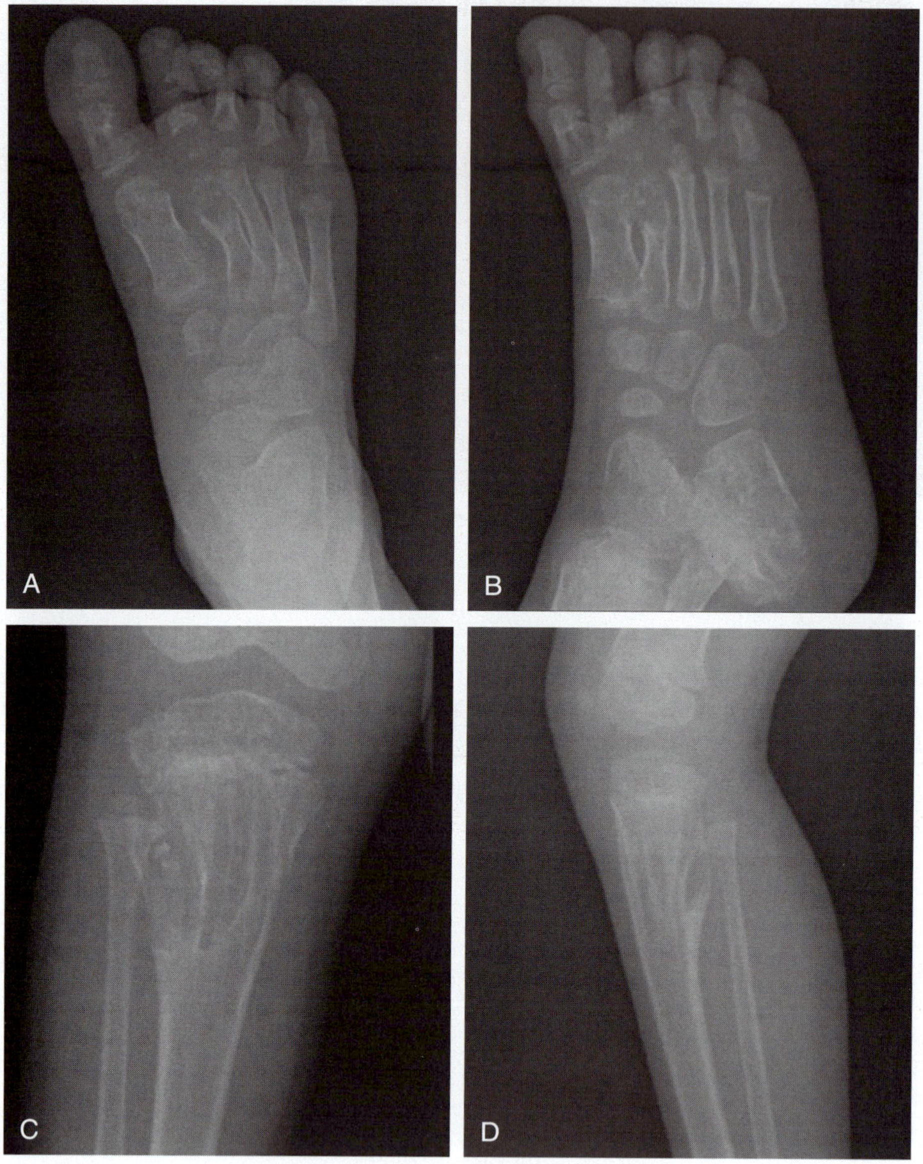

Clinical details: Multiple bony swellings.

1. **Describe the findings in the provided images.**
2. **What is the most appropriate diagnosis?**
3. **What is metachondromatosis?**
4. **What is Maffucci syndrome?**

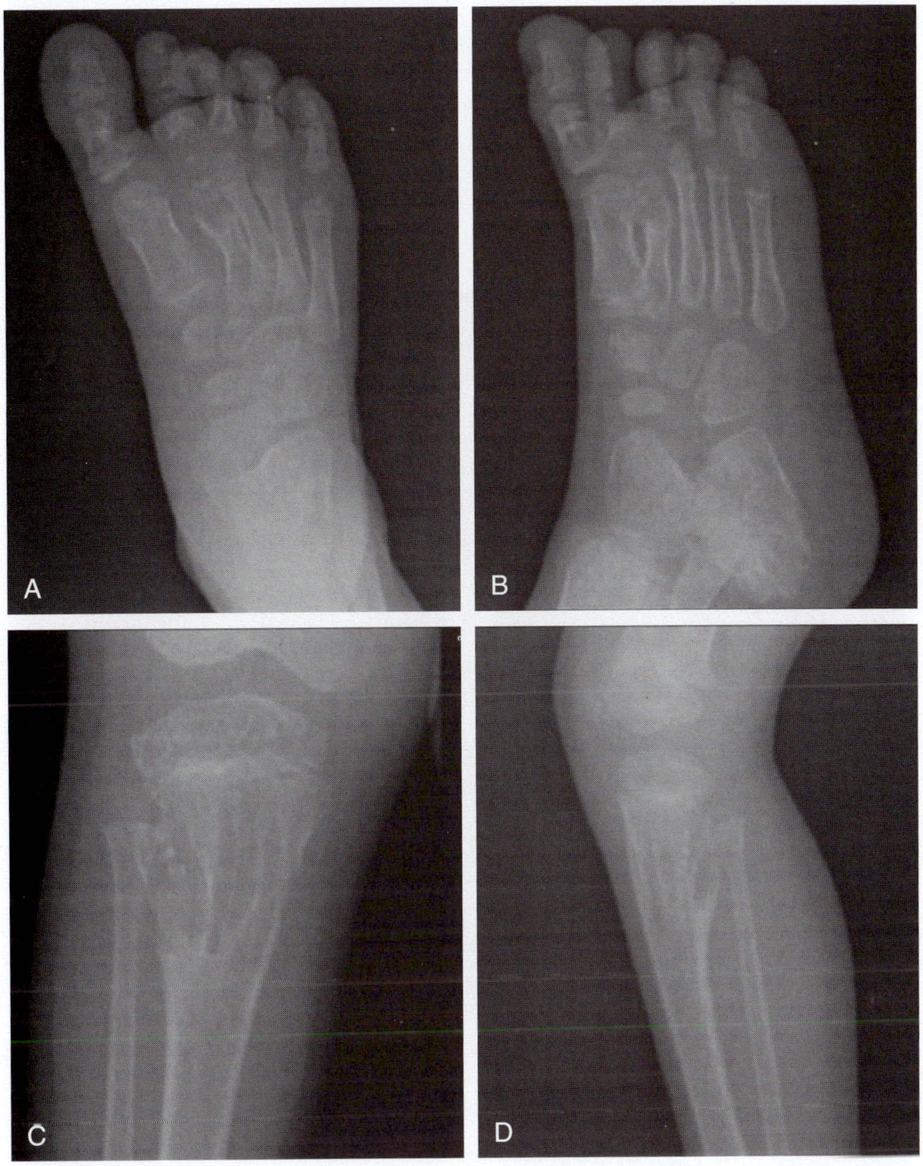

Radiographs of the foot and knee demonstrate multiple enchondromas.

Ollier's Disease

- Ollier's disease is characterized by the presence of multiple enchondromas involving long bone metaphysis. It is also known as enchondromatosis. Ollier's disease increases the risk of development of chondrosarcoma, gliomas and ovarian juvenile granulosa cell tumour.
- Concurrence of multiple osteochondromas with Ollier's disease is known as metachondromatosis.
- On the radiograph, multiple enchondromas are seen within the tubular bones of hands and feet.
- Maffucci syndrome: Multiple enchondromas with soft tissue haemangiomas.

OSCE

66

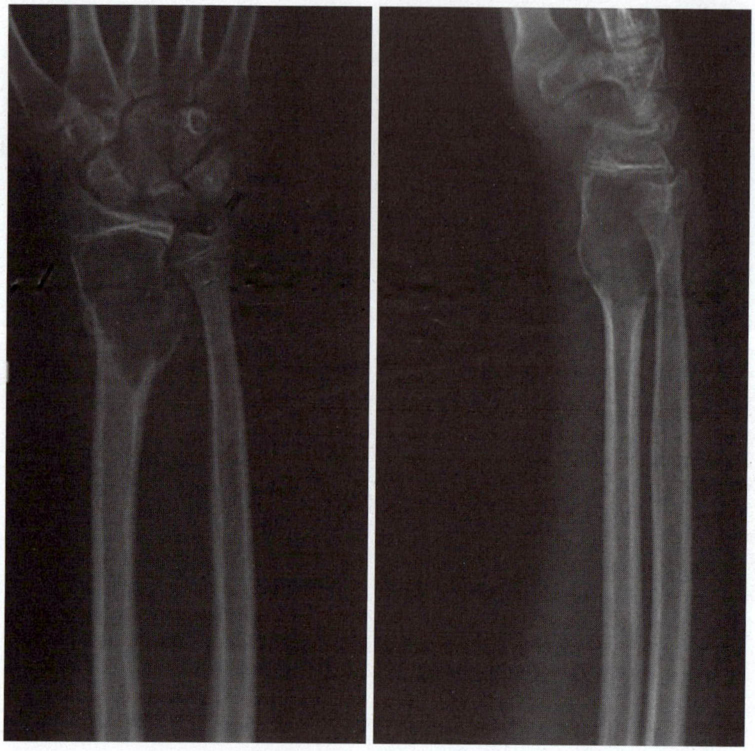

Clinical details: Teenager with pain and swelling over distal forearm.

1. **Describe the findings in the provided images.**
2. **What is the most appropriate diagnosis?**
3. **What are the findings on computed tomography (CT) scan and magnetic resonance imaging (MRI)?**
4. **Which bone malignancy exhibits the doughnut sign?**

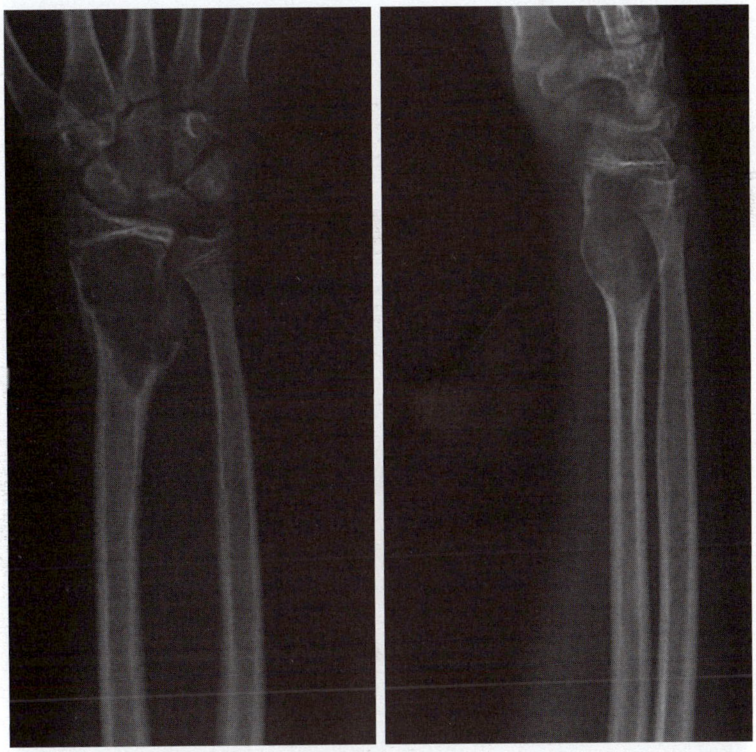

Aneurysmal bone cyst: Distal radial metaphysis shows a well-defined, lytic, expansile lesion with a narrow zone of transition and multiple internal thin-walled cavities. No pathological fracture, no matrix calcification, no periosteal reaction or associated soft tissue mass.

Aneurysmal Bone Cyst

- Aneurysmal bone cyst (ABC) is a benign bone tumour that typically affects children and young adults.
- Location: Most commonly found in the metaphysis of long bones of the limbs and the spine.
- ABC is characterized by a cystic lesion that contains blood-filled spaces and fibrous tissue.

RADIOLOGICAL FEATURES

- Typically presents as an eccentric, expansile lytic on radiographs, with a narrow zone of transition and possible cortical disruption or fracture.
- Magnetic resonance imaging (MRI) is highly sensitive for detecting ABC.
  - T1: Low to intermediate signal intensity
  - T2: Heterogeneous high signal intensity
  - There may also be fluid-fluid levels or septations within the cyst.
- Bone scintigraphy reveals increased peripheral uptake with a photopenic centre, resembling a doughnut (doughnut sign). It can be seen in ABC, giant cell tumour, simple bone cyst and telangiectatic osteosarcoma (malignant cause).

Treatment: Referral to orthopaedic oncologist → curettage/complete en bloc resection + bone grafting

- Causes of fluid-fluid levels and bone tumours are as follows:
  1. Aneurysmal bone cyst
  2. Giant cell tumour
  3. Chondroblastoma
  4. Telangiectatic osteosarcoma
  5. Simple bone cyst

OSCE 67

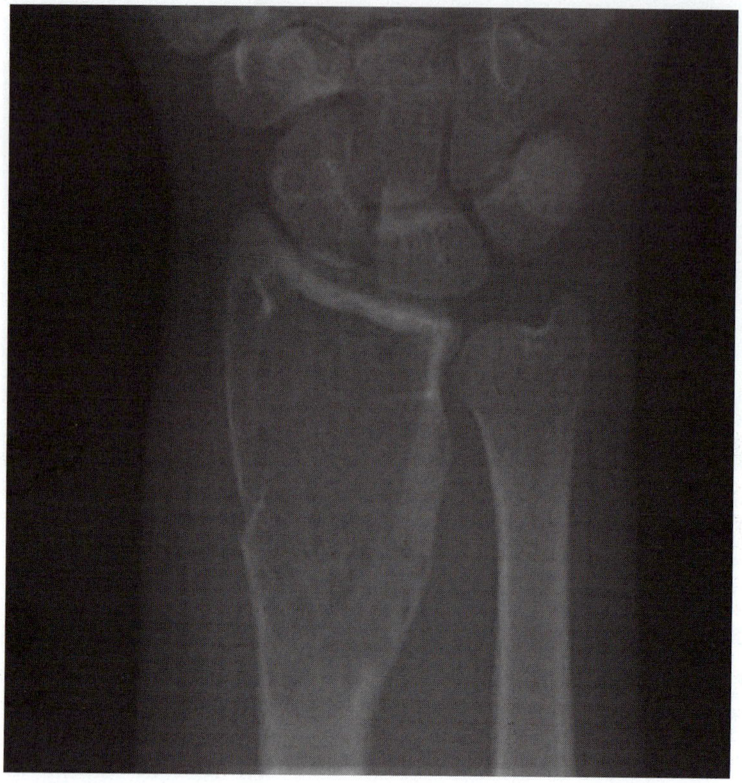

Clinical details: Adult male with pain and swelling over distal forearm.

1. **Describe the findings.**
2. **What is the most appropriate diagnosis?**
3. **What is the treatment of this lesion?**
4. **Which classification is used for this lesion?**

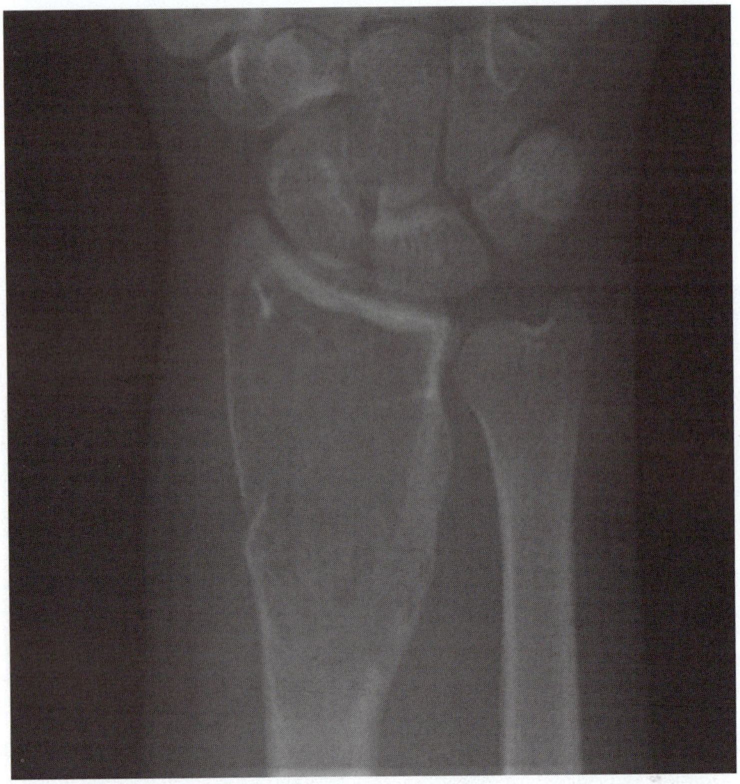

Frontal wrist radiograph of a skeletally mature patient: Well-circumscribed, expansile osteolytic lesion located centrally in the distal metaphysis and epiphysis of the radius with a narrow zone of transition. Multiple septations noted within the lesion. There is a cortical break in the lateral margin of the lesion. No evidence of any matrix calcification, periosteal reaction, soft tissue involvement, skip lesions or satellite lesions noted. With these findings on the radiograph, the impression is of a benign pathology, likely giant cell tumour.

Giant Cell Tumour

Giant cell tumours (GCTs) are locally aggressive bone neoplasms that occur in skeletally mature patients of 20 to 40 years at the epiphysis of long bones. GCTs account for 5% of bone tumours with a slight female predilection.

- Location: Most frequent sites of GCT are the distal femur, proximal tibia and distal radius.

RADIOLOGICAL FEATURES

- GCT usually presents as a lytic epiphyseal expansile lesion, extending to the subchondral bone without surrounding sclerosis. Septations vary from fine striations to coarse trabeculation.
- Campanacci system of grading can be used to characterize plain radiographs.
- Magnetic resonance imaging (MRI) can be used for pre-operative local evaluation and to assess the extraosseous component.
- GCT usually shows a low to intermediate signal on T1-weighted (best to appreciate the intramedullary component) and T2-weighted images (fluid levels and low signal due to haemosiderin deposition with significant enhancement of the solid component after contrast).
- The usual treatment for GCT is curettage with or without bone graft and cement.
- Differentials include chondroblastoma (immature skeleton and epiphyseal location), aneurysmal bone cyst (seen in younger age group than GCT) and chondromyxoid fibroma (bubbly appearance and sclerotic margins).

OSCE

68

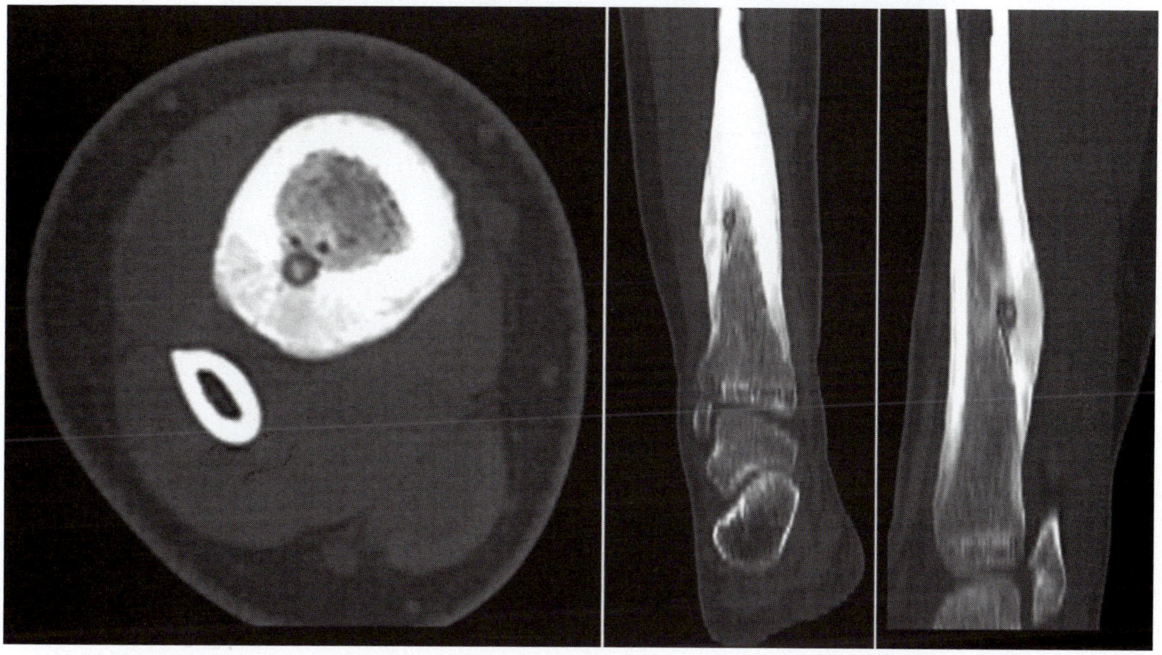

Clinical details: A young boy presented with nocturnal pains in leg relieved by aspirin

1. **Describe your findings.**
2. **What is the diagnosis?**
3. **What is 'double density sign'?**
4. **How is it treated?**

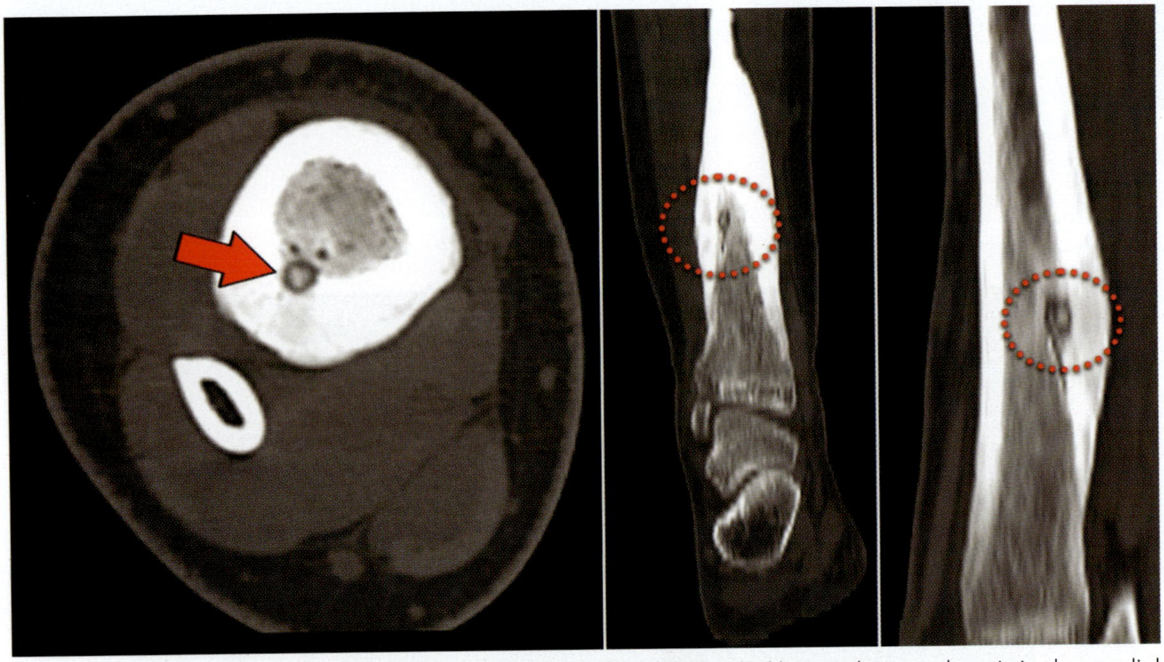

NCCT of the distal tibia: There is a well-defined small radiolucent nidus surrounded by moderate sclerosis in the medial tibial metadiaphyseal cortex. A central region of mineralization is seen within the nidus. No cortical destruction or extraosseous soft tissue extension. Features are in keeping with an osteoid osteoma.

Osteoid Osteoma

Osteoid osteoma is a benign bone tumour that commonly occurs in children and adolescents.

It accounts for approximately 10% of all benign bone tumours.

- Location: Long bones, particularly the femur and tibia, phalanges or vertebrae (lumbar > cervical > thoracic spine).
- Osteoid osteoma is often characterized by dull, aching pain that worsens at night and is relieved by nonsteroidal anti-inflammatory drugs (NSAIDs).

RADIOLOGICAL FEATURES

- On X-ray, osteoid osteomas appear as small, round or oval radiolucent lesions surrounded by a dense sclerotic rim. Narrow zone of transition.
- Computed tomography (CT) is considered excellent for diagnosing osteoid osteomas, as it can detect small lesions and accurately identify their location within the bone. On CT, osteoid osteomas appear as radiolucent nidus with a surrounding reactive sclerotic rim. Central dot may be seen within the nidus.
- Magnetic resonance imaging (MRI) can also be used to diagnose osteoid osteomas, particularly if the lesion is located near a joint or neurovascular bundle.
- On MRI, osteoid osteomas have a low signal intensity on T1-weighted images and a high signal intensity on T2-weighted images. Nidus often enhances post-contrast on MRI.
- **Double density sign:** Also known as 'hotter spot within hot area sign'. It is seen on a bone scintigraphy scan in osteoid osteoma as central higher uptake in the nidus with lesser uptake in the surrounding rim.
- Osteoid osteomas are often treated with surgical excision or minimally invasive techniques, such as radiofrequency ablation. Radiofrequency ablation involves inserting a needle into the centre of the lesion and using heat to destroy the tumour. The success rate for radiofrequency ablation is high with reported cure rates of over 90%.

OSCE

69

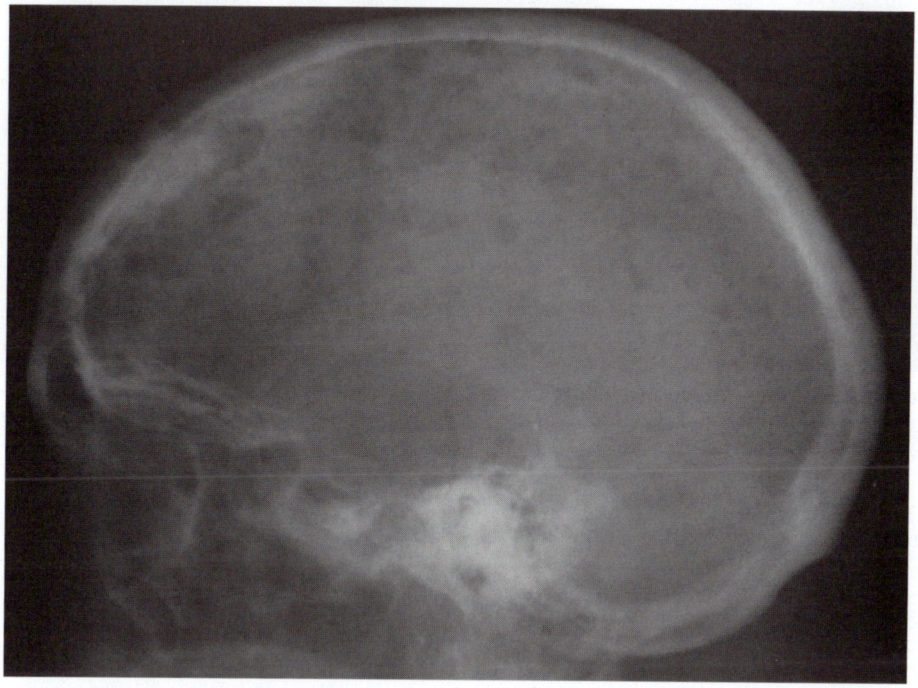

Clinical details: A 70-year-old male with bone pains, anaemia and hypercalcaemia.

1. **What is the characteristic radiological appearance seen in this image?**
2. **What is the most common primary malignant bone neoplasm in adults?**
3. **Give three indications where you will do a 'skeletal survey'?**
4. **What is POEMS syndrome?**

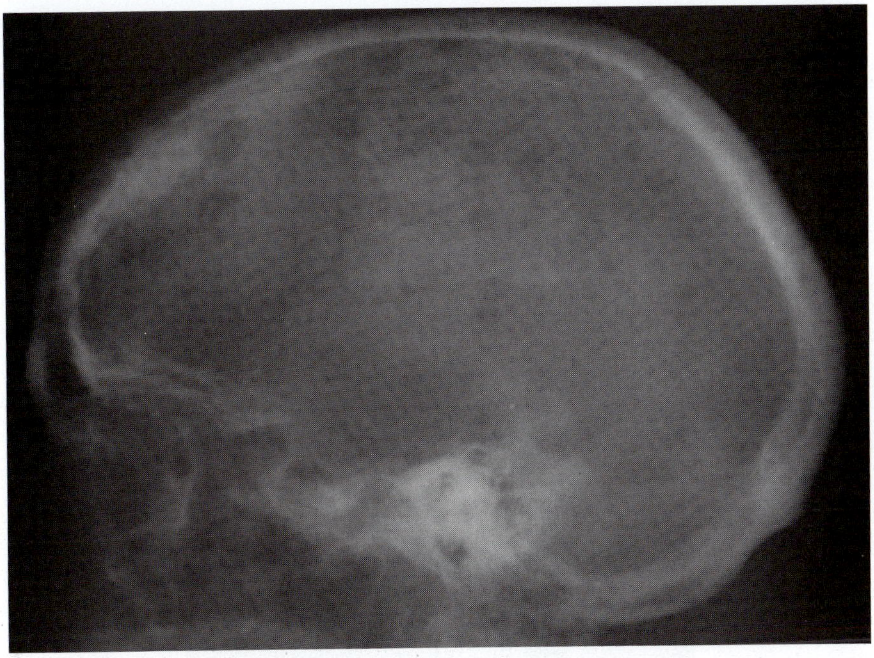

Lateral radiograph of skull: 'Raindrop' skull or 'pepper pot' skull due to numerous radiolucent lesions spread throughout in a case of multiple myeloma.

Multiple Myeloma

Multiple myeloma is a malignant plasma cell disorder characterized by the proliferation of monoclonal plasma cells in the bone marrow, which can result in skeletal lesions and organ damage. It is considered the most common primary malignant bone neoplasm in adults.

RADIOLOGICAL FEATURES

- Most common skeletal manifestation is the presence of numerous, punched-out, lytic lesions, which can be found anywhere in the skeleton, but are more frequently seen in the axial skeleton, including the spine, skull, ribs, pelvis and proximal long bones.
- Generalized skeletal demineralization on plain radiographs (osteopenia).
- Pathologic fractures are common.
- Computed tomography (CT) and magnetic resonance imaging (MRI) are more sensitive than skeletal survey in detecting bone marrow involvement and soft tissue masses, such as plasmacytomas.
- MRI is particularly useful in identifying spinal cord compression due to vertebral involvement.
- Positron emission tomography (PET)/CT is used for staging and monitoring response to treatment.

  Skeletal survey is done in:

  - Multiple myeloma
  - Non-accidental injury (suspected child abuse)
  - Skeletal dysplasia
  - Paget's disease
  - Rickets
  - Scurvy
  - Hyperparathyroidism
  - Renal osteodystrophy

POEMS SYNDROME
- Polyneuropathy
- Organomegaly
- Endocrinopathy
- Monoclonal gammopathy
- Skin changes

OSCE

70

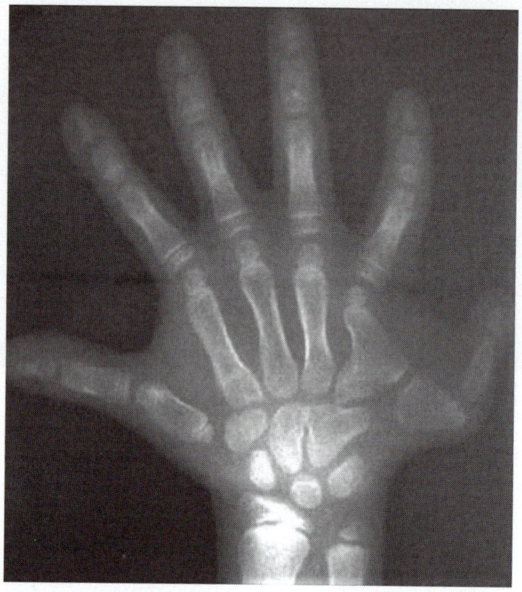

Clinical details: Short stature with cleft lip and congenital polydactyly.

1. **What is the diagnosis?**
2. **Enumerate three findings in this disease.**
3. **Which type of limb shortening is seen in skeletal dysplasia?**
4. **What percentage of cases show cardiac anomalies?**

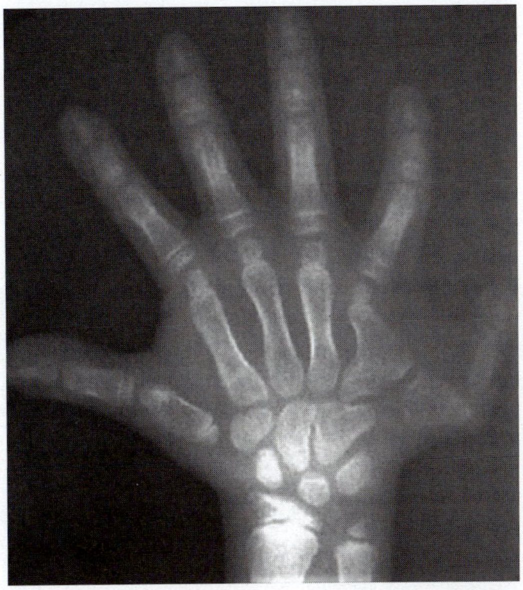

Ellis–van Creveld Syndrome

- Ellis–van Creveld syndrome is also known as chondroectodermal dysplasia.
- It is a rare form of skeletal dysplasia.

Important features include following:

- Short stature with short limbs
- Genu valgum
- Post-axial polydactyly, carpal coalition
- Medial tibial osteochondromas, metaphyseal irregularity
- Mesomelic limb shortening
- Cleft lip or palate
- Cryptorchidism, epispadias
- Dental abnormalities
- Congenital cardiac defects are seen in approximately 50% of the cases

OSCE

71

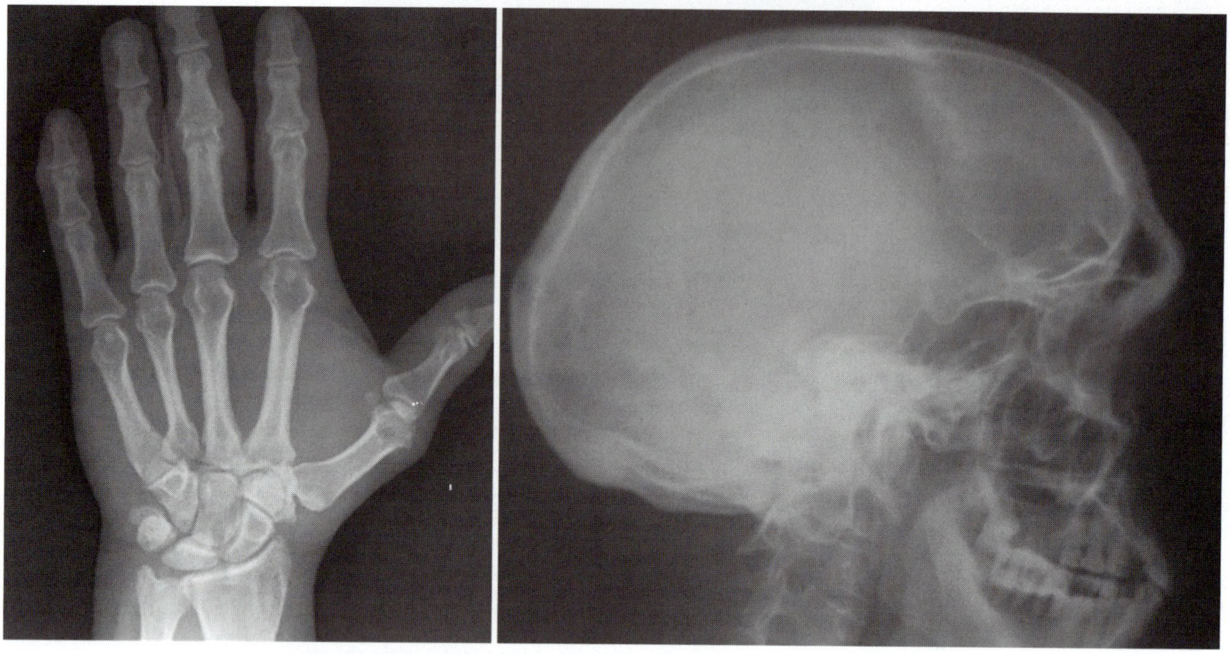

Clinical details: Adult with increasing skull size and frontal bossing.

1. **What is the diagnosis?**
2. **Which brain tumour can be associated with this?**
3. **Read this statement: 'Spine of this patient with show anterior vertebral scalloping'. True or false?**
4. **Provide one feature seen in the foot in this condition.**

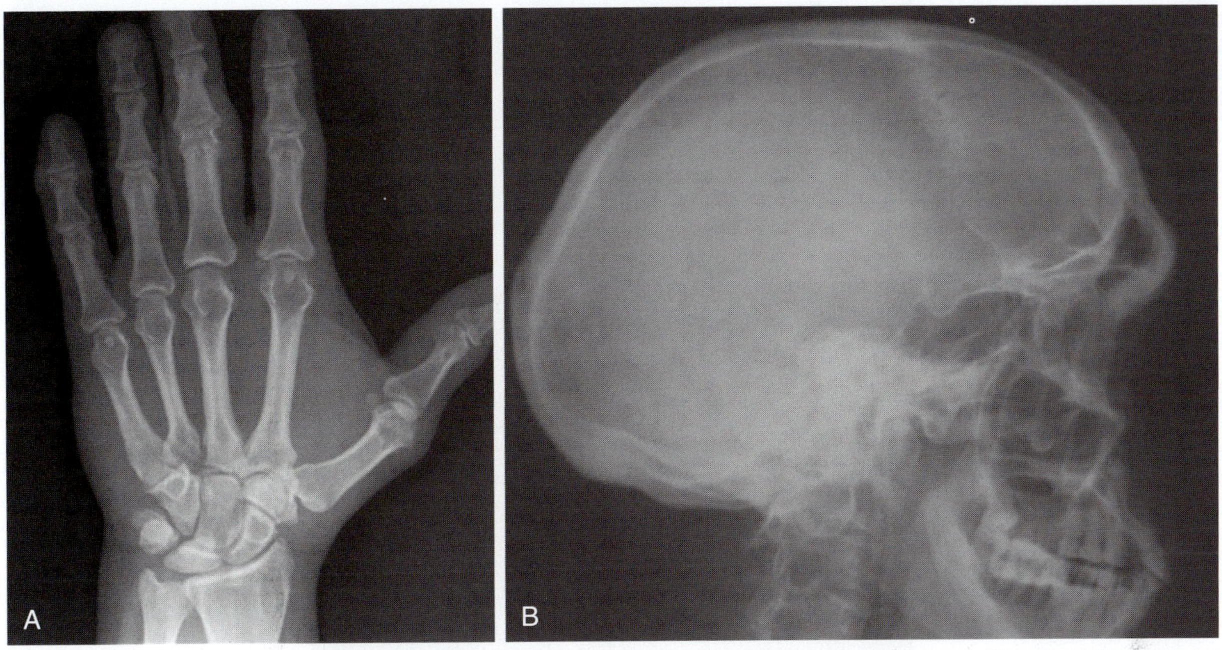

(A) Anteroposterior (AP) radiograph of the hand shows hypertrophied terminal tufts of phalanges with spade-like appearance and soft tissue thickening. (B) Lateral skull radiograph reveals mild scalp thickening, prominent paranasal sinuses.

Acromegaly

Acromegaly is a hormonal disorder caused by excessive growth hormone (GH) production in adults. The condition is often caused by a pituitary adenoma.

RADIOLOGICAL FEATURES

Skull and brain:

- Frontal bossing
- Calvarial thickening (inner table)
- Paranasal sinuses enlargement
- Prognathism
- Enlarged pituitary fossa (sella turcica)
- Pituitary adenoma

Spine:

- Posterior vertebral scalloping
- Enlargement of vertebral bodies

Hands and feet:

- Hypertrophied terminal tufts of phalanges with spade-like configuration (known as 'spade phalanx sign')
- Increased heel pad thickness (more than 25 mm)

OSCE 72

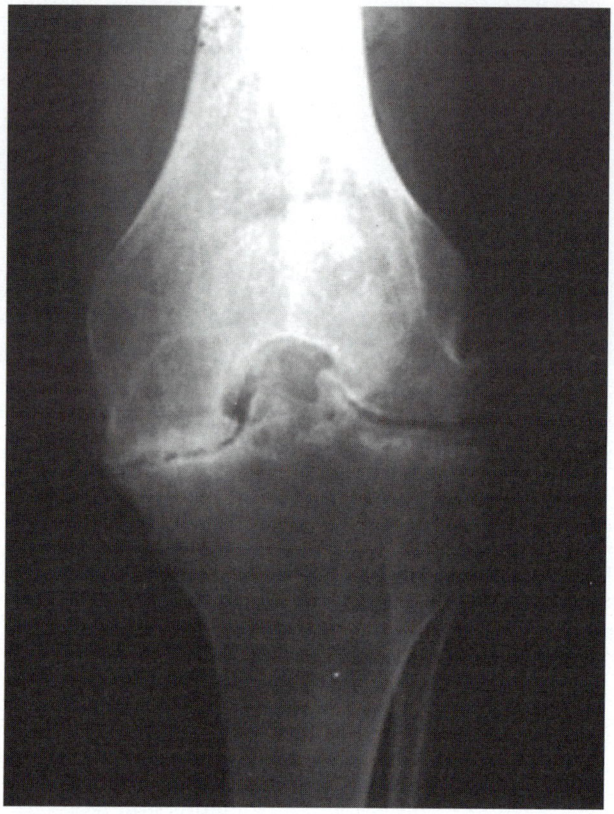

Clinical details: Adult male with severe joint pain with reduced range of motion.

1. **Describe the findings in the given radiograph.**
2. **What is the most appropriate diagnosis?**
3. **Which classification is used to describe the changes in the knee joint?**
4. **What is the inheritance pattern of this disease?**

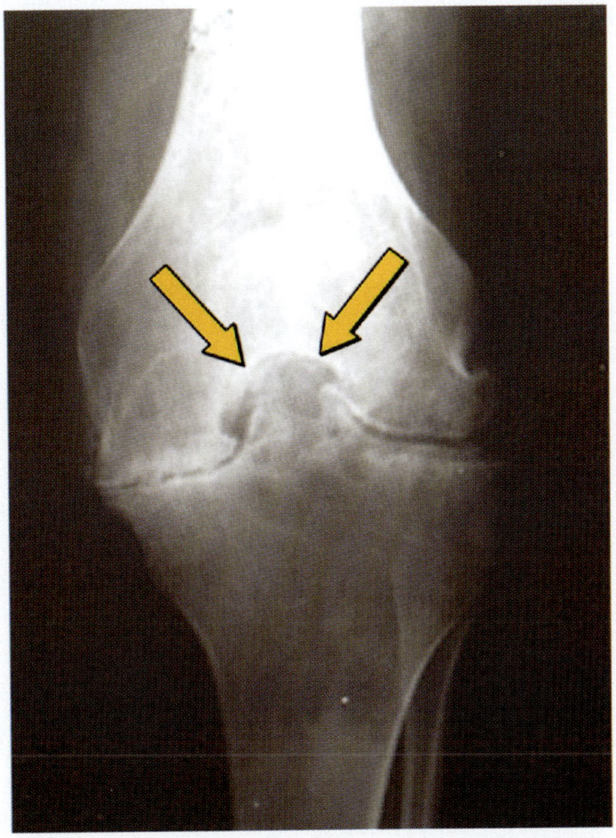

Frontal radiograph of the knee joint reveals bulbous appearance of medial femoral condyle, widening of the intercondylar notch (yellow arrows), severe joint space narrowing and juxtaarticular osteoporosis in a case of haemophilic arthropathy.

Haemophilic Arthropathy

Haemophilic arthropathy is a progressive joint disease characterized by recurrent haemarthrosis that occurs in individuals with haemophilia. Haemophilia is inherited in an X-linked recessive pattern.

RADIOLOGICAL FEATURES

- Synovial hypertrophy due to chronic inflammation
- Effusion into the joint spaces
- Widening of the intercondylar notch of the knee
- Bulbous appearance of the femoral condyles
- Subchondral osteoporosis adjacent to the joint space
- Joint space narrowing with irregularities
- On magnetic resonance imaging (MRI), siderotic synovitis may be seen

Arnold–Hilgartner classification reduced to classify the findings of haemophilic arthropathy in the knee joint.

OSCE

73

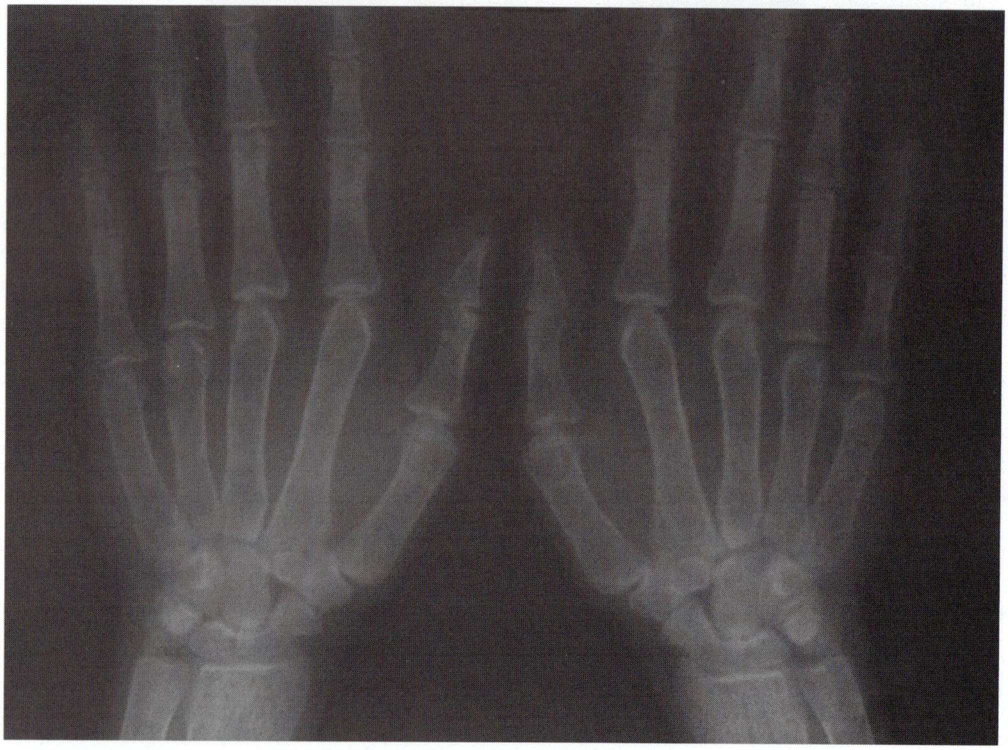

Clinical details: Adult male with severe anaemia and iron overload.

1. Describe your findings.
2. What is the most appropriate diagnosis?
3. Give two causes of hair-on-end appearance.
4. Describe two features you would see in the spine of this patient.

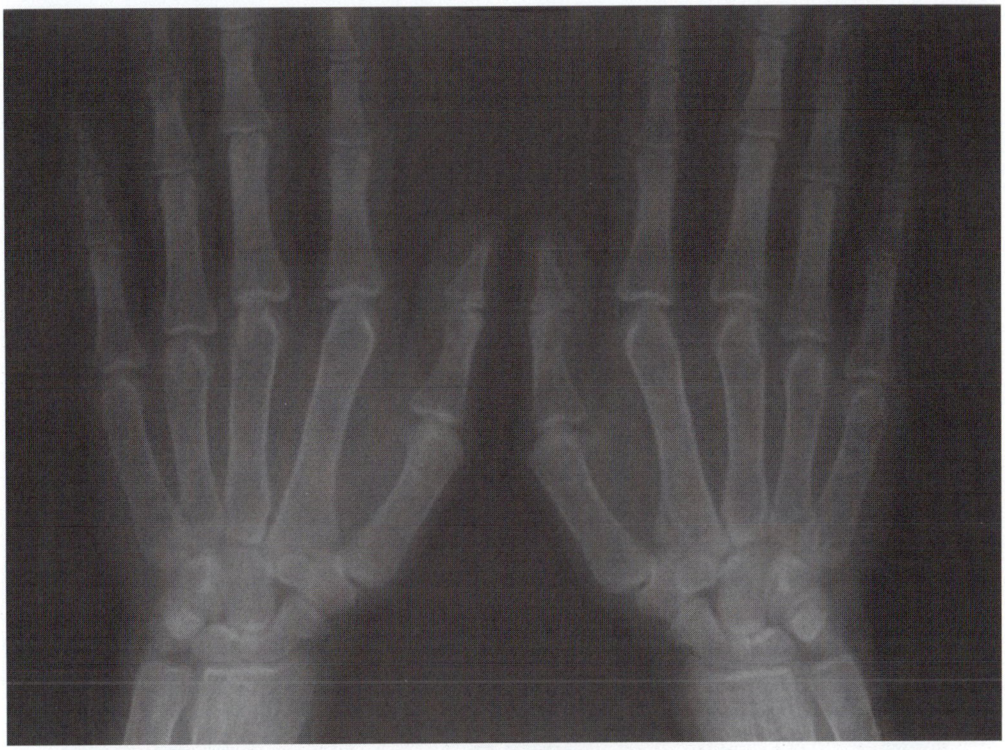

Frontal radiograph of both hands: Widening and expansion of metacarpal shafts with thinning of cortex and coarsened trabecular bone.

Thalassaemia

Thalassaemia is a type of haemoglobinopathy that is inherited in an autosomal recessive pattern.

RADIOLOGICAL FEATURES

Skull and face:

- Hair-on-end appearance (also seen in sickle cell anaemia, hereditary spherocytosis and iron deficiency anaemia).
- Diploic space widening.
- Paranasal sinuses become hypopneumatized and replaced by marrow containing bone. Ethmoidal sinuses are spared as they lack red bone marrow.
- Chipmunk facies or rodent facies: Frontal bossing facial bony overgrowth along with hypopneumatization of paranasal sinuses.
- Dental malocclusion.

Spine and pelvis:

- Scoliosis
- Extramedullary haematopoiesis (lobulated paravertebral soft tissue masses)
- Biconcave appearance of vertebrae or codfish vertebrae
- Erlenmeyer flask deformity

Long bones:

- Widening of the medullary cavities
- Thinning of the cortex with increased risk of fractures

Ribs:

- Rib within a rib appearance

Hands and feet:

- Widening of medullary spaces in metacarpals and metatarsals
- Coarsening of the trabecular pattern

Abdomen:

- Splenomegaly
- Cholelithiasis
- Haemosiderosis

OSCE 74

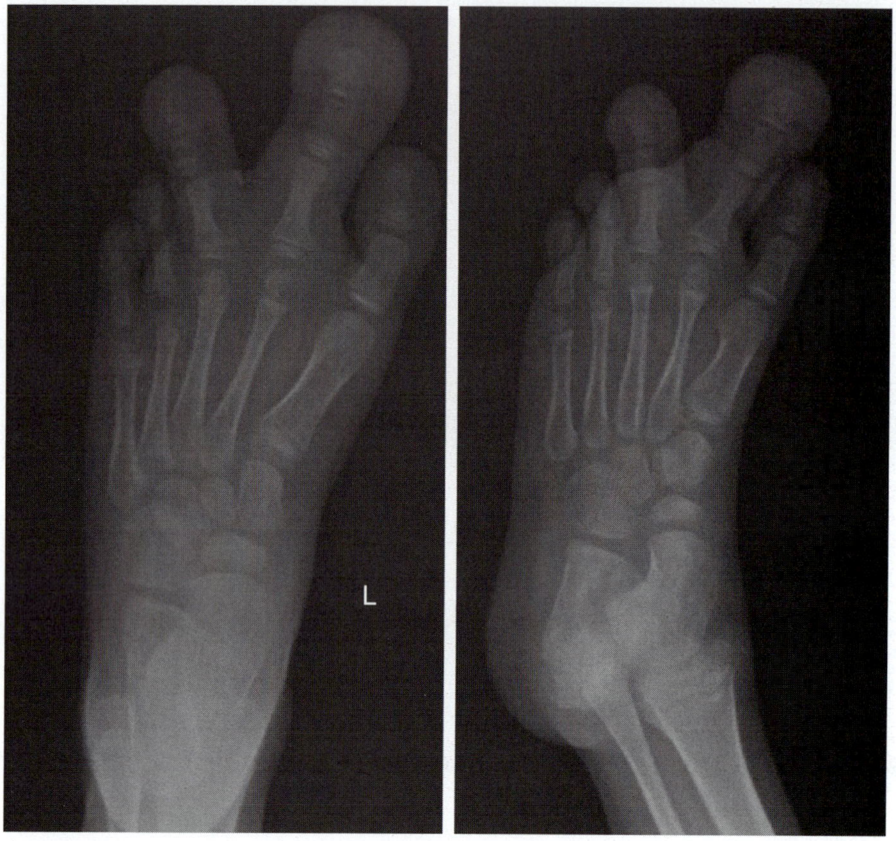

Clinical details: A young boy with painless overgrowth of second and third toes.

1. **Describe the radiological features.**
2. **What is the diagnosis?**
3. **What is Beckwith–Wiedemann syndrome?**

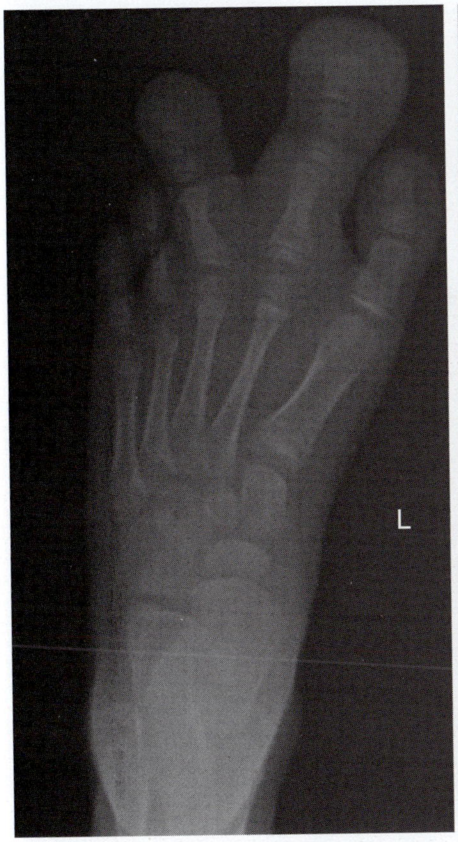

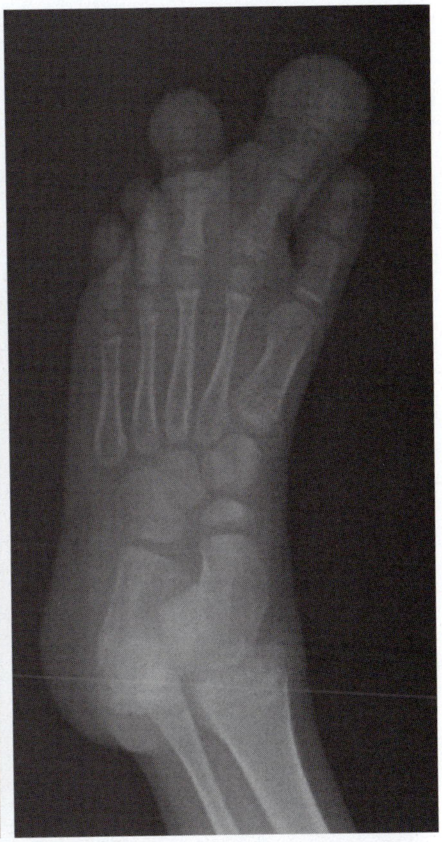

Macrodystrophia Lipomatosa

Macrodystrophia lipomatosa (MDL) is a rare congenital disorder characterized by the overgrowth of bones and soft tissues of a single digit or limb (localized gigantism). The radiological features of MDL are important for diagnosis and management of the condition.

RADIOLOGICAL FEATURES

- Bony overgrowth: Phalanges are expanded, elongated and widened.
- Soft tissue enlargement: The affected digit or limb exhibits increased thickness of soft tissue and fat deposition (fibroadipose tissue).
- Asymmetry: MDL shows asymmetry of the affected digit or limb compared to the normal side.
- Magnetic resonance imaging (MRI) findings: MRI can show the extent of soft tissue involvement and fat deposition in MDL.
- Differential diagnosis: MDL should be differentiated from other conditions such as neurofibromatosis, Proteus syndrome and hemihypertrophy (Beckwith–Wiedemann syndrome).
- Beckwith–Wiedemann syndrome is a rare congenital disorder characterized by:
  - Omphalocele
  - Macroglossia
  - Hemihypertrophy
  - Organomegaly
  - Cardiac anomalies
  - Hypoglycaemia

OSCE

75

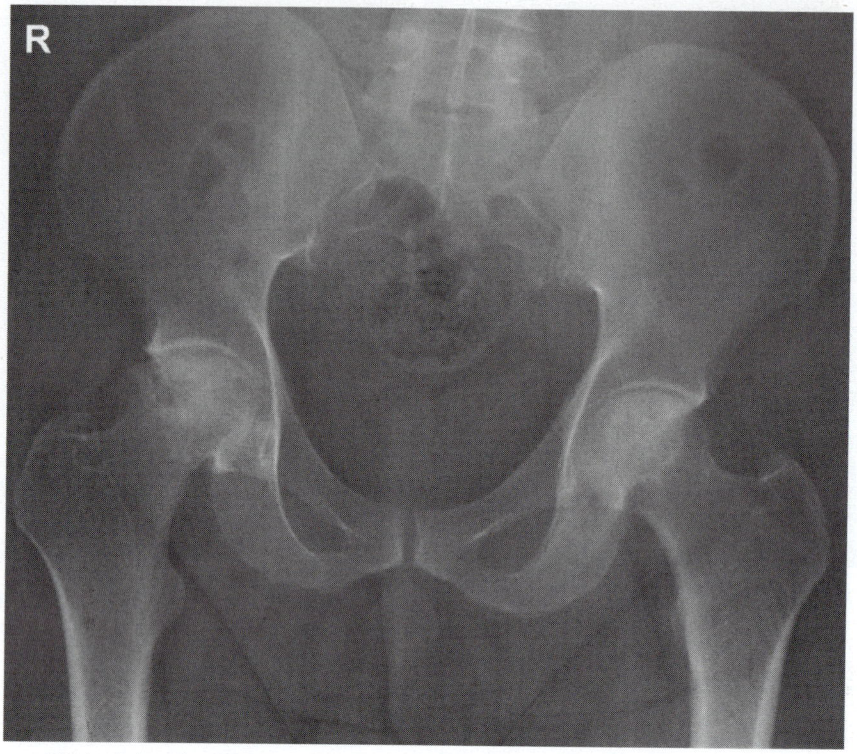

Clinical details: A patient on steroids developing pain at right hip joint.

1. **Describe the findings.**
2. **What is the most appropriate diagnosis?**
3. **What is 'crescent sign'?**
4. **Describe the features found in stage IV of Ficat and Arlet staging classification.**

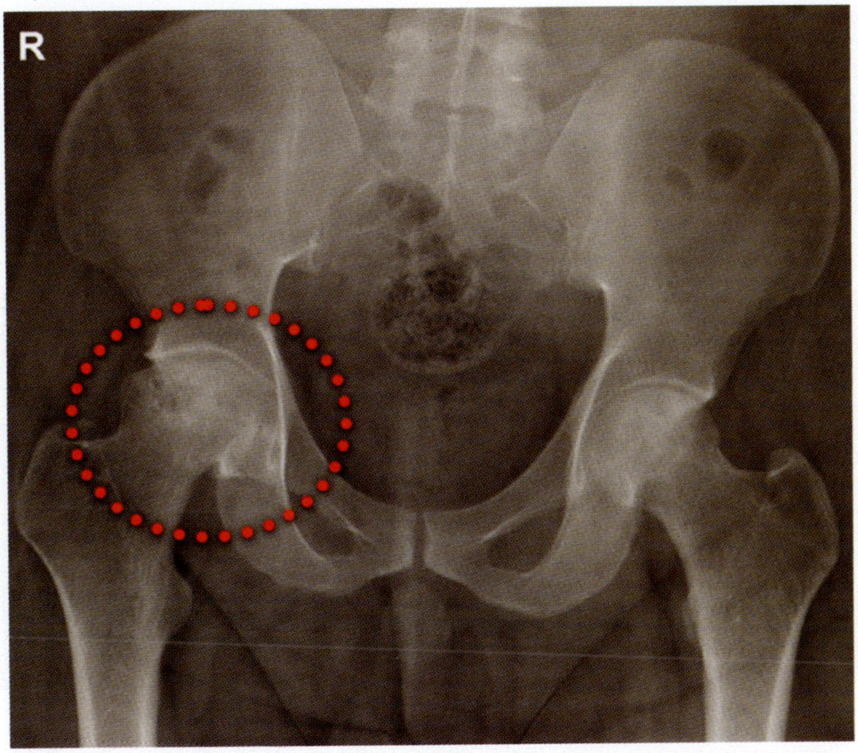

Frontal radiograph of pelvis reveals irregularity and sclerosis of the right femoral head with structural collapse.

Avascular Necrosis of Hip

- Avascular necrosis (AVN) of hip is defined as osteonecrosis or ischaemic necrosis of the femoral head and often extending to the subchondral plate. It can be traumatic or non-traumatic. AVN due to traumatic cause is usually unilateral, whereas non-traumatic AVN is more commonly bilateral (~80%).

Causes of non-traumatic AVN include following:

- Sickle cell anaemia
- Chronic corticosteroid use
- Chronic alcoholism
- Gaucher disease

Ficat and Arlet classification system is a widely used grading system for AVN of the femoral head, which is a type of AVN that commonly affects the hip joint. The grading system is based on the radiological features seen on X-rays and other imaging studies.

FICAT AND ARLET GRADING SYSTEM

Stage 0: Preclinical or normal

- No radiographic or clinical signs of AVN

Stage I:

- Normal X-ray or may show osteopenia
- Magnetic resonance imaging (MRI) may show areas of hyperintensity signifying oedema
- Bone scan shows increased uptake

Stage II:

- X-ray shows the presence of osteopenia with or without the presence of sclerosis
- MRI shows a geographical defect, double line sign: Serpiginous hypointense line with adjacent hyperintense rim of oedema
- Bone scan shows increased uptake

Stage III.

- X-ray shows crescent sign (curvilinear subchondral lucency most commonly seen in the anterolateral portion of the proximal femoral head)
- MRI also shows the crescent sign as low signal intensity line which parallels the subarticular region

Stage IV:

- X-ray shows complete collapse of the femoral head with deformation of the head and acetabulum
- MRI may show fragmentation or disappearance of the femoral head

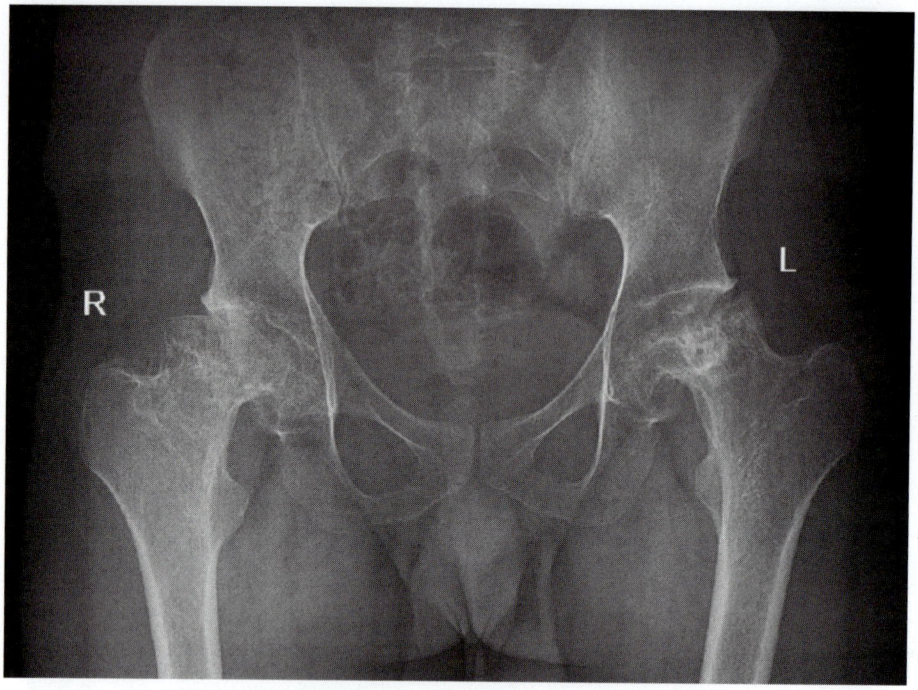

Bilateral hip AVN in a patient with sickle cell anaemia.

OSCE

76

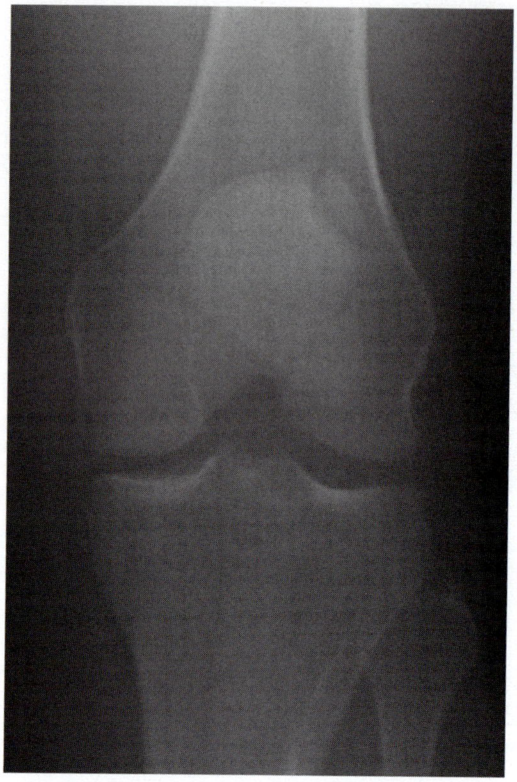

Clinical details: Young athlete with knee pain.

1. **Describe the findings.**
2. **What is the most appropriate diagnosis?**
3. **What is the most common location of this entity?**

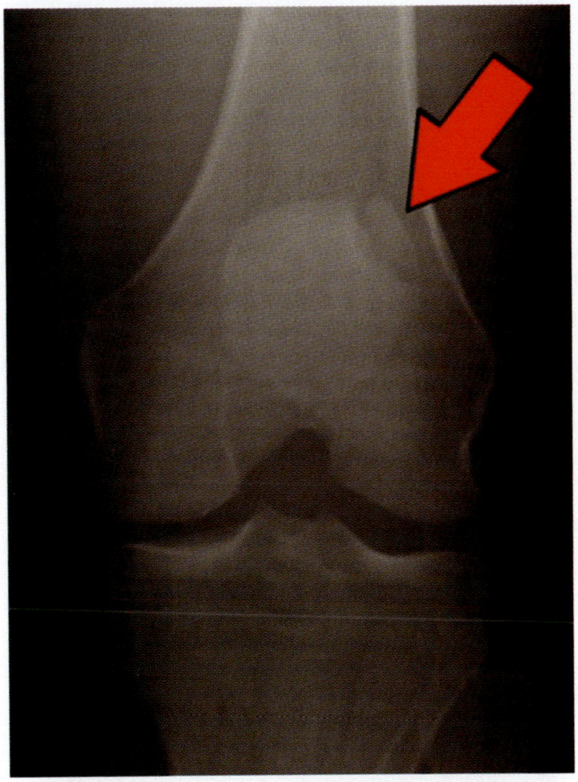

Bipartite Patella

Bipartite patella is a normal variant of the patellar bone of the knee. It can be seen in up to 2%–3% of the population. The patella develops from a cartilaginous precursor that ossifies into a single bone during early childhood. However, in cases of bipartite patella, this fusion process does not occur completely, resulting in the formation of two separate bones.

It is bilateral in approximately 43% of the cases and is more common in men.

Common locations of the unfused secondary ossification centre are as follows:

1. Superolateral (75%)
2. Lateral (20%–25%)
3. Inferior (1%–5%)

Bipartite patellae might be wrongly interpreted as a patellar fracture. A bipartite patella has a large radiolucent line dividing the two parts of bone with smooth, corticated borders.

Because they are sometimes bilateral, a view of the other knee can be beneficial.

OSCE 77

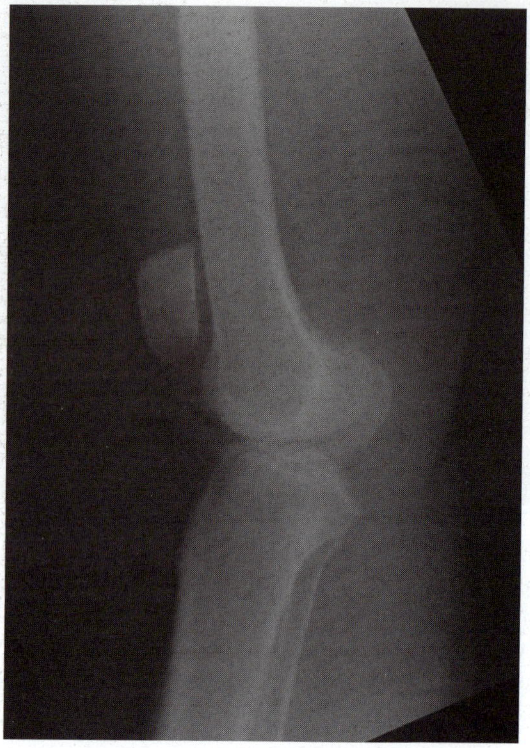

Clinical details: A young male with sensation of anterior knee pain on physical activity.

1. **Describe your findings.**
2. **What is the most appropriate diagnosis?**
3. **How do you measure the Insall–Salvati ratio?**
4. **What is the normal Insall–Salvati ratio?**

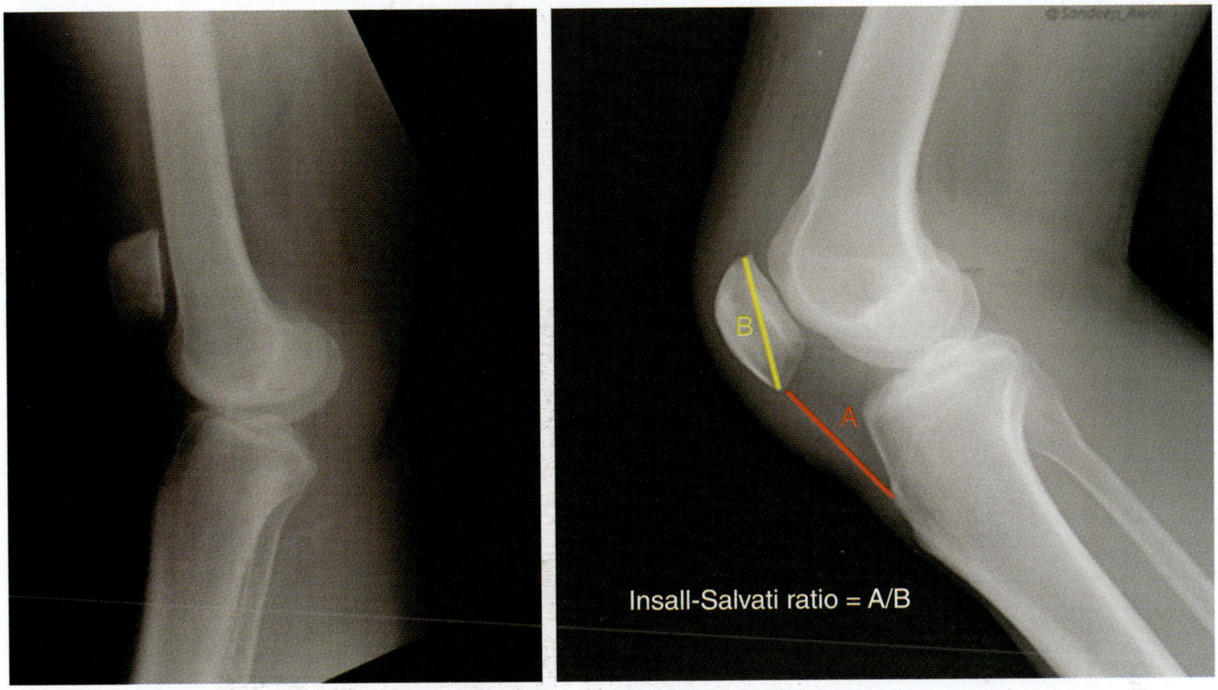

Patella Alta

- Patella alta refers to the abnormally elevated location of the patella within the knee joint, that is, high riding patella. It may be idiopathic or can be caused by rupture of the patellar tendon.
- It can be associated with chondromalacia patellae, recurrent patellar dislocation.
- The Insall–Salvati ratio is a radiographic measurement used to determine patella height. It is calculated by dividing the length of the patellar tendon (from the inferior pole of the patella to the tibial tuberosity) by the length of the patella (from the superior to the inferior pole).

INSALL–SALVATI RATIO (A/B)	
1.0	Normal
>1.2	Patella alta
<0.8	Patella baja

Major risk factors for patellar instability are as follows:

1. Patella alta
2. Trochlear dysplasia (flattening of trochlear surface)
3. Increased tibial tuberosity to trochlear groove distance (TT–TG distance)

OSCE

78

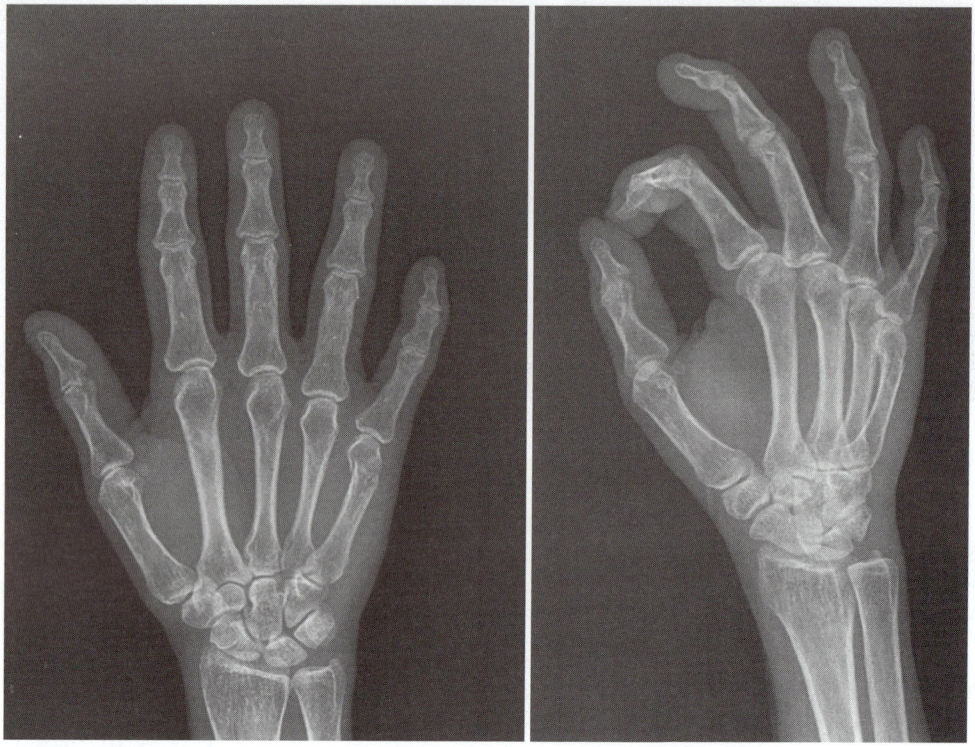

Clinical details: History of trauma due to punching wall after losing a poker game.

1. **Where is the abnormality?**
2. **What is the eponymous name of this fracture?**
3. **What is gamekeeper's thumb?**
4. **What is the difference between Bennett and Rolando fractures?**

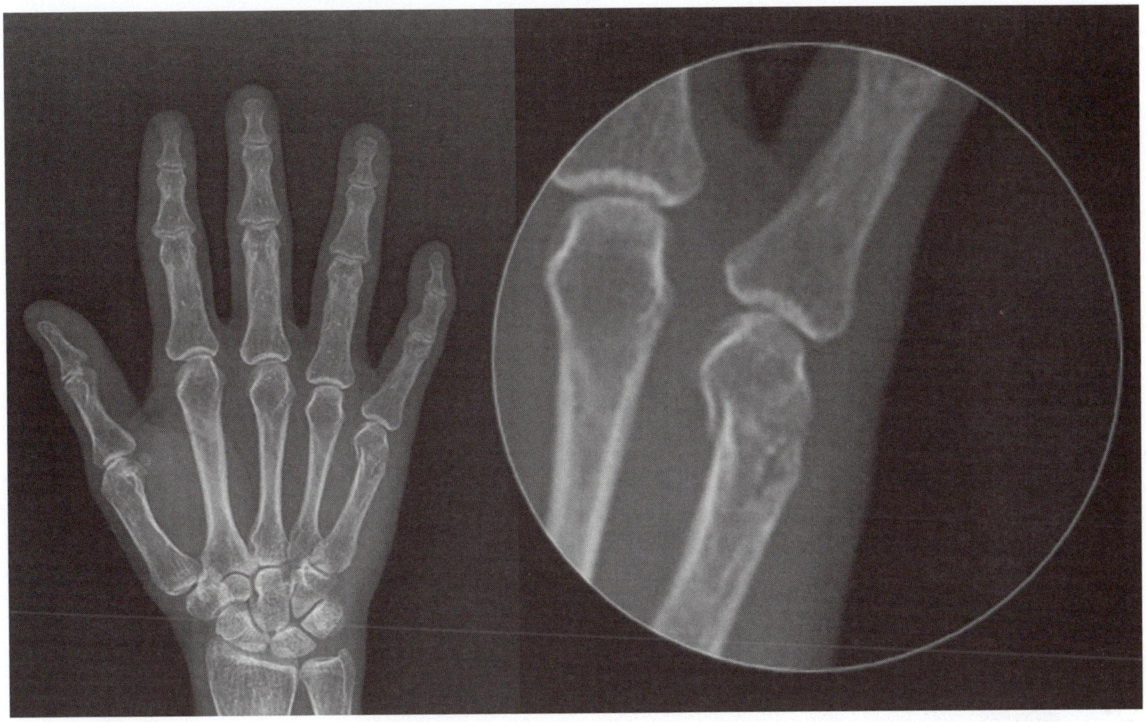

Frontal radiograph and zoomed image demonstrate a fracture through the neck of the fifth metacarpal (Boxer fracture).

Eponymous Upper Limb Fractures

Colles' fracture	Distal radius fracture with dorsal displacement and angulation.
Smith's fracture	Distal radius fracture with volar displacement of the distal fragment.
Boxer's fracture	Fracture of the fifth metacarpal neck, often due to direct impact with a clenched fist.
Barton's fracture (dorsal Barton)	Intraarticular fracture of the distal radius with *dorsal* dislocation of the radiocarpal joint.
Reverse Barton fractures (volar Barton)	Intra-articular fracture of the distal radius with *volar* displacement.
Mallet finger (baseball finger)	Avulsion fracture at the base of the distal phalanx, often involving the extensor tendon.
Gamekeeper's thumb or skier's thumb	Ulnar collateral ligament avulsion injury of the first metacarpophalangeal joint with avulsion fracture at the base of the proximal first phalanx.
Bennett's fracture	Intra-articular two-part fracture at the base of the first metacarpal. (NOT *comminuted.*)
Rolando's fracture	Intra-articular three-part or *comminuted* fracture at the base of the first metacarpal.
Monteggia fracture	Fracture of the proximal ulna with dislocation of the radial head. (Mnemonic to remember Monteggia and Galeazzi fractures = MU——GR.)
Galeazzi fracture	Fracture of distal radial shaft with dislocation of the distal radioulnar joint.
Bankart fracture	Fracture of the anteroinferior glenoid rim in the shoulder joint, typically associated with anterior shoulder dislocation or instability.
Hill–Sachs defect	Impaction fracture on the posterolateral humeral head due to anterior shoulder dislocation, resulting from the humeral head impacting against the glenoid during dislocation.
Chauffeur fracture	Intra-articular fracture of the radial styloid process. Also called backfire fracture or Hutchinson fracture.
Essex-Lopresti fracture	Combination of radial head fracture, dislocation of the distal radioulnar joint and rupture of the interosseous membrane.

PART G

Neuroradiology—Head and Neck

OSCE

79

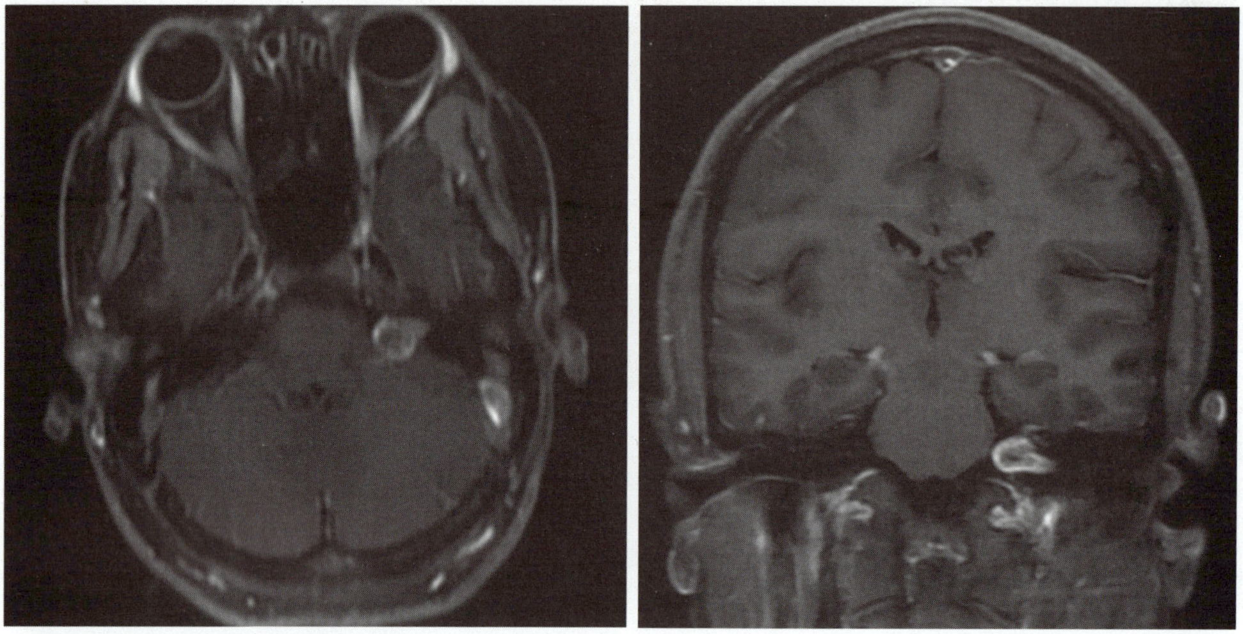

Clinical details: A 35-year-old female with left-sided hearing loss and tinnitus.

1. **What are the differentials for a mass in this location?**
2. **Which is the most common tumour in this location?**
3. **How do you differentiate between a cerebellopontine (CP) angle schwannoma and a meningioma?**
4. **Which characteristic sign is seen here?**

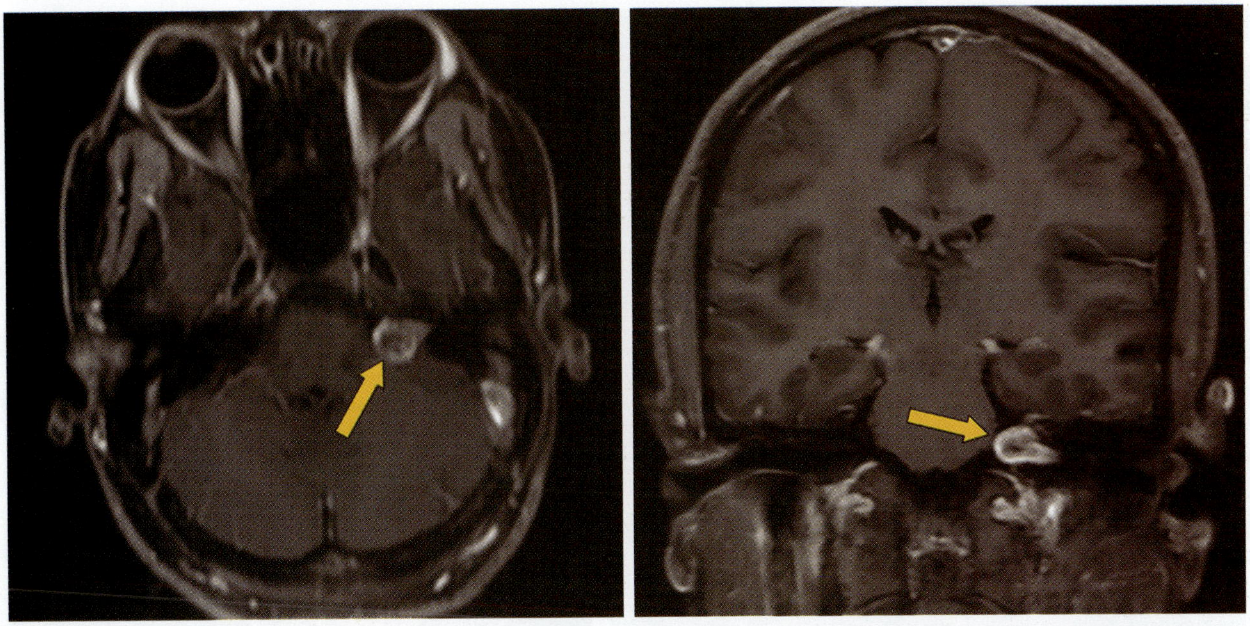

Axial T2 and coronal T1 C+ magnetic resonance imaging (MRI) brain images reveal a well-defined heterogeneously enhancing extra-axial mass (*yellow arrows*) with internal non-enhancing areas in the left cerebellopontine angle. It is extending into the porous acusticus laterally with resultant widening of the right internal auditory meatus.

Cerebellopontine Angle Schwannoma

Vestibular schwannoma is the most common tumour in the cerebellopontine (CP) angle region.

RADIOLOGICAL FEATURES

- On computed tomography (CT), majority schwannomas appear hypodense to isodense on non-contrast imaging with post-contrast enhancement. The tumour, often forming an acute angle with the petrous bone, can widen the internal auditory meatus, creating a characteristic 'ice-cream cone' appearance on imaging.
- Magnetic resonance imaging (MRI): T1-weighted imaging shows isointensity or hypointensity, T2-weighted imaging displays high signal intensity and Gadolinium-enhanced T1-weighted imaging reveals marked enhancement, solid in the majority cases and sometimes exhibiting heterogeneous enhancement.
- A simple mnemonic for CP angle masses is SAME:

  S – Schwannoma

  A – Arachnoid cyst

  M – Meningioma

  E – Epidermoid cyst

CP Angle Schwannoma	CP Angle Meningioma
1. Heterogeneous with cystic areas	1. More likely to be homogenous
2. Extension into internal acoustic meatus – 'ice-cream cone' appearance	2. Broad base with dura
3. Calcifications less common	3. Calcifications more common
4. Acute angle with petrous bone	4. Obtuse angle with petrous bone
5. No dural tail	5. Dural tail

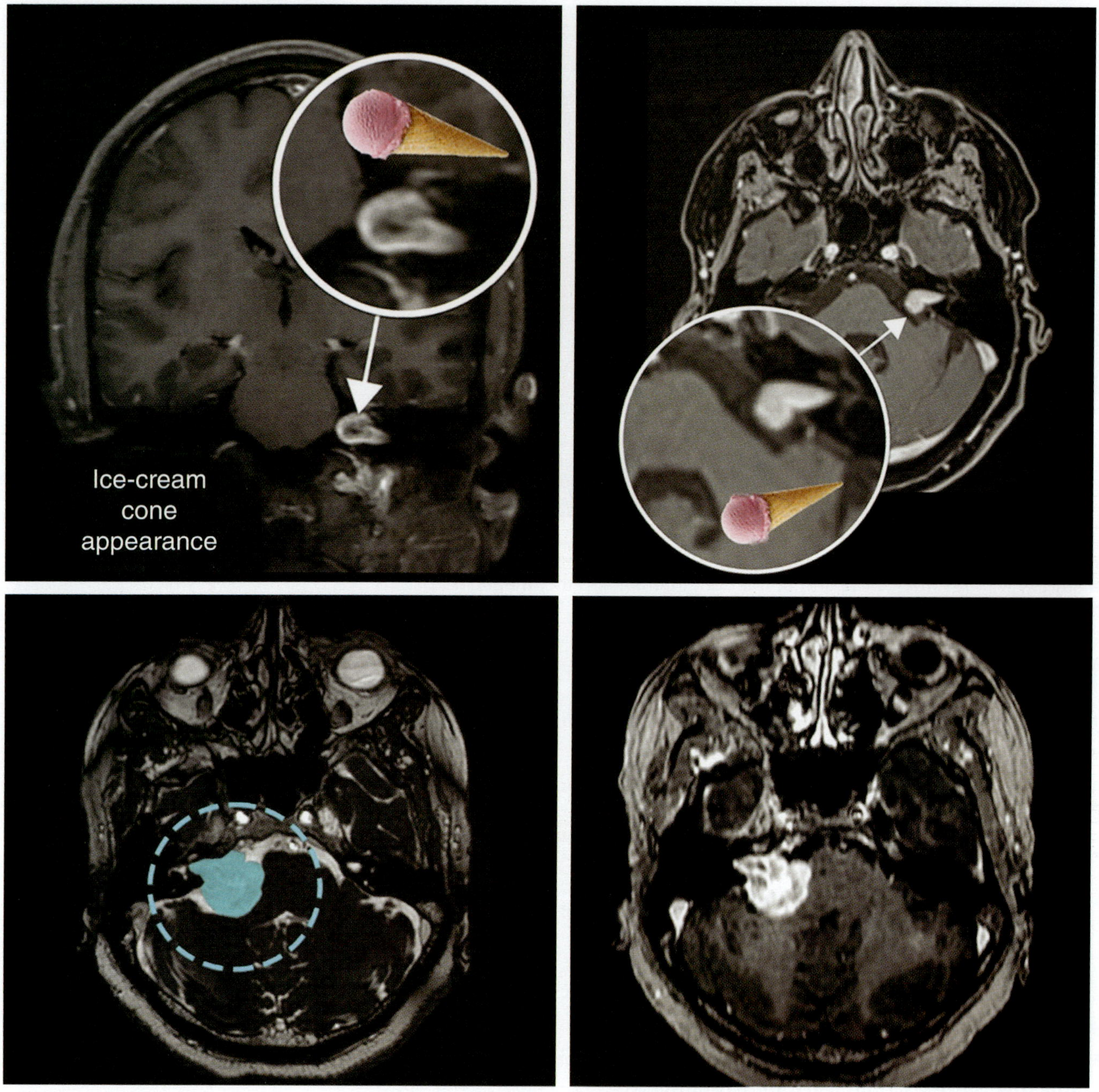
Ice-cream
cone
appearance

OSCE

80

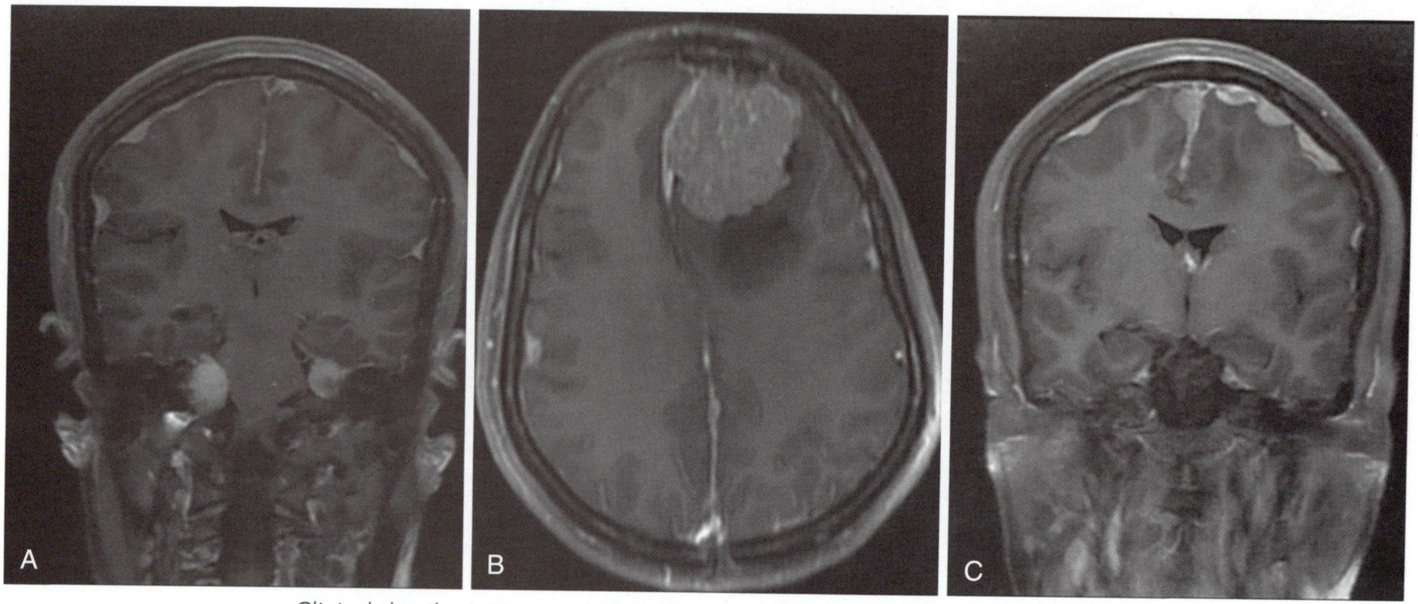

Clinical details: A 40-year-old female presented with headache and seizures.

1. **What is the most appropriate diagnosis for the cerebellopontine (CP) angle lesions?**
2. **In image two, which characteristic sign is seen?**
3. **What is the syndrome which shows this constellation of findings?**
4. **What investigation would you do next?**

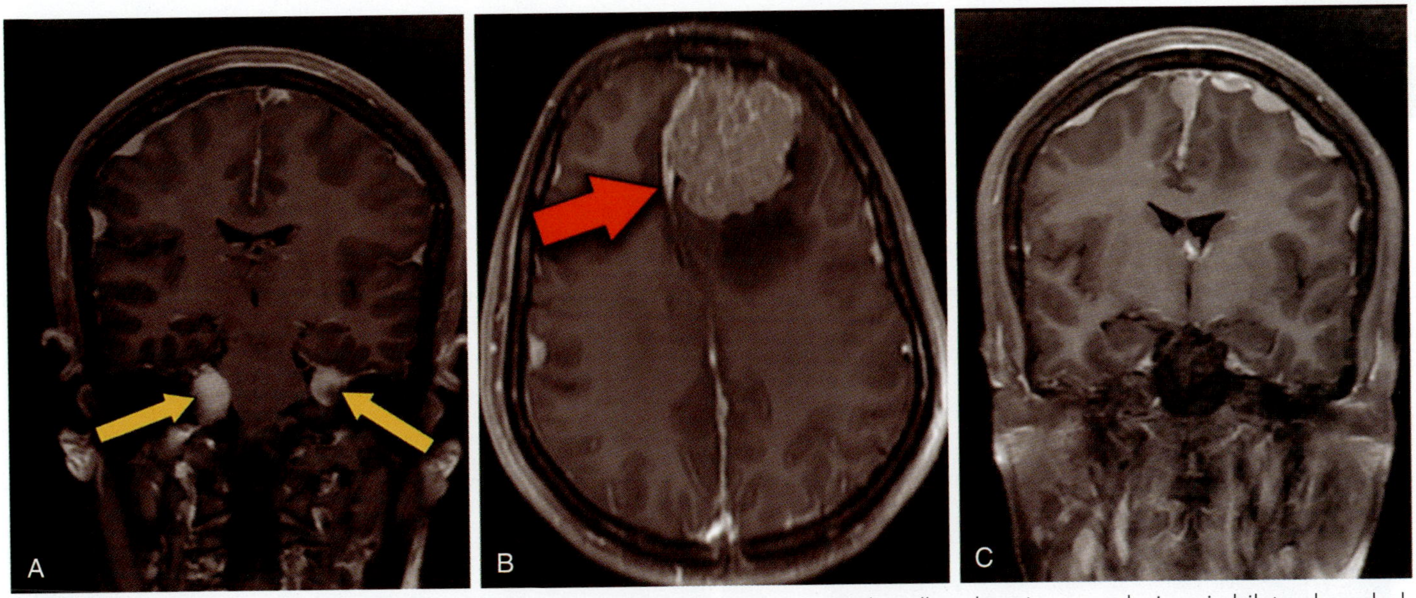

Axial and coronal T1 C+ magnetic resonance imaging (MRI) brain images reveal avidly enhancing mass lesions in bilateral cerebellopontine (CP) angle cisterns – bilateral acoustic schwannomas (*yellow arrows*).

Multiple lobulated avidly enhancing extra-axial masses scattered in bilateral cerebral hemispheres – meningiomas. Largest meningioma in left frontal lobe shows 'dural tail sign' (*red arrow*).

MISME Syndrome (Neurofibromatosis Type 2)

- Neurofibromatosis type 2 (NF-2) is an autosomal dominant phakomatosis characterized by multiple inherited schwannomas, meningiomas and ependymomas (MISME). Neurofibromas are not seen in NF-2 and are part of the NF I spectrum.
- It occurs due to a defect in the NF-2 gene located on the chromosome 22q12. Bilateral vestibular schwannomas form the hallmark of NF-2 and are seen in up to 90% of patients. Spinal tumours are common in NF-2. Hence, the entire neuraxis including spine should be imaged. Screening of family members and genetic counselling is required.
- The fifth cranial nerve (CN V) is the second most common site of schwannomas in NF-2 patients. NF-2 patients may also have posterior sublenticular capsular cataracts.

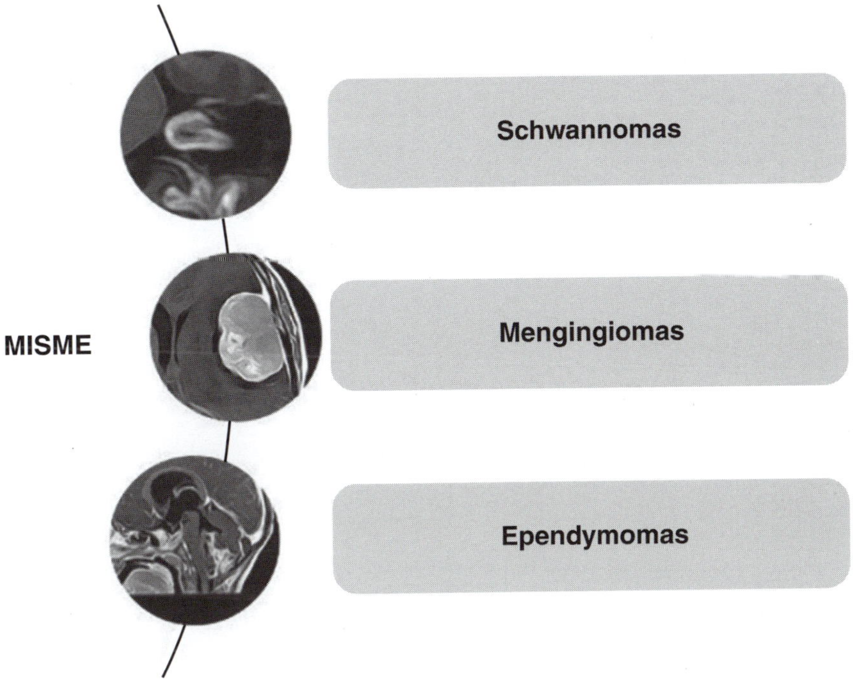

OSCE

81

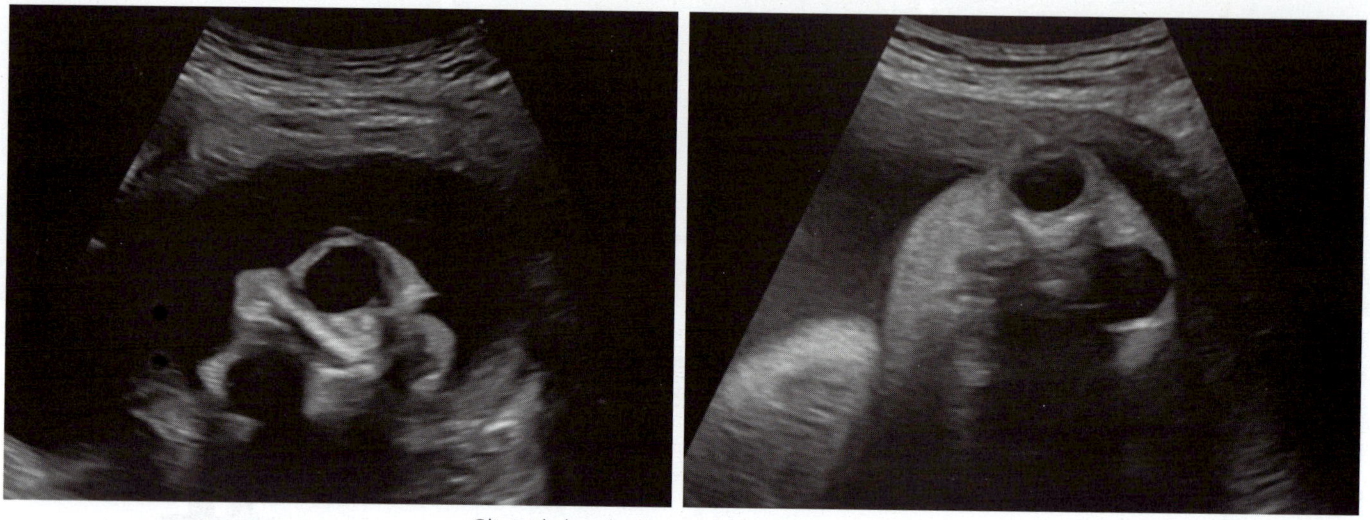

Clinical details: Routine antenatal scan.

1. What is the most appropriate diagnosis?
2. Name two associations with this entity.
3. What is the classic radiological sign seen here?
4. How can the risk of this entity be reduced antenatally?

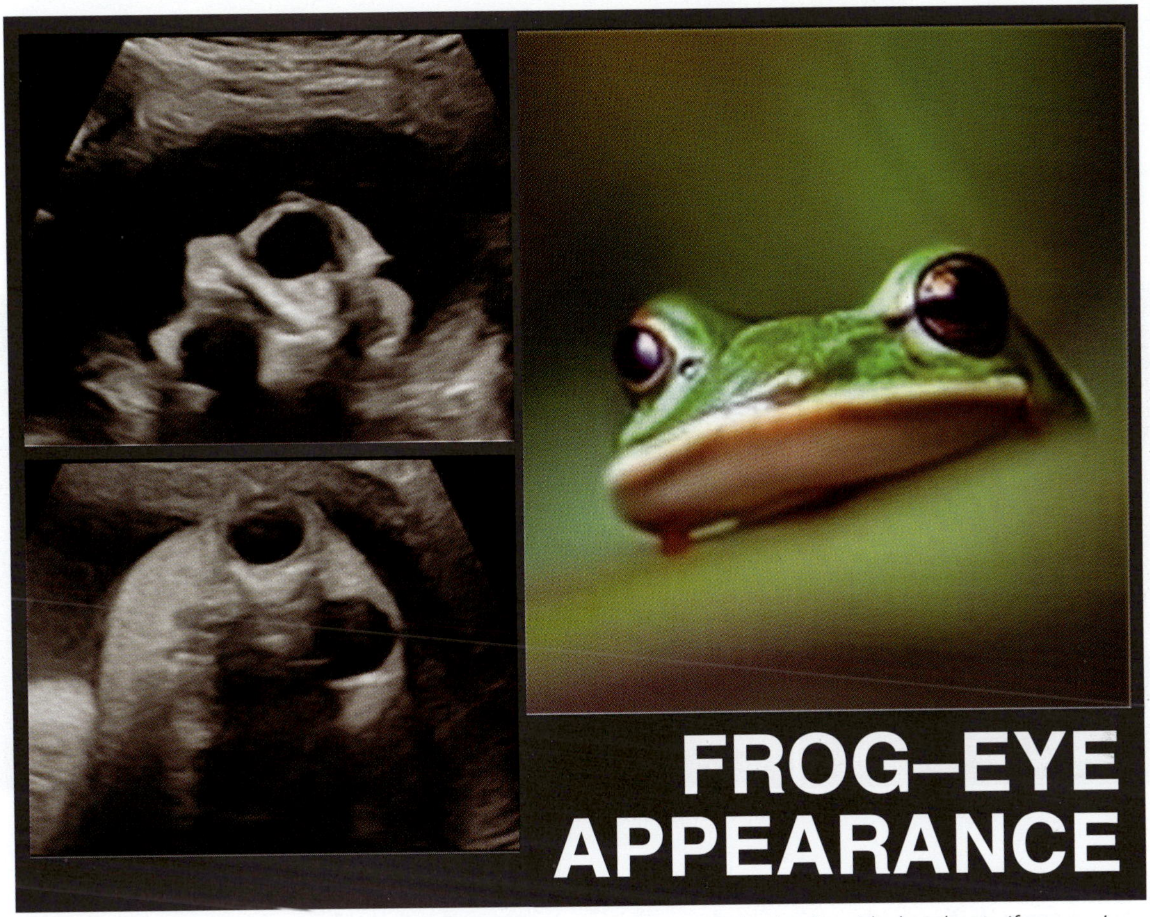

Ultrasound of the foetal head shows absence of foetal brain parenchyma and calvaria with the classic 'frog-eye' appearance.

Anencephaly

- Anencephaly is a neural tube defect (NTD) characterized by the absence of a well-formed brain parenchyma and absent calvaria. It can be detected sonologically as early as 10–13 weeks of pregnancy.
- Associations with other anomalies is reported such as – spina bifida, congenital heart defects (CHDs), clubfoot, cleft lip or palate and diaphragmatic defect/hernia.
- Antenatal ultrasonography (USG) shows absent calvaria with little to no brain tissue giving the foetal head the classic 'frog-eye' appearance.
- Alpha-fetoprotein levels in maternal serum (MSAFP) levels are elevated. Anencephaly is a highly lethal anomaly. Daily supplementation of 400 micrograms (mcg) of folic acid by the mother in the first trimester of pregnancy helps in reducing the risk of NTDs like anencephaly and spina bifida.

OSCE

82

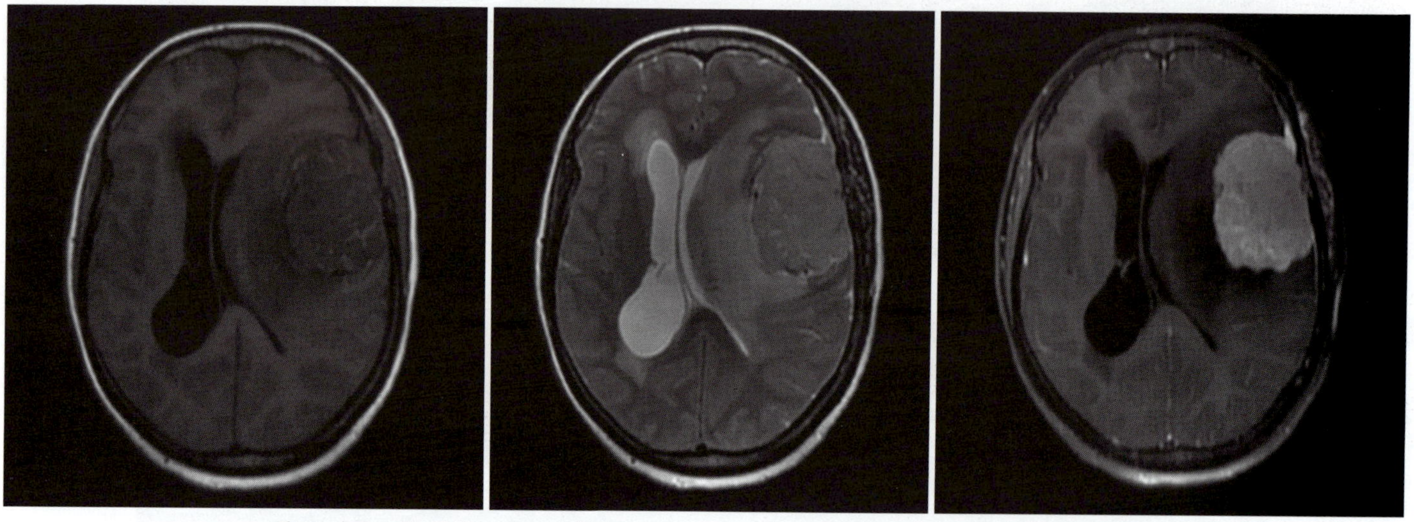

Clinical details: A 44-year-old female presented with history of chronic headache.

1. **What is the most appropriate diagnosis?**
2. **Enumerate four different locations where this lesion can be found.**
3. **Name one syndrome associated with this.**
4. **Which peak is elevated in magnetic resonance (MR) spectroscopy in this lesion?**

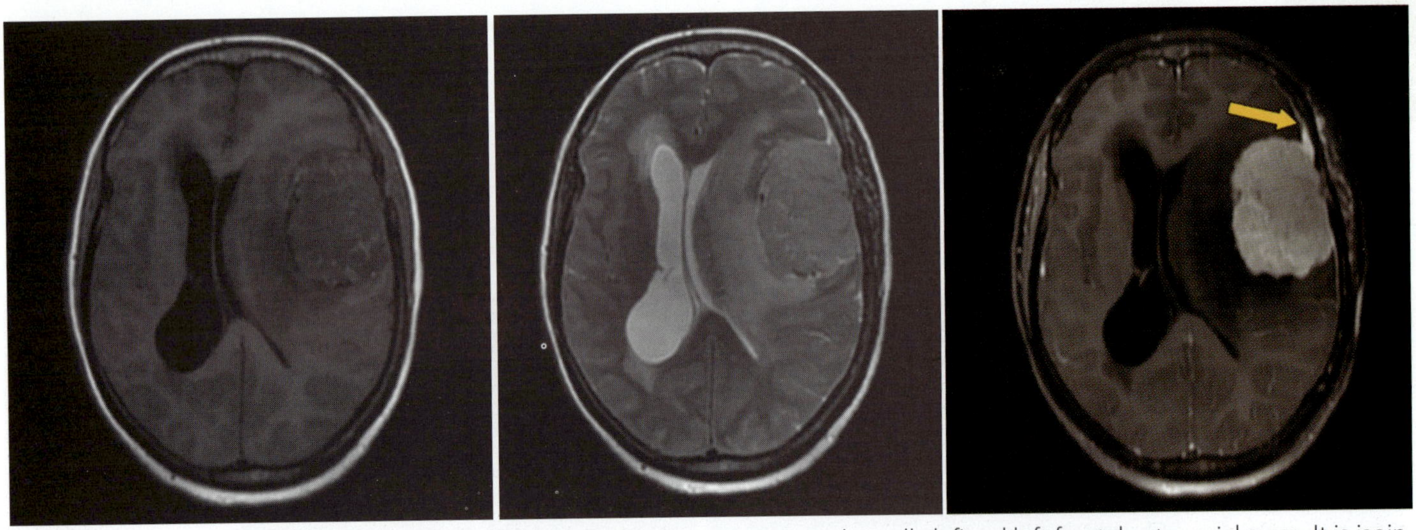

Axial T1, T2 and T1 C+ magnetic resonance imaging (MRI) brain images reveal a well-defined left frontal extra-axial mass. It is isointense on T1 and T2 WI. It shows marked homogenous enhancement with a 'dural tail' (*yellow arrow*). It is broad-based with dura, shows cerebrospinal fluid (CSF) cleft sign, vasogenic oedema, significant mass effect and midline shift. Findings are suggestive of meningioma.

Meningioma

- Meningioma is the most common extra-axial tumour of the central nervous system (CNS). It arises from arachnoid cap cells. It can occur in brain and spine, but most is commonly found in supratentorial compartment with parasagittal/convexity meningioma being most common. Other common locations include olfactory groove, planum sphenoidale, cerebellopontine angle cistern, pituitary fossa, intraventricular, optic nerve and spinal regions.
- It is more common in females. Syndromic association in neurofibromatosis II (multiple inherited schwannomas, meningiomas and ependymomas [MISME] syndrome) is well-known.

RADIOLOGICAL FEATURES

- Meningiomas typically appear as extra-axial masses on imaging, with a broad dural base. On non-contrast computed tomography (CT), they are often slightly hyperdense to normal brain, with variable adjacent oedema. Post-contrast CT shows homogeneous enhancement in the majority of cases.
- Magnetic resonance imaging (MRI) reveals well-circumscribed masses with T1 and T2 isointensity, and intense and homogeneous enhancement on post-contrast images. Helpful signs include the dural tail, cerebrospinal fluid (CSF) cleft sign and sunburst/spoke wheel vessel pattern. Angiography is rarely used diagnostically but may be employed for preoperative embolization.
- Apart from the findings described above, it can show hyperostosis on CT brain.
- On magnetic resonance (MR) spectroscopy, an alanine peak is found (1.3–1.5 ppm).
- Pertinent differentials include dural metastasis and solitary fibrous tumour (SFT) of the dura.

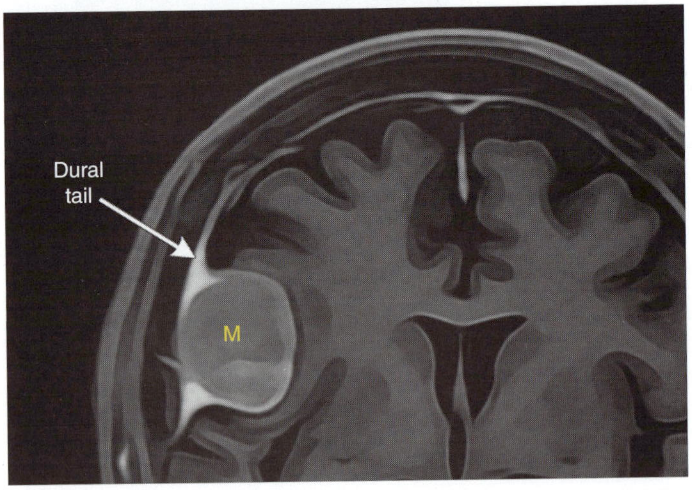

Signs	Extra-Axial Masses	Intra-Axial Masses
CSF cleft sign	+	–
Displaced subarachnoid vessels	+	–
Cortical grey matter between mass and white matter	+	–
Displaced and expanded subarachnoid spaces	+	–
Broad dural base	+	–
Adjacent bony changes like hyperostosis/bony reaction	+	–

OSCE

83

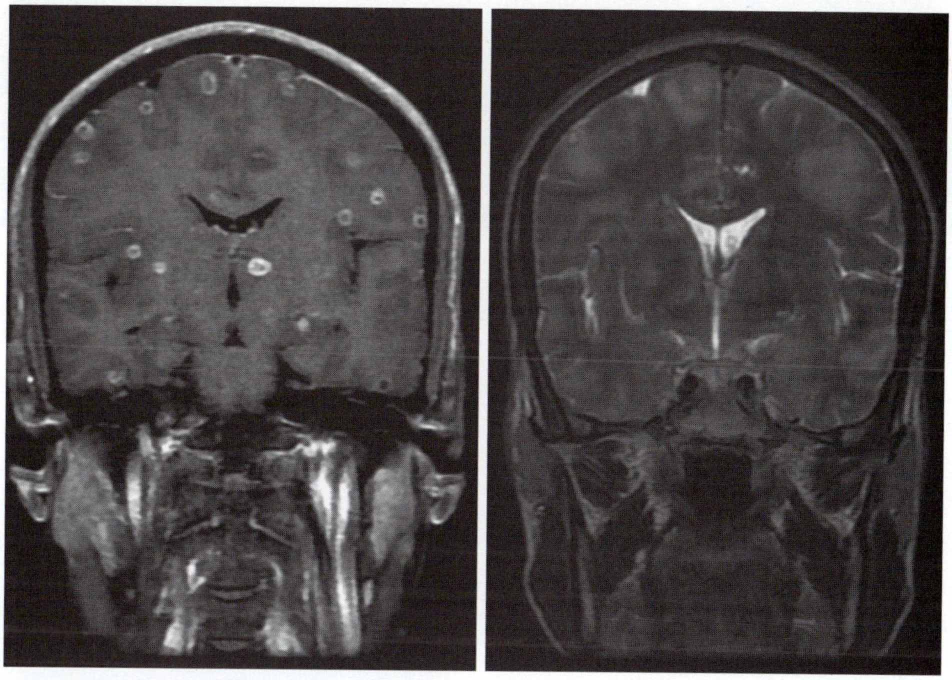

Clinical details: A young male with recurrent episodes of seizures.

1. Describe the findings in the provided images.
2. What is the most appropriate diagnosis?
3. What are the different stages seen in this pathology?
4. Provide two appropriate differentials.

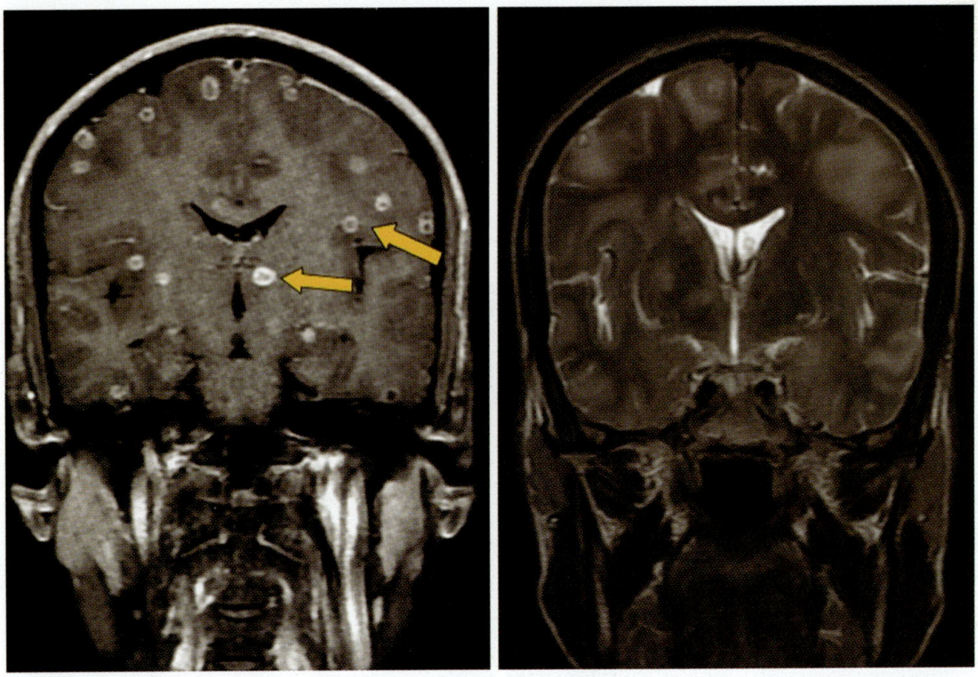

Coronal T1 C+ and coronal T2 WI show multiple ring-enhancing lesions scattered in bilateral cerebral hemispheres with perilesional vasogenic oedema – neurocysticercosis.

Neurocysticercosis

- Neurocysticercosis (NCC) is a common parasitic infection of the central nervous system (CNS) caused by the pork tapeworm – *Taenia solium*. It is a common cause of seizures in endemic population. Infection occurs through the faeco-oral route. Its life cycle consists of four stages – vesicular, colloidal vesicular, granular nodular and nodular calcified. 'Cyst with a dot' sign is a characteristic feature of NCC and is commonly seen in the vesicular stage.

STAGE: VESICULAR
- Small (<2 cm) cystic lesion with a thin, smooth and well-defined cyst wall
- Central hyperdense/hyperintense scolex within the cyst
- Absence of perilesional oedema
- Little or no enhancement post-contrast

STAGE: COLLOIDAL VESICULAR
- Enlarged cyst with irregular cyst wall
- Degenerated scolex or nodule with surrounding oedema
- Ring enhancement post-contrast
- Perilesional oedema extending beyond the cyst

STAGE: NODULAR CALCIFIED
- Small calcified nodules (1–2 mm)
- Decreasing oedema and enhancement

STAGE: GRANULAR NODULAR
- End-stage calcified stage
- No oedema or enhancement

- Antiepileptic drugs with anthelmintic drugs like albendazole form the mainstay of management.

- Differentials of ring-enhancing lesions can be memorized by the mnemonic – DR MAGIC.

M – Metastasis

A – Abscess

G – Glioblastoma multiforme

I – Infarction (subacute phase)

C – Contusion

D – Demyelination lesions

R – Radiation necrosis

OSCE 84

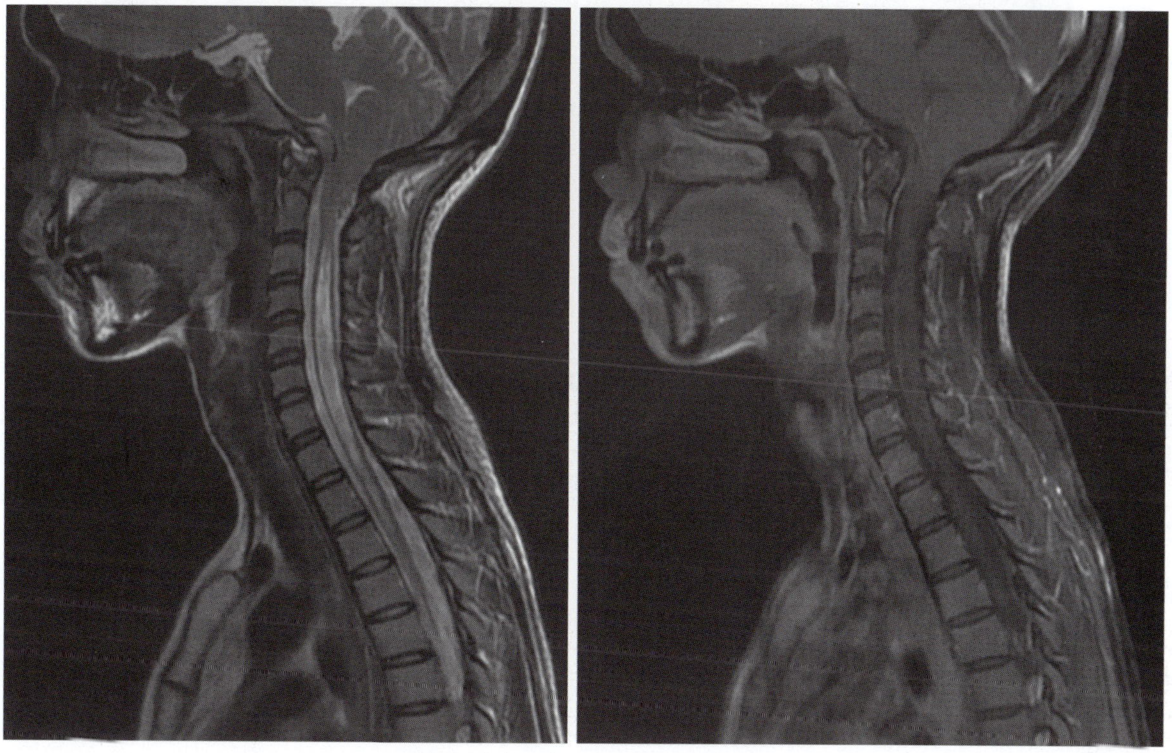

Clinical details: History withheld.

1. Identify the sequences and describe your findings.
2. What is the most appropriate diagnosis?
3. What another investigation/s would be recommended?
4. Provide one differential for low-lying cerebellar tonsils.

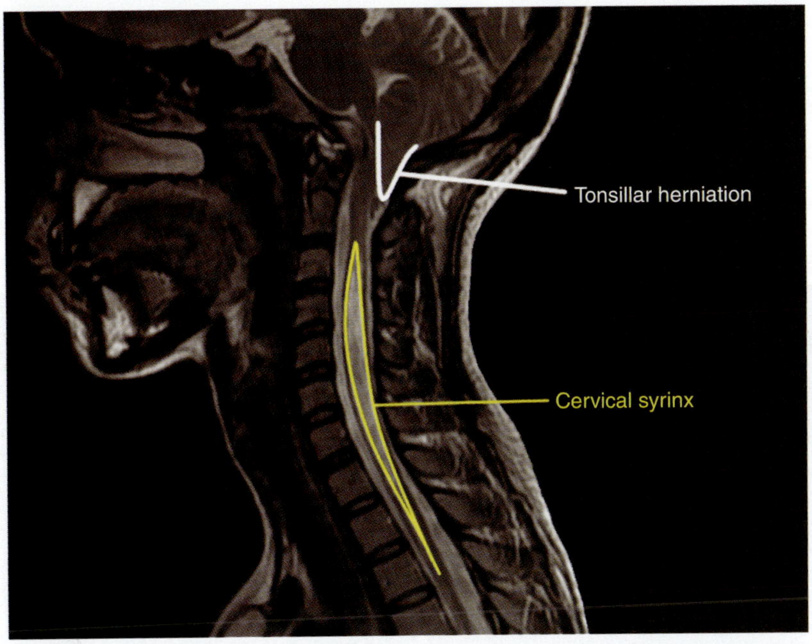

Peg-like tonsillar herniation through the foramen magnum with T2 hyperintense cervical cord syrinx in a patient with Chiari I malformation. On post-contrast imaging, no enhancement was observed in the syrinx.

Chiari I Malformation

- Chiari malformations are a group of hind-brain malformations first described by Hans Chiari, an Austrian pathologist.
- Chiari I malformation is the most common type, characterized by peg-like caudal descent of the cerebellar tonsils of more than 5 mm through the foramen magnum. It can be associated with a cervical cord syrinx in 30%–50% of cases. Abnormal cerebrospinal fluid (CSF) flow can lead to hydrocephalus. 'Crowded foramen magnum' can be seen on axial computed tomography (CT)/magnetic resonance images (MRI) images.
- Imaging the brain to rule out hydrocephalus and CSF flow studies are the important imaging methods to aid in the workup of a Chiari I malformation case.
- Other associations are Klippel–Feil anomaly, basilar invagination, atlanto-occipital assimilation and platybasia.
- Differential diagnosis includes acquired tonsillar herniation due to elevated intracranial pressure (ICP) or due to intracranial hypotension and other types of Chiari malformations.

Chiari 1	• Most prevalent type. • Characterized by the downward displacement of cerebellar tonsils into the upper cervical canal through the foramen magnum.
Chiari 1.5	• Manifests as downward descent of cerebellar tonsils and brainstem.
Chiari 2	• Involves displacement of the medulla, fourth ventricle and cerebellar vermis through the foramen magnum. • Typically associated with lumbosacral spinal myelomeningocele.
Chiari 3	• Involves displacement of the medulla, fourth ventricle and cerebellar vermis through the foramen magnum. • Additionally presents with occipital and/or high cervical encephalocele.

OSCE

85

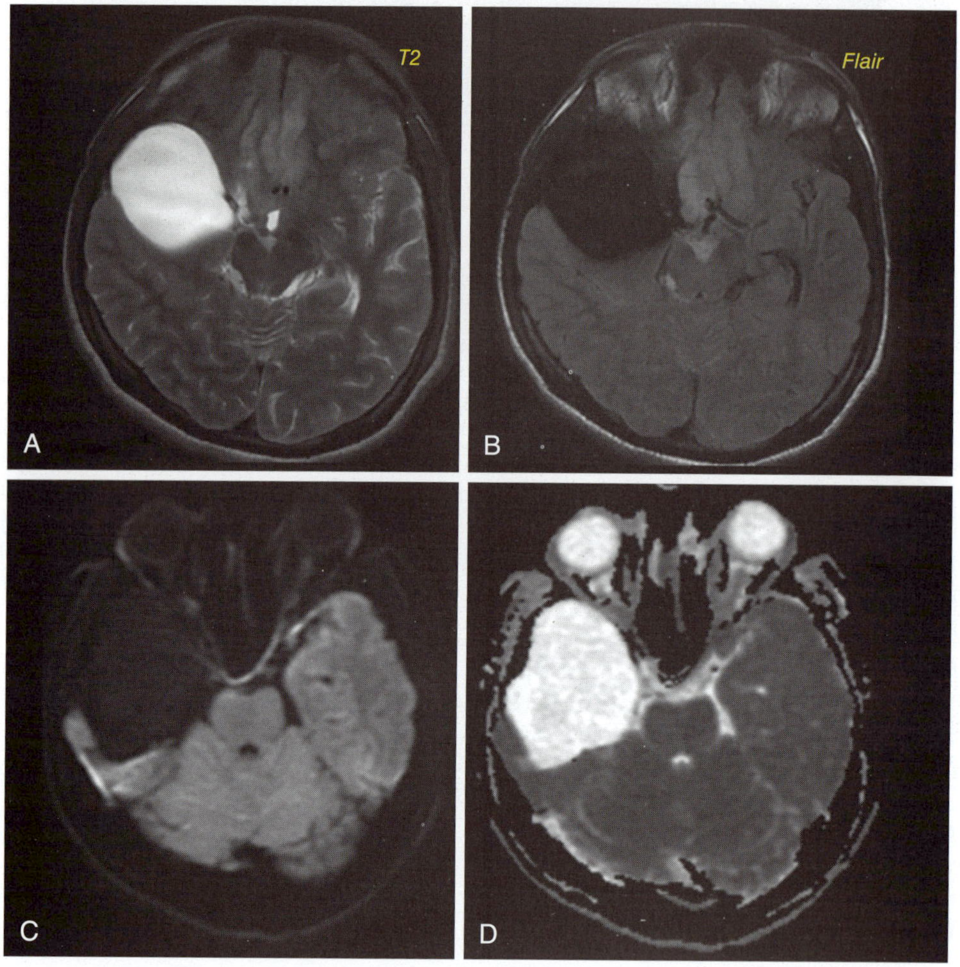

Clinical details: Middle-aged man presented with slowly progressive chronic headache.

1. **Identify the sequences C and D.**
2. **Describe your findings in the provided images.**
3. **What is the most appropriate diagnosis?**
4. **Enumerate one apt differential which shows restricted diffusion.**

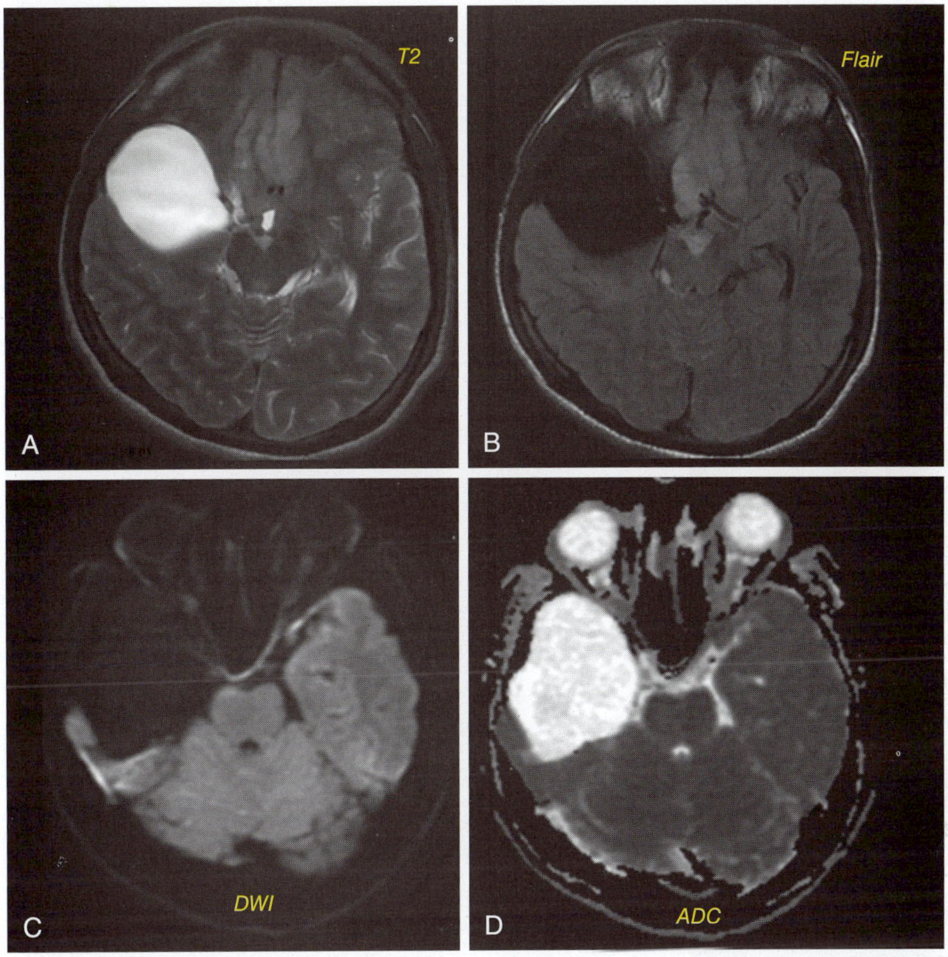

Axial magnetic resonance imaging (MRI) brain images: Large extra-axial cystic lesion in the right middle cranial fossa. It follows cerebrospinal fluid (CSF) signal on sequences. No diffusion restriction. Features are consistent with arachnoid cyst.

Arachnoid Cyst

- Arachnoid cyst (AC) is a common benign cystic lesion of the central nervous system (CNS) and contains cerebrospinal fluid (CSF). Smaller ACs are usually asymptomatic but larger lesions can cause symptoms due to mass effect.

RADIOLOGICAL FEATURES

- On computed tomography (CT), AC is well-circumscribed with a thin wall and may cause adjacent bone remodelling if large. On magnetic resonance imaging (MRI), it shows cerebrospinal fluid (CSF) signal intensity on all sequences. It completely suppresses on FLAIR sequence and does not show restricted diffusion. AC does not show enhancement on post-contrast images.
- The major differential diagnosis of an AC is epidermoid cyst. Epidermoid cyst does not completely suppress on FLAIR and typically demonstrated restricted diffusion on diffusion-weighted imaging (DWI).
- Middle cranial fossa at ACs are classified by the Galassi classification.

MIDDLE CRANIAL FOSSA ARACHNOID CYSTS—GALASSI CLASSIFICATION

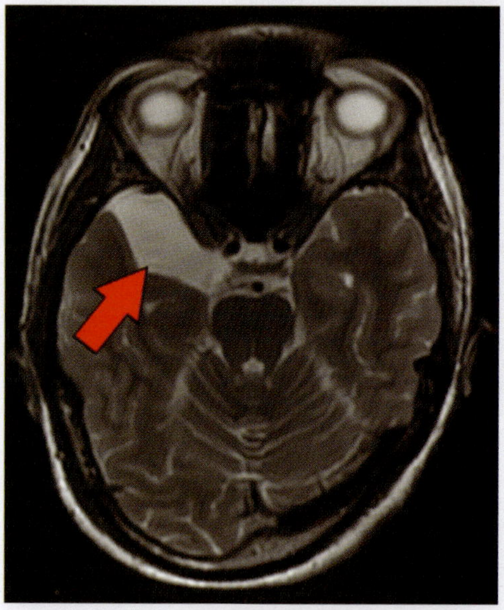

Type I

- Small in size
- Occupies the anterior temporal region

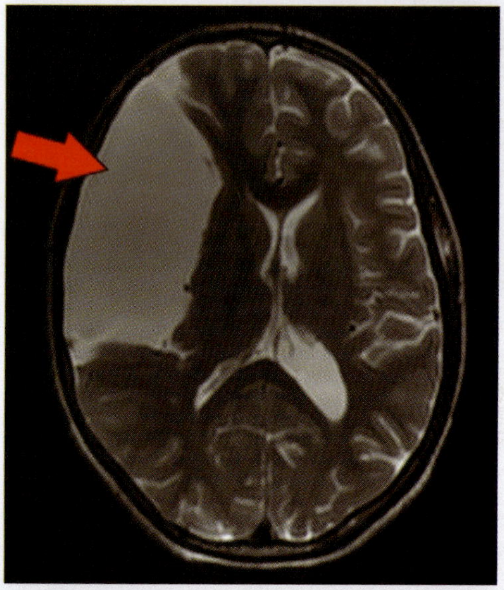

Type II

- Larger than type I
- Occupies both the anterior and middle temporal regions
- Causes displacement of the temporal lobe

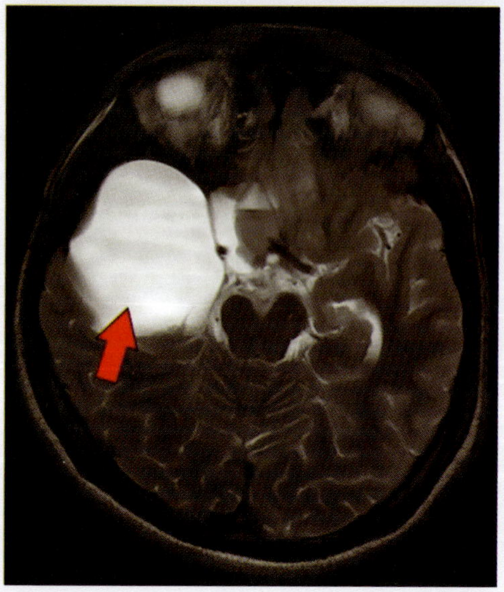

Type III

- Large in size
- Significant mass effect
- Fills the entire temporal fossa and extends into the fronto-parietal regions

OSCE

86

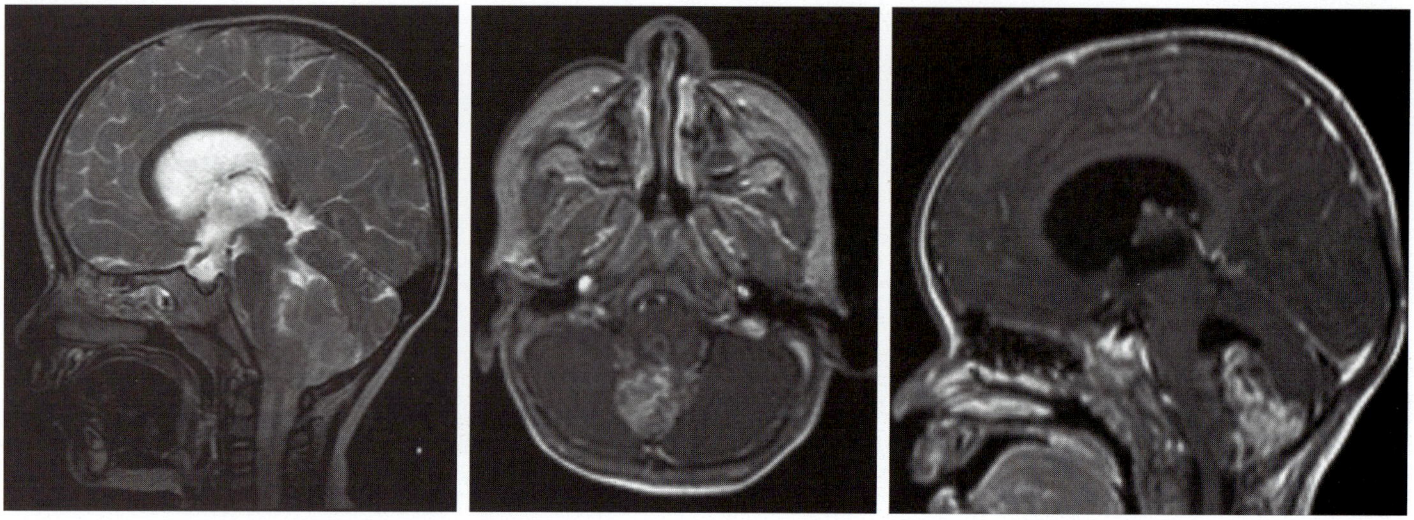

Clinical details: A young male presented with blurring of vision.

1. **Identify the sequences and describe your findings.**
2. **What is the most appropriate diagnosis?**
3. **Give one differential diagnosis.**
4. **What should be the next step?**

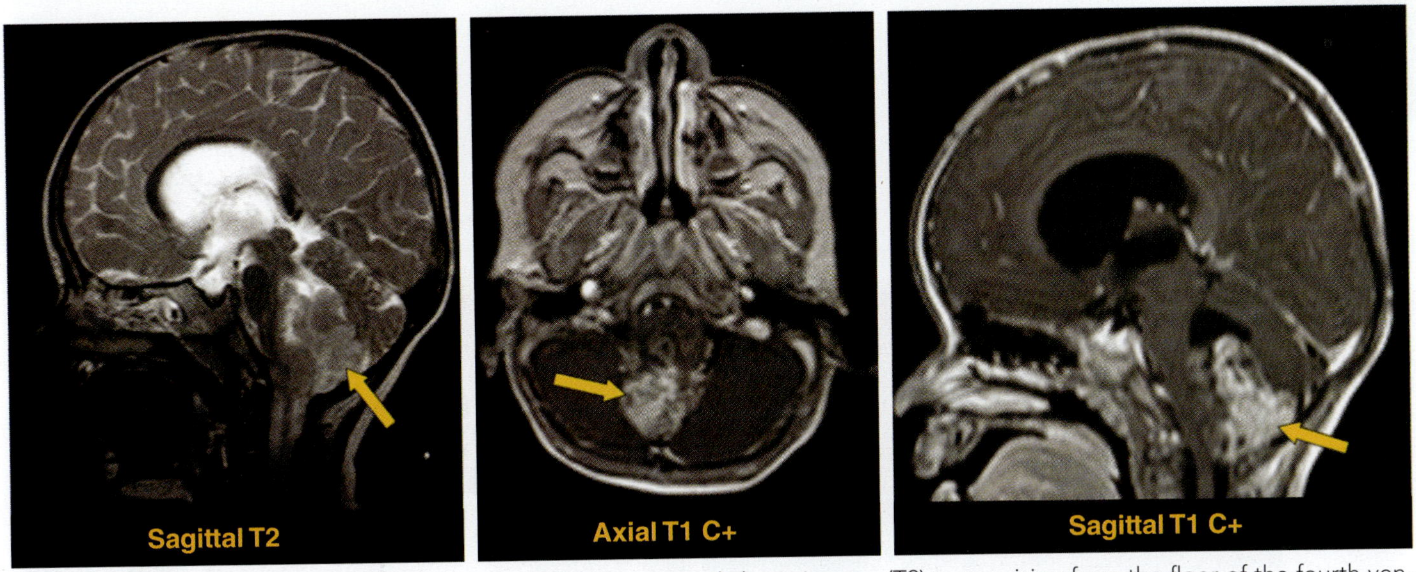

Magnetic resonance imaging (MRI) brain images: Heterogeneously hyperintense (T2) mass arising from the floor of the fourth ventricle, extending into the foramina of Luschka and showing post-contrast enhancement – posterior fossa ependymoma. Hydrocephalus is evident.

Posterior Fossa Ependymoma

Posterior fossa ependymoma is an ependymal central nervous system (CNS) neoplasm. It is usually found in children but be seen in any age group.

RADIOLOGICAL FEATURES

- Posterior fossa ependymoma arises from the floor of the fourth ventricle. They can be seen extending through the foramina of Luschka and Magendie. Due to this feature of extension through adjacent foramina, ependymoma are known as 'plastic tumours'.
- On imaging, they appear as heterogenous lesions and they show cystic necrotic areas, haemorrhage and calcification.
- On computed tomography (CT), calcification and haemorrhage are well seen, with the lesion showing heterogenous post-contrast enhancement. Magnetic resonance imaging (MRI) demonstrates the lesion as the heterogenous posterior fossa mass arising from the floor of the fourth ventricle, again with heterogenous enhancement. Ependymoma may show restricted diffusion.
- As cerebrospinal fluid (CSF) seeding may be seen in posterior fossa ependymomas, imaging the entire neuraxis is necessary.
- Differential diagnosis includes medulloblastoma (arises from roof of the fourth ventricle) and subependymoma (older demographics).

OSCE

87

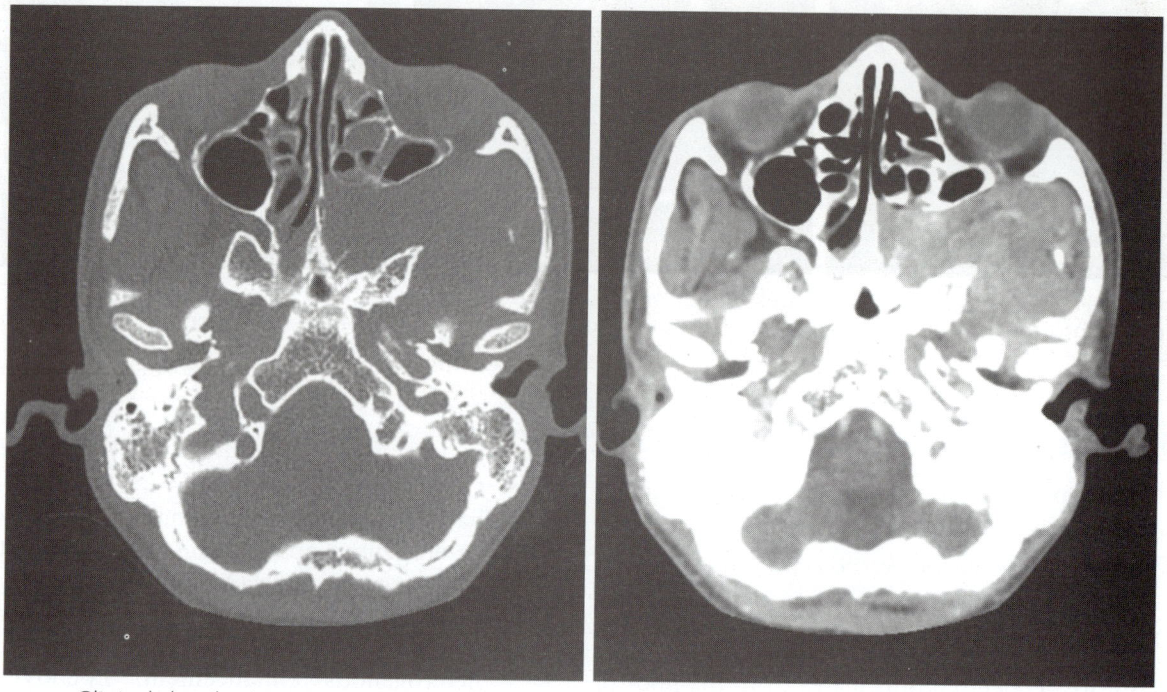

Clinical details: A teenager presented with a history of recurrent epistaxis and nasal stuffiness.

1. **What is the most appropriate diagnosis?**
2. **Which radiological sign do you see here (with respect to the posterior left maxillary sinus wall)?**
3. **Which is the age group in which this pathology commonly occurs in?**
4. **Which procedure is recommended preoperatively?**

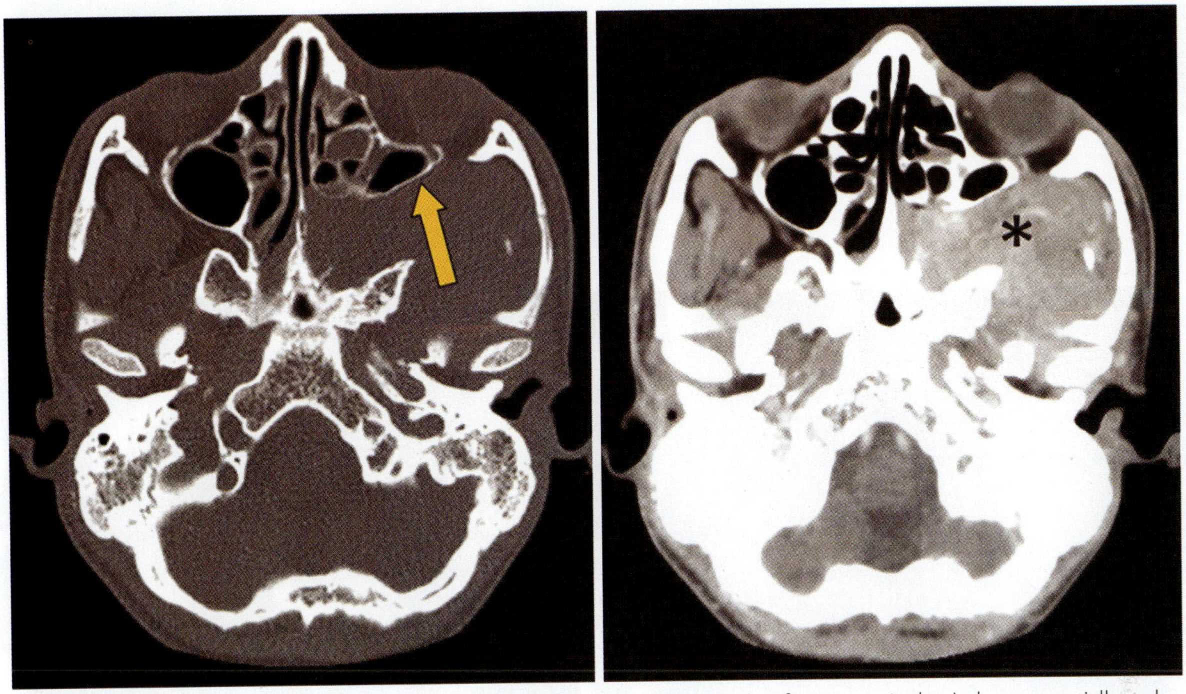

Axial contrast-enhanced computed tomography (CT) images (bony window and soft tissue window) show an avidly enhancing mass (*) centred on the widened left sphenopalatine foramen. On bony window, anterior bowing of the posterior wall of left maxillary sinus is evident (*yellow arrow*).

Juvenile Nasopharyngeal Angiofibroma

- Juvenile nasopharyngeal angiofibroma (JNA) is a highly vascular tumour which commonly occurs in adolescent males. Recurrent epistaxis is a common presentation. JNA is a benign tumour but is locally aggressive.

RADIOLOGICAL FEATURES

- On contrast-enhanced computed tomography (CT) of the paranasal sinus (PNS), JNA is seen as a heterogeneous mass which is centred on the sphenopalatine foramen. Sphenopalatine foramen widening is often seen. On bony windows, the mass causes mass effect on the posterior wall of the ipsilateral maxillary antral wall, resulting in its bowing. This is known as 'Holman-Miller sign' or the 'antral bow sign'. On magnetic resonance imaging (MRI), JNAs show vivid post-contrast enhancement and 'salt-and-pepper appearance' (due to vessels causing multiple flow voids). Selective angiography can be used to delineate the feeling vessels.
- Preoperative embolization of the feeding vessels is recommended to reduce blood loss during surgery.
- Differential diagnosis includes nasopharyngeal carcinoma, rhabdomyosarcoma and olfactory neuroblastoma.

OSCE

88

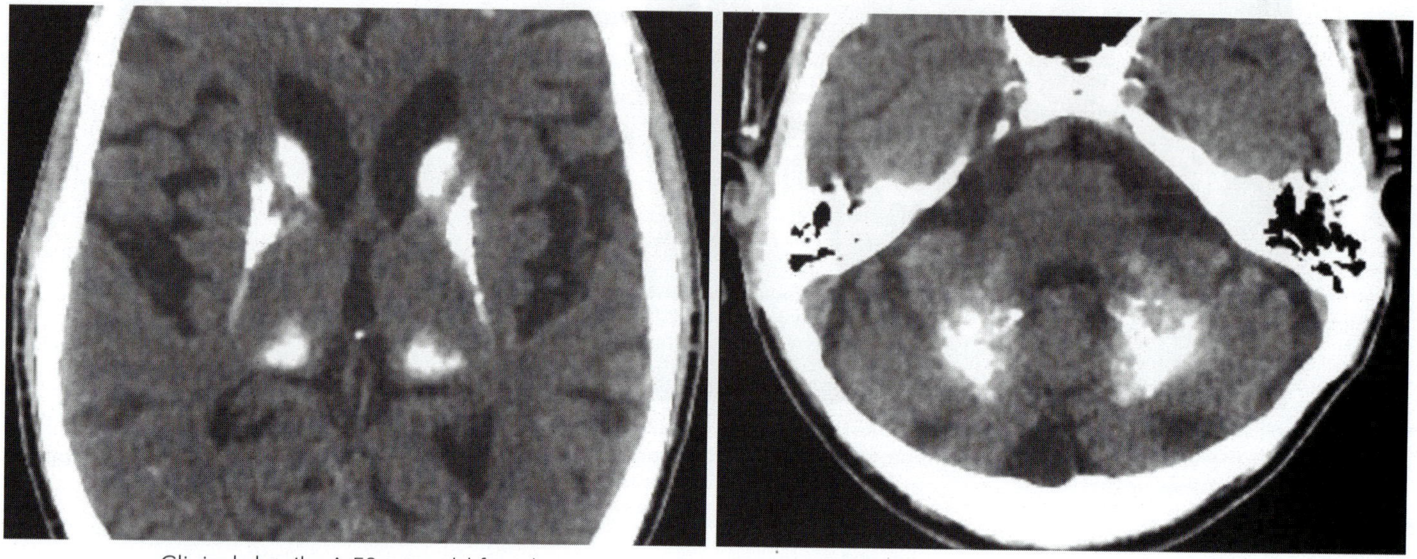

Clinical details: A 50-year-old female presented with progressive psychosis and cognitive impairment.

1. **Describe your findings.**
2. **What is the most appropriate diagnosis?**
3. **Which endocrinopathy can cause similar imaging findings?**
4. **Name one inherited cause of basal ganglia calcification.**

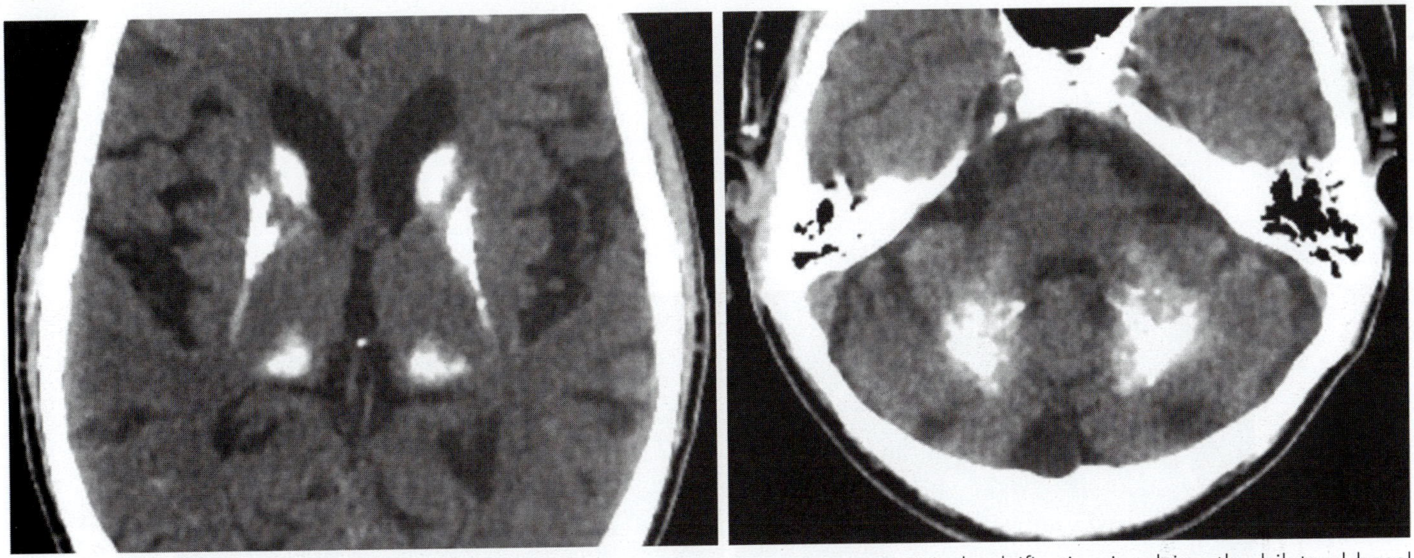

Axial non-contrast computed tomography (NCCT) brain images: Extensive symmetrical calcification involving the bilateral basal ganglia, thalami and dentate nuclei (of cerebellum) – in keeping with Fahr disease.

Fahr Disease

- Fahr disease is characterized by excessive deposition of calcium in the basal ganglia structures, dentate nuclei and subcortical white matter.
- Diagnostic criteria include basal ganglia calcifications, absence of features suggesting mitochondrial or metabolic aetiology, family history, absence of trauma, infection or toxins as an aetiology, progressive central nervous system (CNS) dysfunction and presentation in the fourth or fifth decade of life.
- Secondary causes of basal ganglia calcifications include endocrinopathies (hypoparathyroidism, pseudo-hypoparathyroidism and pseudo-pseudo-hypoparathyroidism), inherited causes like mitochondrial disorders and CNS infections.

OSCE

89

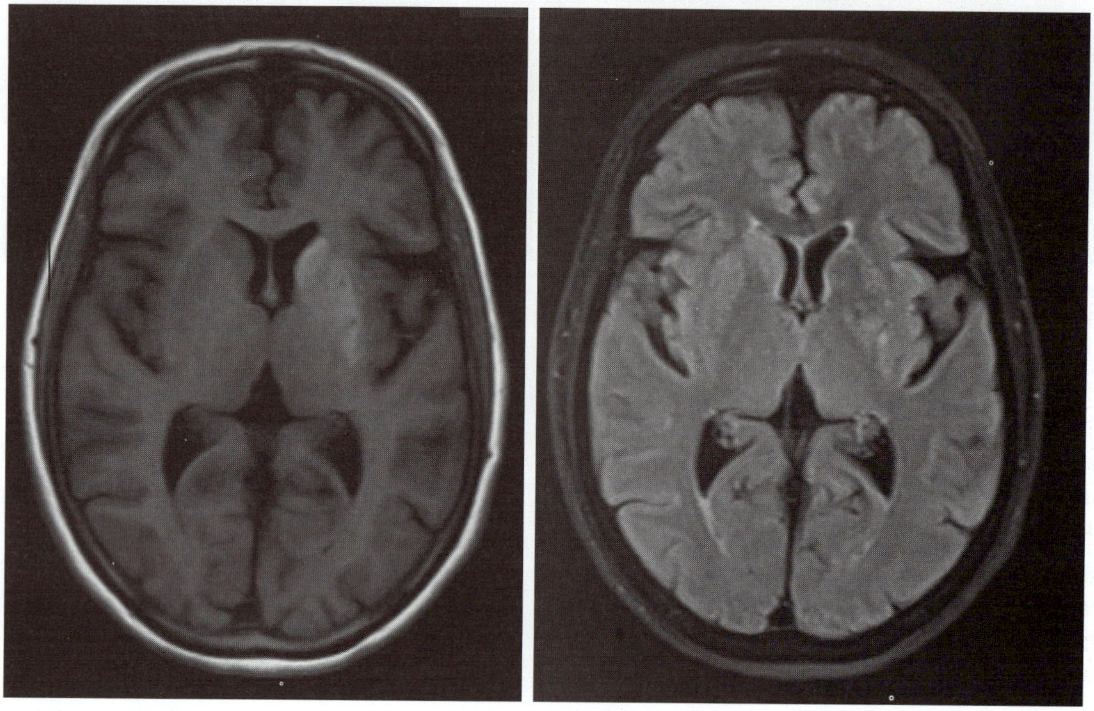

Clinical details: A 60-year-old diabetic lady presented with rapid development of chorea and hemiballismus.

1. **Identify the sequences.**
2. **What is the most appropriate diagnosis?**
3. **Which underlying metabolic disease is this associated with?**
4. **Which syndrome does it cause?**

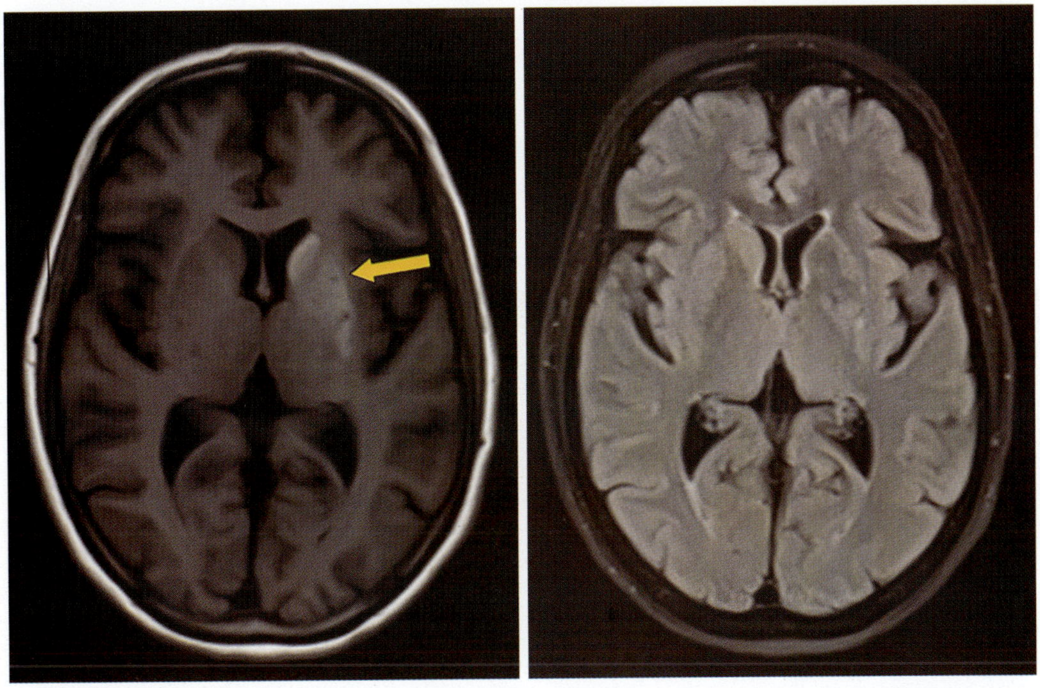

Axial non-contrast T1 and FLAIR sequences: Axial T1 image reveals hyperintensity in the right lentiform and caudate nucleus. No significant signal changes seen on the FLAIR image. Findings are in keeping with non-ketotic hyperglycaemic hemichorea (NKHH).

Non-Ketotic Hyperglycaemic Hemichorea

- Non-ketotic hyperglycaemic hemichorea (NKHH) or diabetic striatopathy is a rare complication affecting patients with poorly controlled diabetes.
- Clinically it presents with chorea and hemiballismus and is called hemichorea-hemiballismus syndrome, when unilateral.

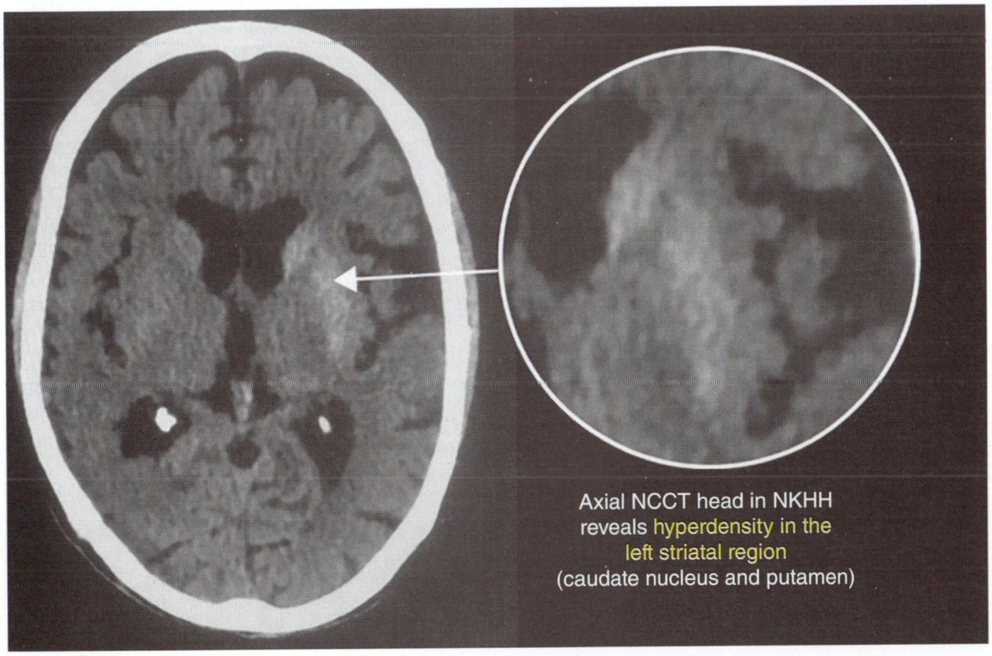

RADIOLOGICAL FEATURES

- Computed tomography (CT) brain can be normal or may show subtle unilateral hyperdensity involving the caudate and putamen (striatum). Magnetic resonance imaging (MRI) typically shows T1 hyperintensity involving the stratum. Findings are known to resolve after controlling hyperglycaemia.

CAUSES OF BASAL GANGLIA T1 HYPERINTENSITY

- Paramagnetic substances like calcification (Fahr and hypoparathyroidism), methaemoglobin (haemorrhage) and manganese (liver failure and haemodialysis)
- Wilson's disease (copper deposition)
- Diabetic striatopathy (NKHH)
- Fabry disease
- Neurofibromatosis I
- Chronic bilirubin encephalopathy

OSCE

90

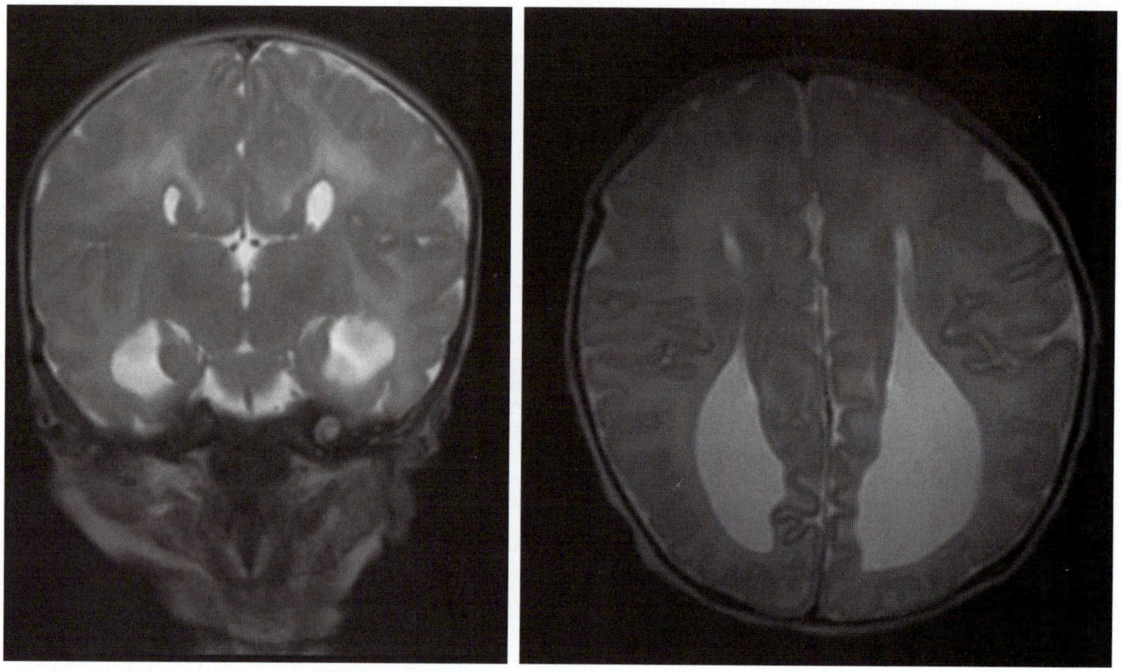

Clinical details: Child with global developmental delay.

1. **Identify the sequences.**
2. **What is the most appropriate diagnosis?**
3. **Which characteristic radiological sign is seen in the first image?**
4. **Enumerate two associated central nervous system (CNS) anomalies?**

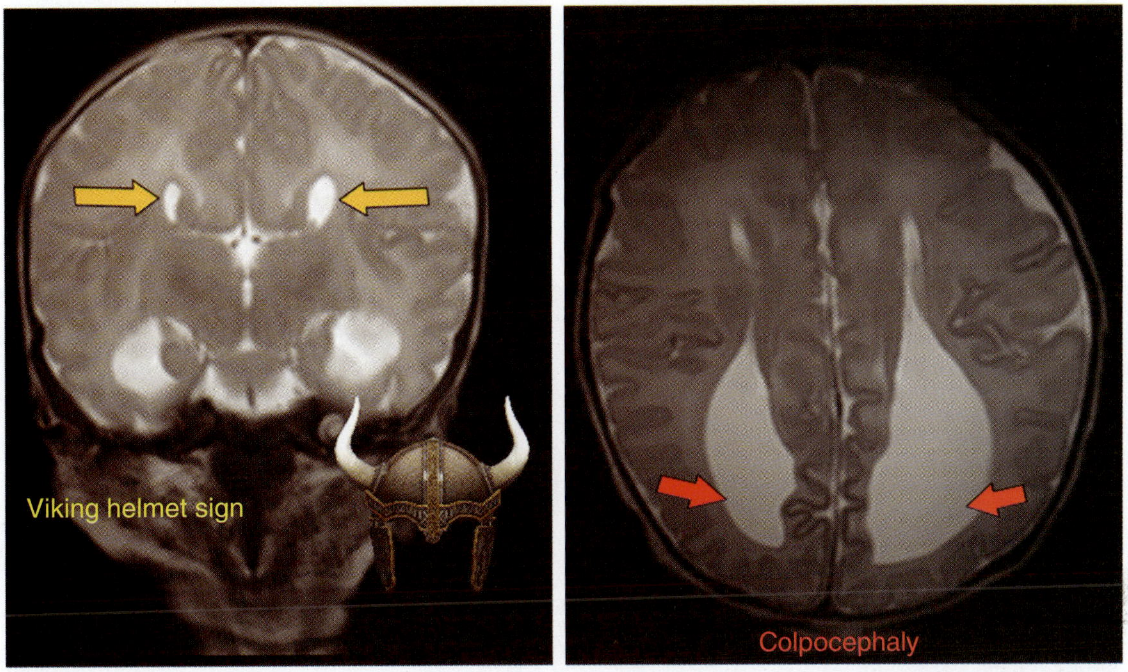

Coronal and axial T2-weighted images demonstrate corpus callosum agenesis. Widely spaced, vertically oriented lateral ventricles demonstrating the characteristic 'Viking helmet sign' is evident in first image. Lateral ventricles appear widely separated, with absent corpus callosum and dilated occipital horns (colpocephaly).

Corpus Callosum Agenesis

Complete absence of the corpus callosum is termed as 'corpus callosum agenesis'. It is the most common malformation of the central nervous system (CNS). Maternal consumption of alcohol during pregnancy is a known risk factor.

RADIOLOGICAL FEATURES

- Computed tomography (CT) and magnetic resonance imaging (MRI) brain show widely spaced and parallelly oriented lateral ventricles with absent corpus callosum. On sagittal imaging, cerebral gyri appear to be radiating towards the third ventricle.
- On coronal images, the characteristic 'Viking helmet' or 'moose head' appearance is seen. 'Racing car' appearance is characteristically demonstrated on axial images.
- Several associated CNS anomalies may be seen, some of which include – Chiari II malformations, hydrocephalus, grey matter heterotopia, interhemispheric cysts and lipoma, schizencephaly and porencephaly.

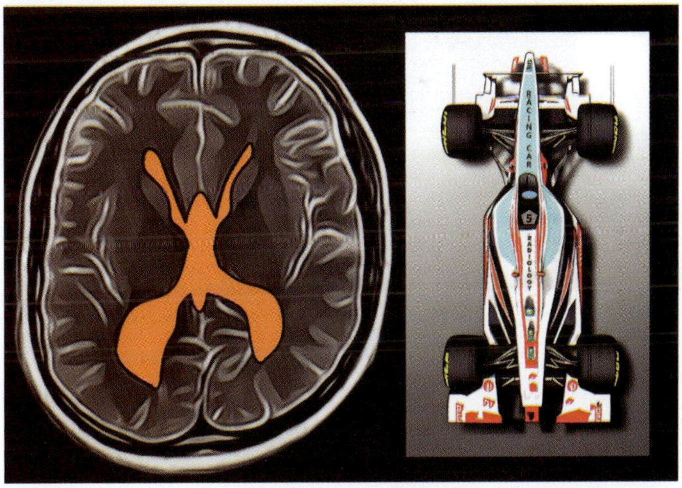

Racing car sign

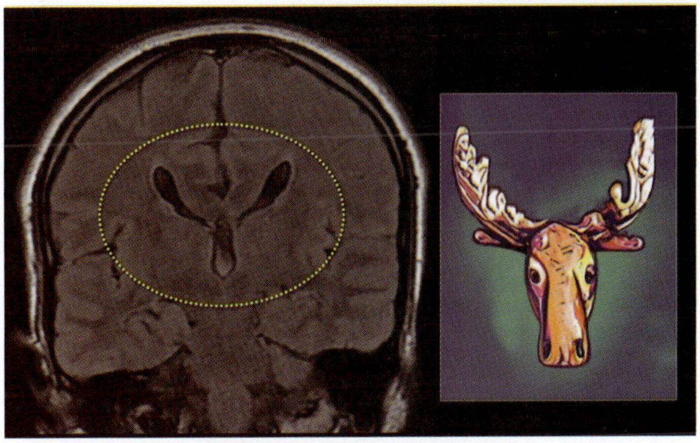

Moose head appearance

OSCE

91

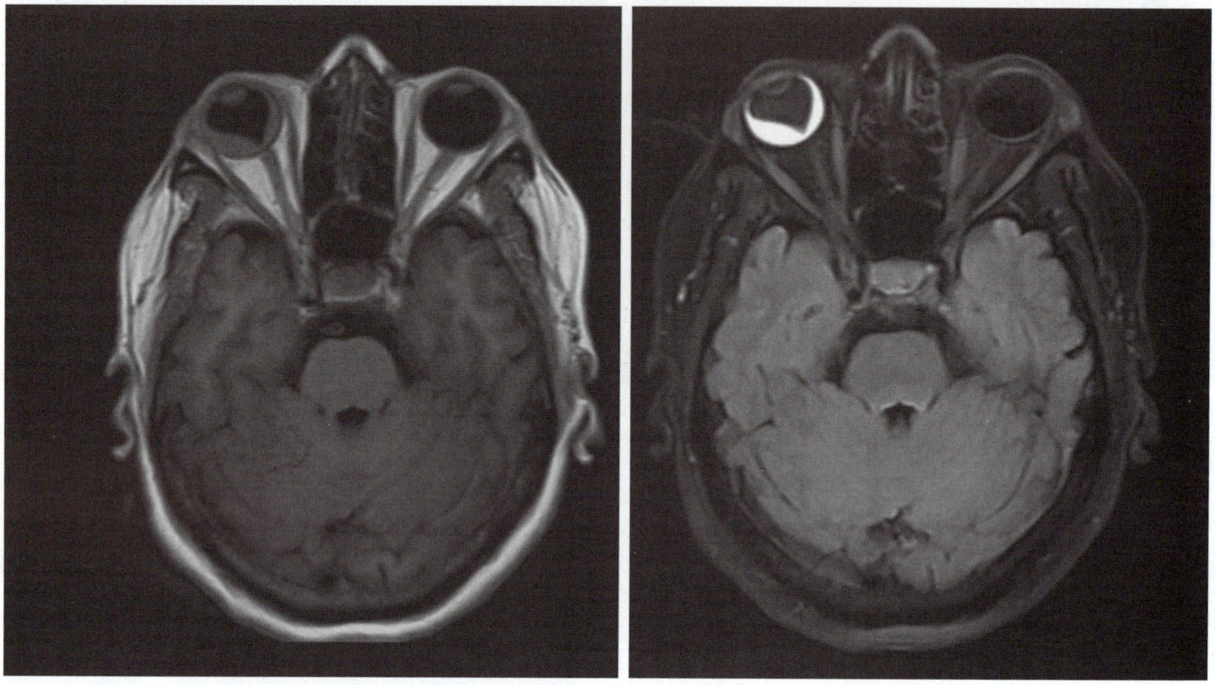

Clinical details: Sudden loss of vision following motor vehicle accident.

1. Identify the sequences.
2. What is the most appropriate diagnosis?
3. Which imaging modality is commonly used as a primary investigative tool?
4. Enumerate two differential diagnoses.

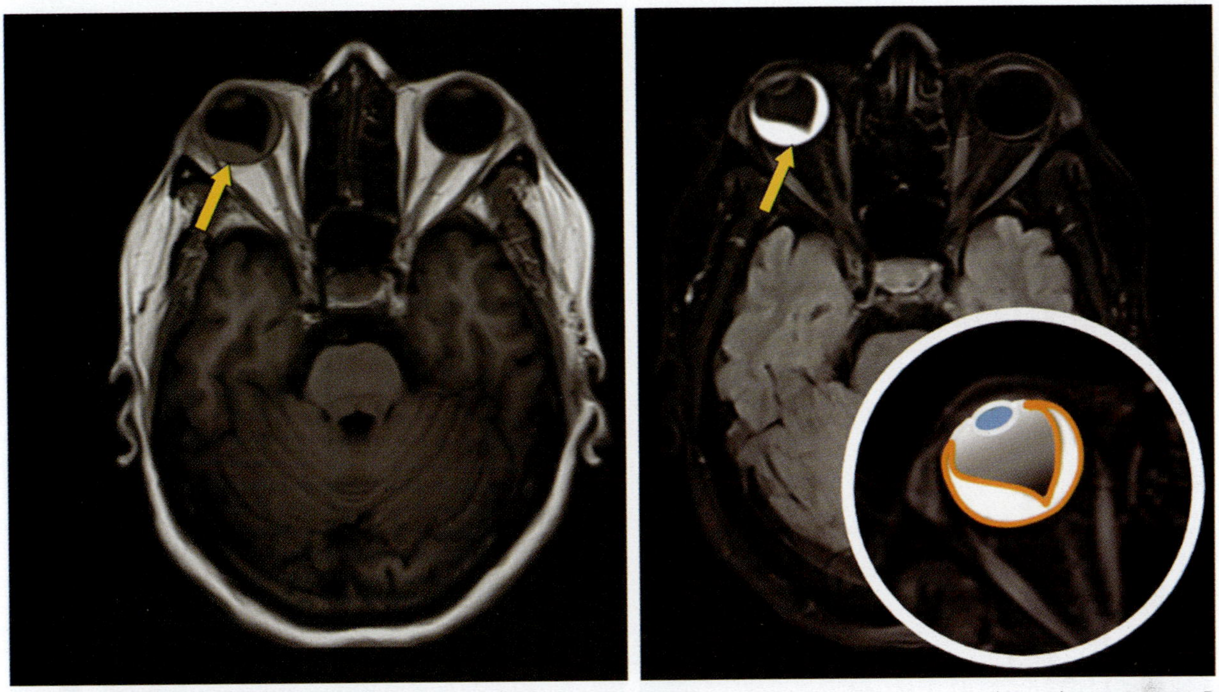

Axial T1 and FLAIR images, respectively, demonstrate retinal detachment in the right eyeball in a V-shaped orientation. Posteriorly the detachment is seen to converge on the optic disc and anterior it is limited by the ora serrata on both sides.

Traumatic Retinal Detachment

- Traumatic retinal detachment is an ophthalmic emergency and needs urgent intervention. Imaging may not always be required.
- High-frequency ultrasonography of the eye is usually the primary imaging modality used to evaluate cases of eyeball trauma.
- Differential diagnosis on imaging includes vitreous detachment and choroidal detachment.

OSCE

92

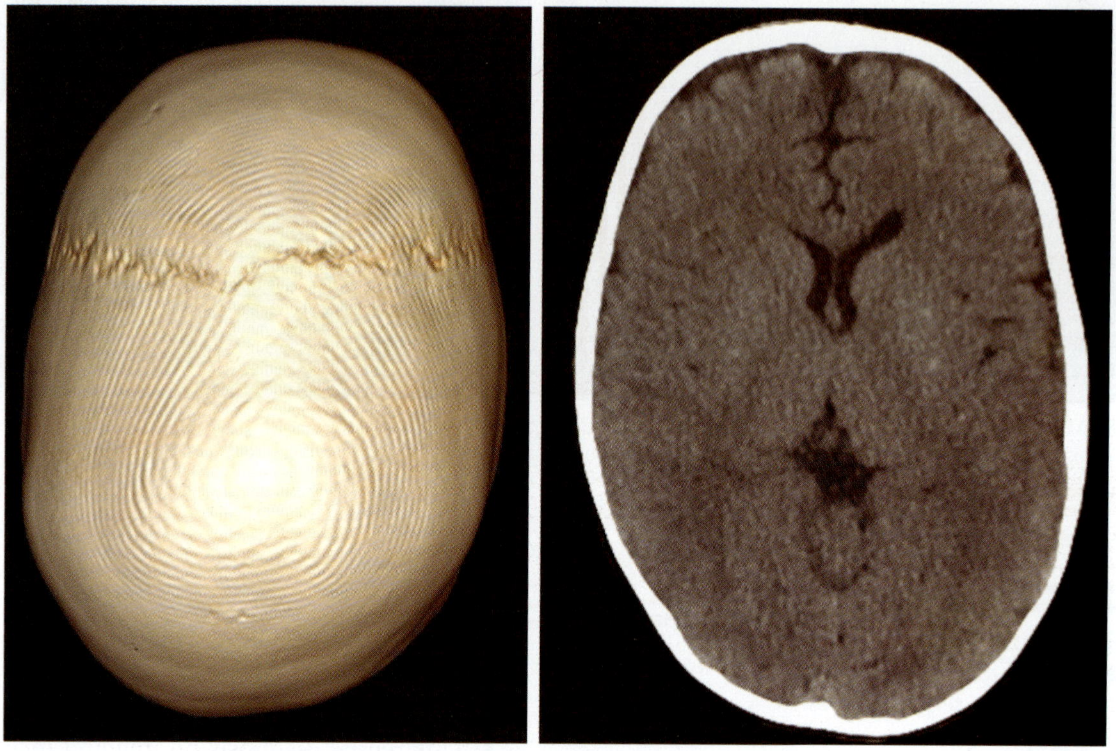

Clinical details: Child with abnormal head shape.

1. **Describe your findings in the provided images.**
2. **What is the most appropriate diagnosis?**
3. **Enumerate one syndromic association.**
4. **Which is the most common type of craniosynostosis?**

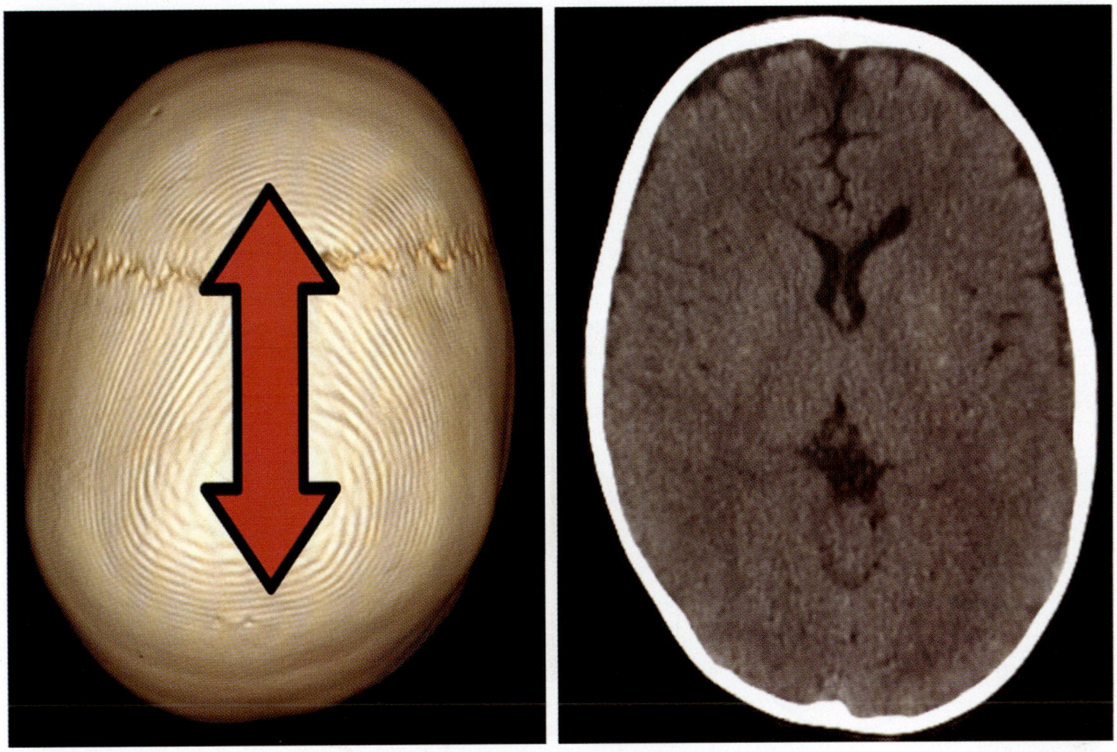

VRT and axial non-contrast computed tomography (NCCT) skull: Premature fusion of sagittal suture with anteroposterior elongation of skull – dolichocephaly/scaphocephaly. Brain parenchyma is normal without hydrocephalus.

Craniosynostosis can be associated with Marfan syndrome, Apert syndrome, Pfeiffer syndrome, Carpenter syndrome, etc.

Craniosynostosis

- Craniosynostosis is defined as the premature fusion of skull sutures. There are various types of craniosynostosis:

- Scaphocephaly/dolichocephaly (most common type) – sagittal suture
- Brachycephaly – bicoronal/bilambdoid sutures
- Anterior or posterior plagiocephaly – unilateral coronal/lambdoid suture
- Trigonocephaly – metopic suture
- Oxycephaly

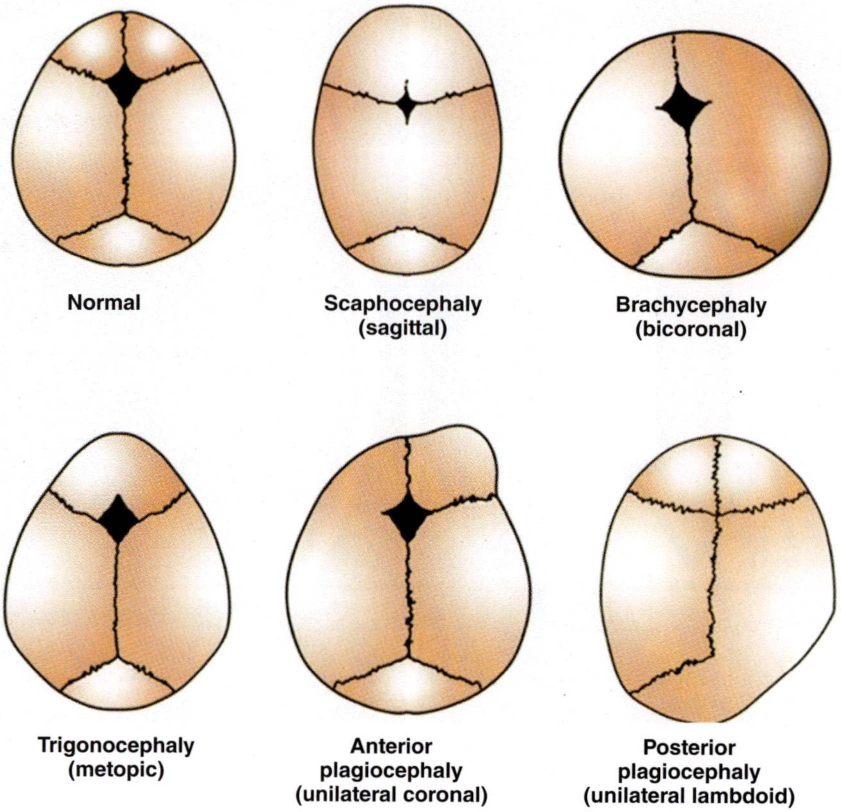
Normal
Scaphocephaly (sagittal)
Brachycephaly (bicoronal)
Trigonocephaly (metopic)
Anterior plagiocephaly (unilateral coronal)
Posterior plagiocephaly (unilateral lambdoid)

OSCE

93

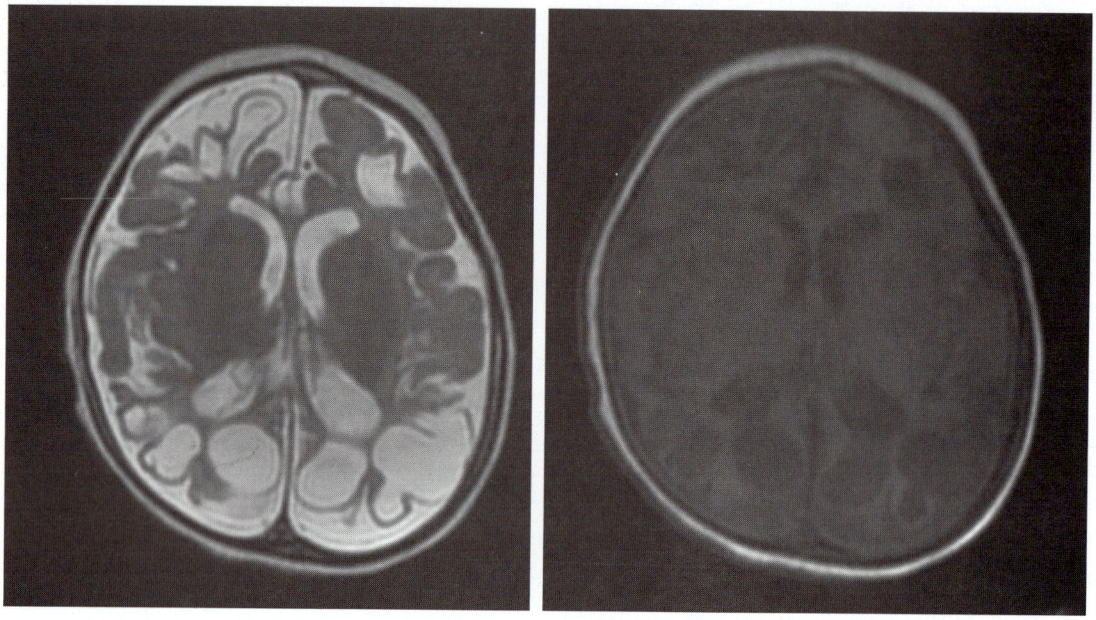

Clinical details: Child with a history of severe birth asphyxia.

1. **Identify the sequences.**
2. **Describe your findings in the provided images.**
3. **What is the most appropriate diagnosis?**
4. **What is the underlying aetiopathology?**

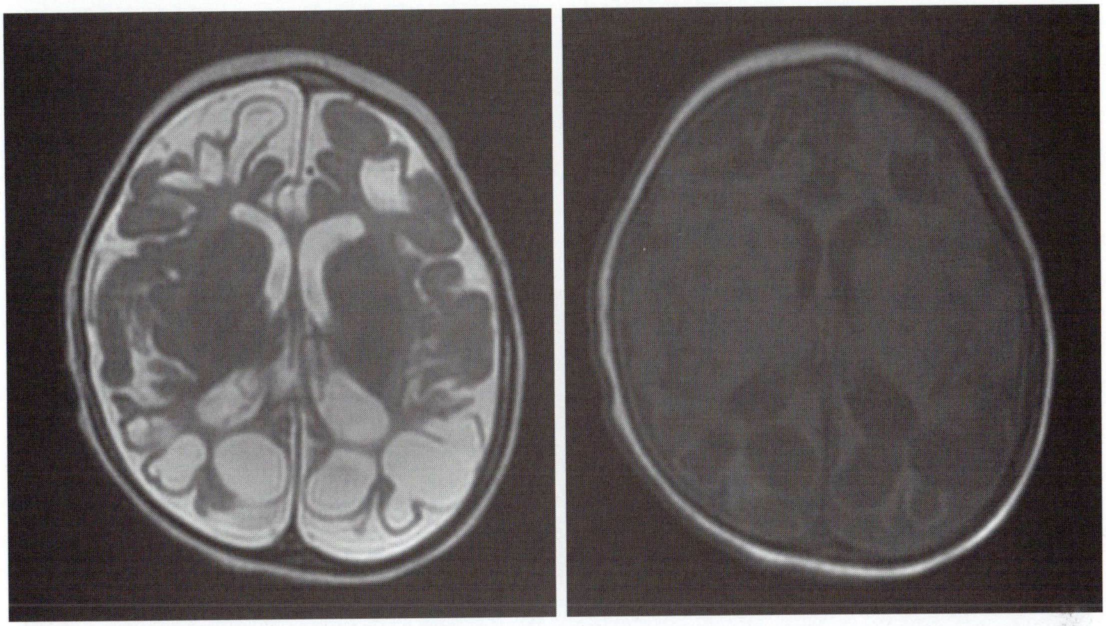

Axial T2 WI and axial T1 WI: Multiple cystic areas of varying sizes within the cortex and white matter of bilateral cerebral hemispheres with atrophy. Cystic areas follow cerebrospinal fluid (CSF) attenuation on all sequences. Basal ganglia structures are spared.

Multicystic Encephalomalacia

- Multicystic encephalomalacia seen in neonates with perinatal hypoxic-ischaemic encephalopathy. It may also be seen as an end-stage finding in non-accidental injury.

RADIOLOGICAL FEATURES

- Computed tomography (CT) and magnetic resonance imaging (MRI) brain reveal numerous cystic spaces of variable sizes seen scattered in bilateral cerebral hemispheres with cerebral atrophy. Posterior fossa, basal ganglia structures and parts of temporal lobe are relatively spared.

OSCE

94

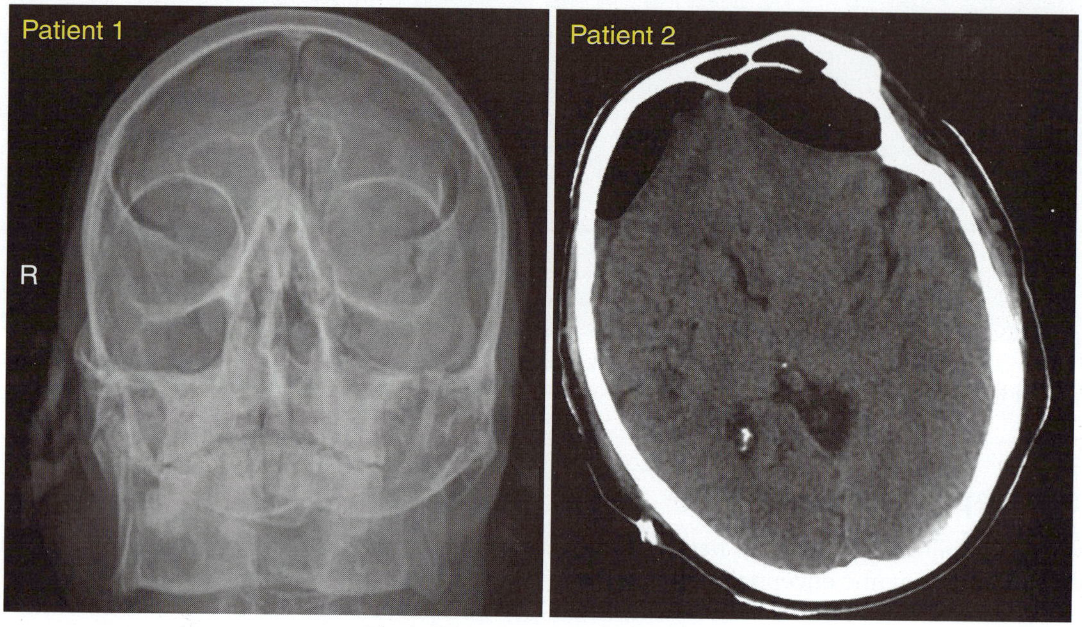

Clinical details: History withheld.

1. **Describe your findings in both cases.**
2. **What is the most appropriate diagnosis?**
3. **What is the most common cause?**
4. **Name the radiological sign associated with this.**

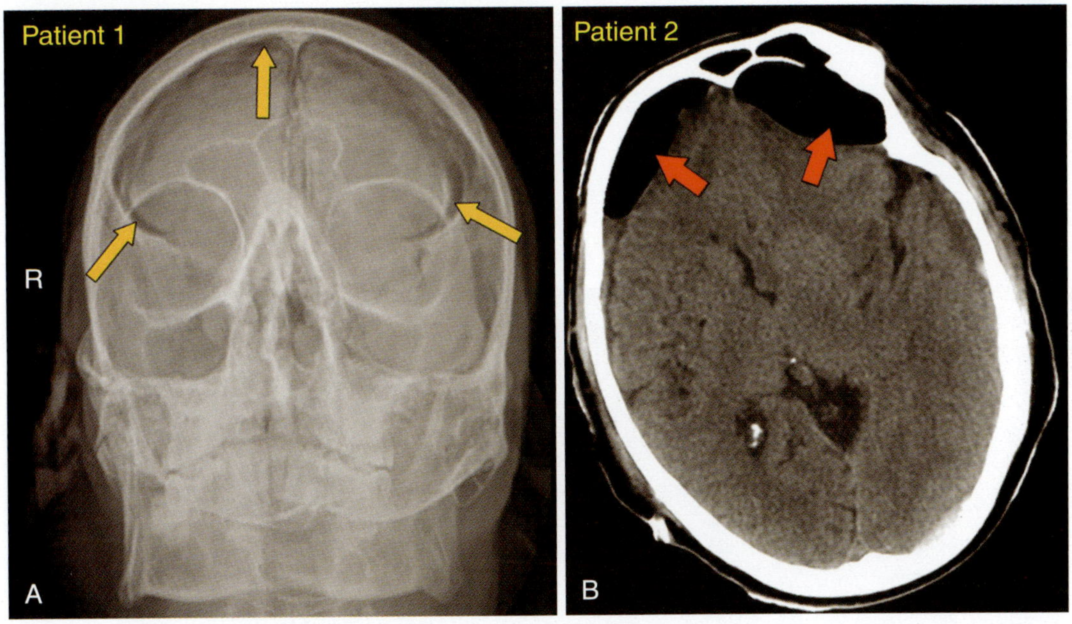

(A) Frontal skull radiograph demonstrates pneumocephalus as curvilinear lucencies (*yellow arrows*) in a patient who suffered from a road traffic accident. (B) Axial non-contrast computed tomography (NCCT) brain shows low density intracranial air in extra-axial compartment of bilateral frontal regions (*red arrows*) in a case of traumatic pneumocephalus.

Pneumocephalus

- Pneumocephalus is the presence of air within the intracranial compartment. It is commonly caused by head trauma but can also be iatrogenic (post-neurosurgery), due to barotrauma or infective causes.
- Pneumocephalus can be intra-axial or extra-axial. Computed tomography (CT) can help differentiate between intracranial air and fat, as air will show a lower density (around –1000 HU) than fat density (–120 to –90 HU).
- Mount Fuji sign is seen on axial CT images in tension pneumocephalus. It is seen as low attenuating subdural air collections in bilateral frontal regions with widened interhemispheric fissure. Tension pneumocephalus is an emergency and needs urgent surgical decompression.

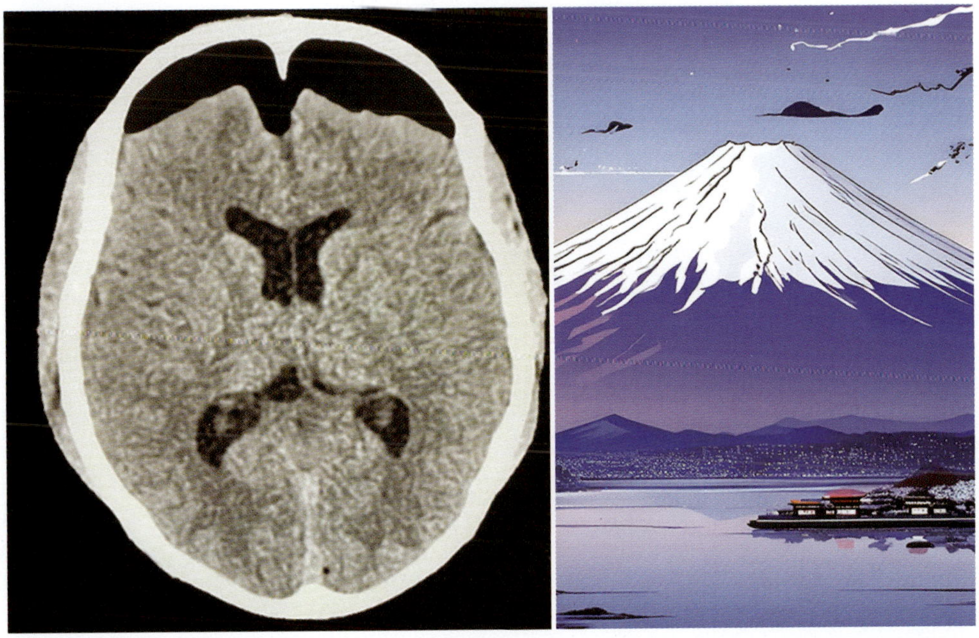

Mount fuji sign.

OSCE

95

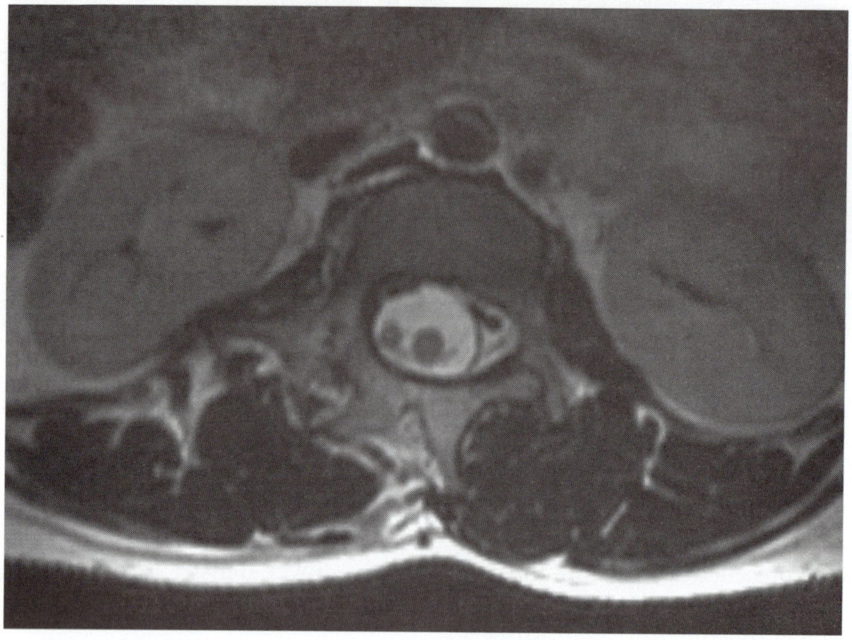

Clinical details: A 10-year-old girl child presented with inability to walk.

1. **Describe the findings in the provided image.**
2. **What is the most appropriate diagnosis?**
3. **How many types are there?**
4. **Provide two points to differentiate between the types.**

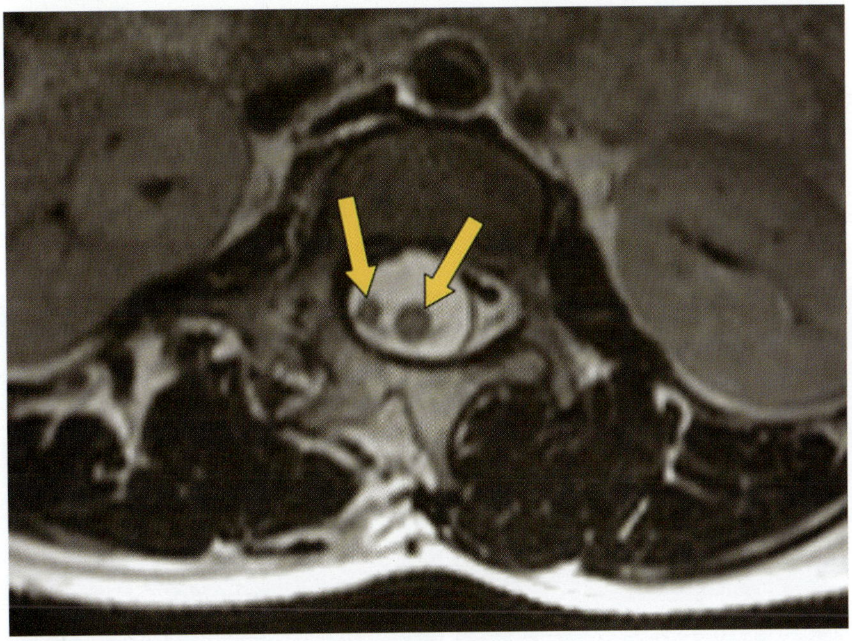

Axial T2 magnetic resonance imaging (MRI) of lumbar spine in a case of type II diastematomyelia: Uneven splitting of spinal cord into two hemicords (*yellow arrows*), with single dural sac containing both hemicords. No evidence of dividing septum or spur.

Diastematomyelia

- Diastematomyelia is a type of spinal dysraphism and is also known as split cord malformation. It is characterized by a cleft/split in the spinal cord. Thoracolumbar spine is the most common affected spinal segment.
- Diastematomyelia may be associated with other anomalies such as meningocele, myelomeningocele and spinal lipoma.
- It is classified into two types – type I and type II.

Type I Diastematomyelia	Type II Diastematomyelia
Separate dural sacs for the two hemicords	Single dural sac containing the two hemicords
Hemicords separated by an osseocartilaginous or fibrous midline septum	No midline septum
More commonly symptomatic	Less commonly symptomatic/ asymptomatic

OSCE

96

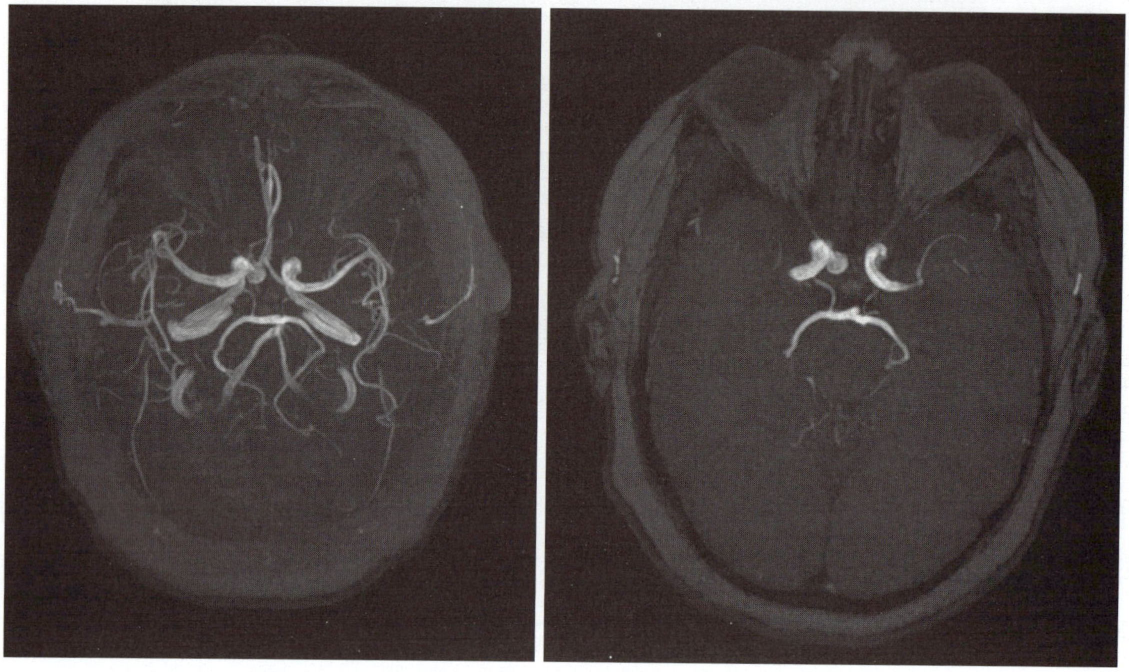

Clinical details: A 31-year-old-lady with pulsatile headache.

1. What is the most appropriate diagnosis?
2. Enumerate the most common locations.
3. What are the complications and available management options?
4. List three associations.

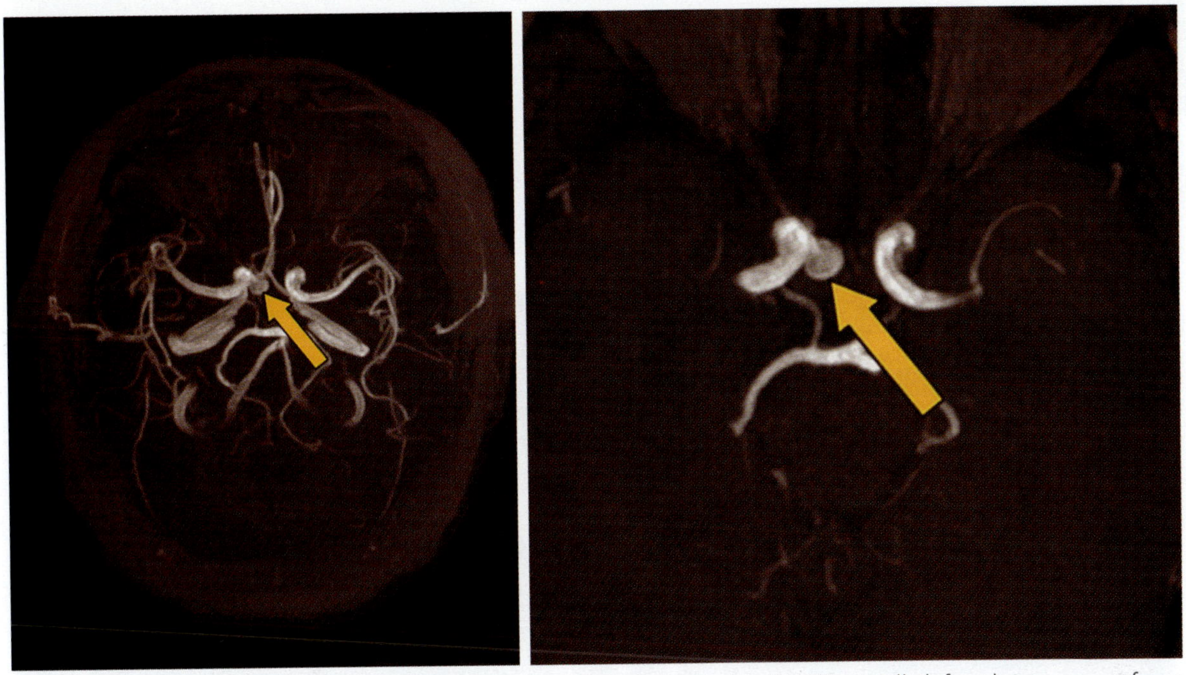

Selected images of a magnetic resonance angiogram at the level of the circle of Willis: Well-defined aneurysm of approximately 4 mm observed arising from the A1 segment of the right anterior cerebral artery. No evidence of rupture. Imaging findings are suggestive of aneurysm arising from the A1 segment of the right anterior cerebral artery.

Cerebral Aneurysms

- Anterior circulation aneurysms are the commonest and account for 90% of all cerebral aneurysms, while the posterior circulation aneurysms account for only 10% of all cerebral aneurysms.
- The anterior cerebral artery aneurysms/ACoA are asymptomatic and account for approximately 30%–40% of the anterior cerebral aneurysms.
- Aneurysms **more than 25 mm** in size are more prone to rupture.
- The complication of cerebral aneurysm is rupture and non-traumatic intracranial subarachnoid haemorrhage.

- Commonest associations are as follows:
  1. Connective tissue disorders like Ehlers–Danlos syndrome
  2. Autosomal dominant polycystic kidney disease
  3. Hereditary haemorrhagic telangiectasia
  4. Bicuspid aortic valve
  5. Coarctation of aorta (CoA)

- Further referral to interventional radiology department is indicated for digital subtraction angiography and endovascular management such as (1) balloon-assisted coiling, (2) stent-assisted coiling, (3) flow diverters and (4) intrasaccular devices.
- The usual interval follow-up is performed using digital subtraction angiography at 12 months interval, if the patient is asymptomatic.

OSCE

97

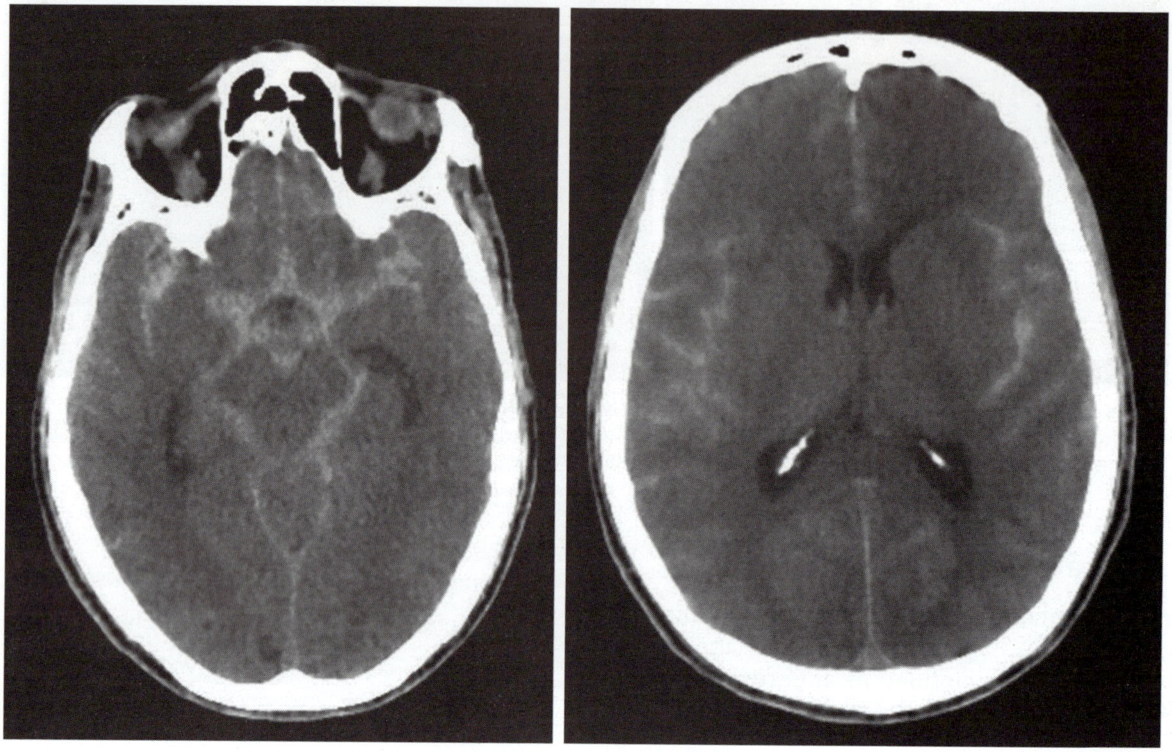

Clinical details: A middle-aged male presented with severe headache.

1. **What is the most appropriate diagnosis?**
2. **What is the investigation of choice?**
3. **What are the types of this pathology?**
4. **What is the most common spontaneous cause of this entity?**

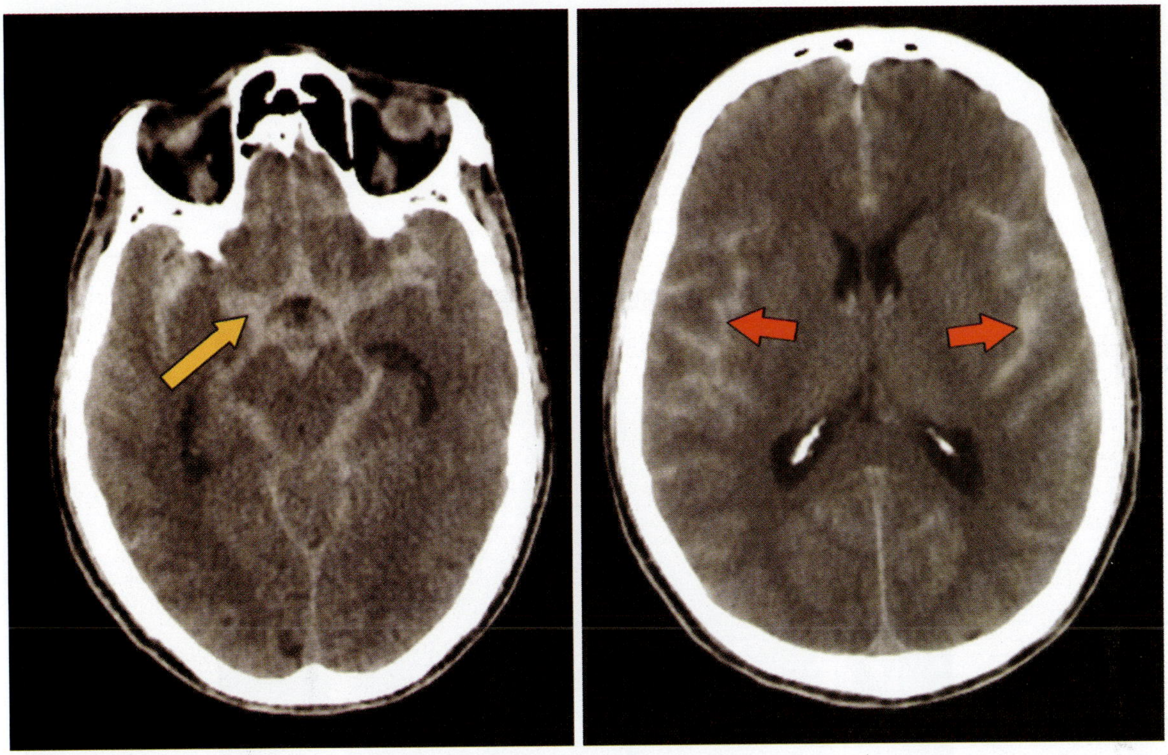

Axial non-contrast computed tomography (NCCT) brain: Hyperdensities of blood attenuation observed along the cortical sulci along the basal cisterns, bilateral Sylvian fissure and interhemispheric fissure – suggestive of diffuse subarachnoid haemorrhage.

Subarachnoid Haemorrhage

- Subarachnoid haemorrhage (SAH) is a haemorrhage within the subarachnoid space between the arachnoid and the pia mater.
- There are non-traumatic and traumatic causes of subarachnoid haemorrhage.
- The most common non-traumatic cause (spontaneous case) of a subarachnoid haemorrhage is rupture of a saccular aneurysm.
- Approximately 10% of spontaneous subarachnoid bleeds are due to benign venous bleeding known as non-aneurysmal perimesencephalic haemorrhage.
- Common causes of subarachnoid haemorrhage are trauma, rupture of aneurysms, vascular malformation, arterial dissection, tumour, vasculitis, reversible cerebral vasoconstriction syndrome, posterior reversible encephalopathy syndrome, cerebral venous thrombosis, septic embolism, septic aneurysm, coagulopathy and Moyamoya disease.

RADIOLOGICAL FEATURES

- Non-contrast computed tomography (NCCT) scan of brain and FLAIR sequences are most sensitive in diagnosis of acute subarachnoid haemorrhage.
- Gradient echo sequences are sensitive to diagnosis of chronic haemorrhage due to haemosiderin deposition.
- Further management in a non-traumatic subarachnoid haemorrhage is a CT angiogram or magnetic resonance imaging (MRI) angiogram to rule out an aneurysm. If an aneurysm is detected, further management is DSA with endovascular management by an interventional radiologist.

OSCE

98

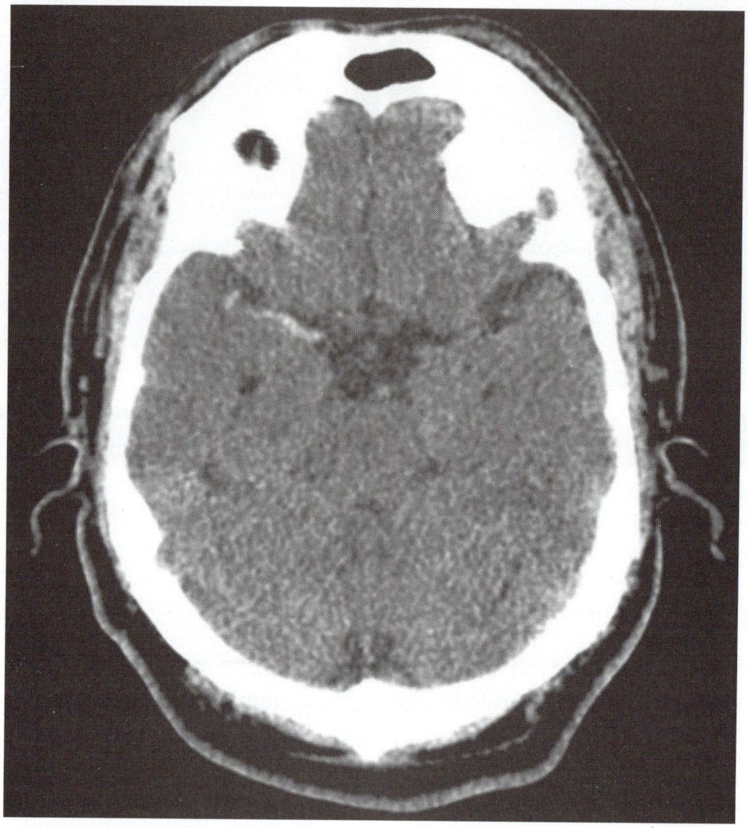

Clinical details: A middle-aged patient with left-sided hemiparesis.

1. **Describe the sign.**
2. **What is the significance of sign.**
3. **What is the next appropriate investigation?**
4. **What is 'insular ribbon sign'?**

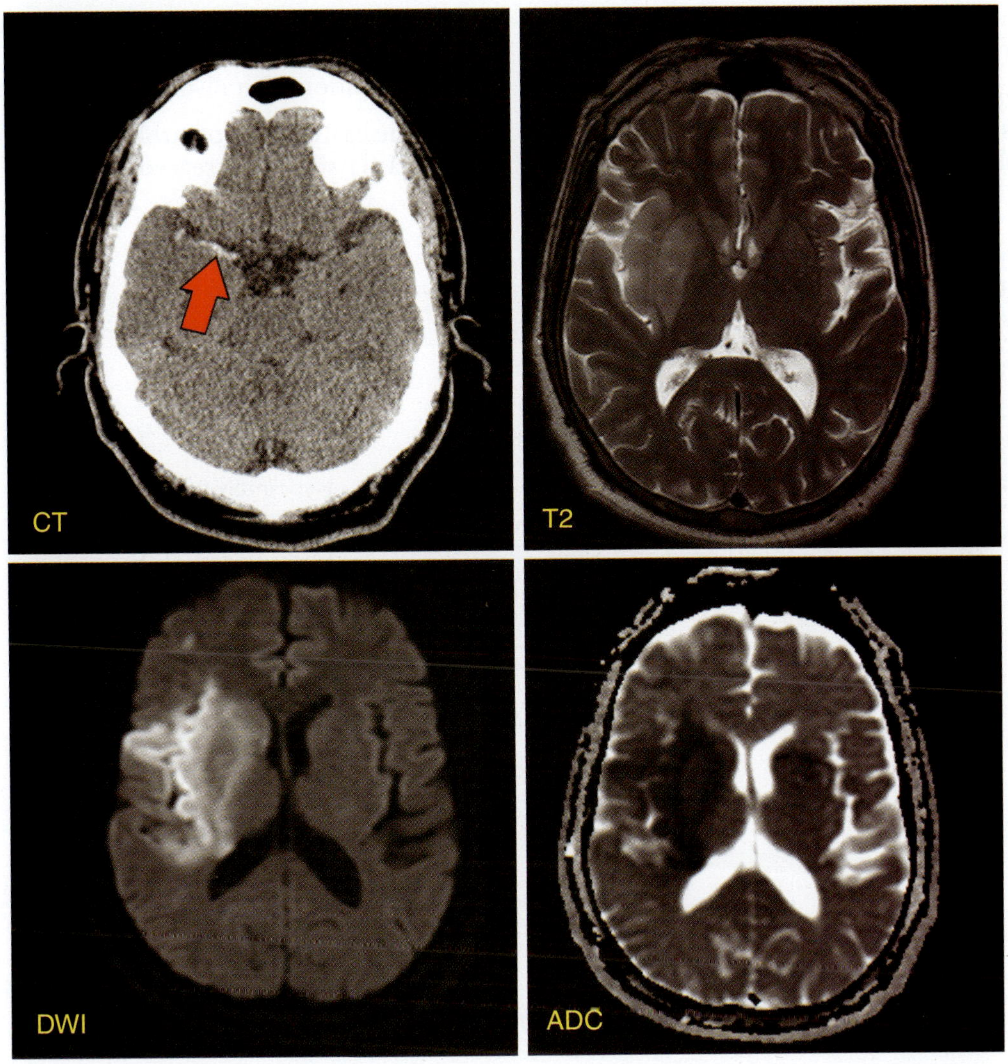

Axial non-contrast computed tomography (NCCT) head demonstrates increased attenuation of the right middle cerebral artery (M1 segment), indicating a hyperdense *MCA sign*.

Magnetic resonance imaging (MRI) brain: Increased signal intensity of the right caudate nucleus, lentiform nucleus and insular cortex on axial T2W sequences of brain with diffusion restriction on diffusion-weighted imaging (DWI)/ADC images, in keeping with a right MCA territory acute infarct.

Dense MCA Sign/Cerebral Infarction

- The hyperdense middle cerebral artery (MCA) sign is observed on non-contrast computed tomography (NCCT) scans of the brain and is an indicator for ischaemic stroke.

RADIOLOGICAL FEATURES

- On NCCT scans of the brain, the hyperdense MCA sign manifests as hyperattenuation in the M1 segment of the middle cerebral artery (MCA). This becomes evident as a thrombus begins to develop in the artery, leading to an increase in attenuation from less than 40 Hounsfield units (HU) in circulating blood to approximately 80 HU in the thrombosed vessel.
- The hyperdense MCA sign appears within 90 minutes of the onset of an acute ischaemic stroke, making it one of the earliest imaging indicators of the condition. Optimal detection of early ischaemic changes and the hyperdense vascular sign can be achieved by utilizing stroke window settings on NCCT (Width:8 Level:32 or Width:40 Level:40).
- Similar hyperdense vascular signs may be observed in other intracranial arteries affected by acute ischaemic stroke. The MCA 'dot' indication describes hyperdensity in the MCA branches (M2 or M3) beyond the MCA bifurcation within the Sylvian fissure. The hyperdense vessel sign may be confused with vascular calcification, but confirmation is usually

straightforward due to the distinct CT attenuation of calcified cerebral arteries.

- Other early signs of MCA infarction include the insular ribbon sign and disappearing basal ganglia sign. **Insular ribbon sign** is the loss of normal insular cortex definition. The **disappearing basal ganglia sign** is characterized by the loss of basal ganglia definition with ill-defined hypodensity.

In the early stages of stroke, diffusion-weighted imaging (DWI) shows increased signal and decreased ADC values.

MRI FINDINGS IN ISCHEMIC STROKE

	DWI	ADC	T1	T2	FLAIR
Hyperacute (<6 hours):	Hyperintense	Hypointense	–	–	–
Acute (6 to 24 hours)	Hyperintense	Hypointense	Hypointense	Hyperintense	Hyperintense
Subacute (1–7 days)	High intensity (T2 shine through)	Pseudo-normalization	Hypointense	Hyperintense	Hyperintense
Chronic	High intensity (T2 shine through)	High	Hypointense	Hyperintense	Variable

OSCE

99

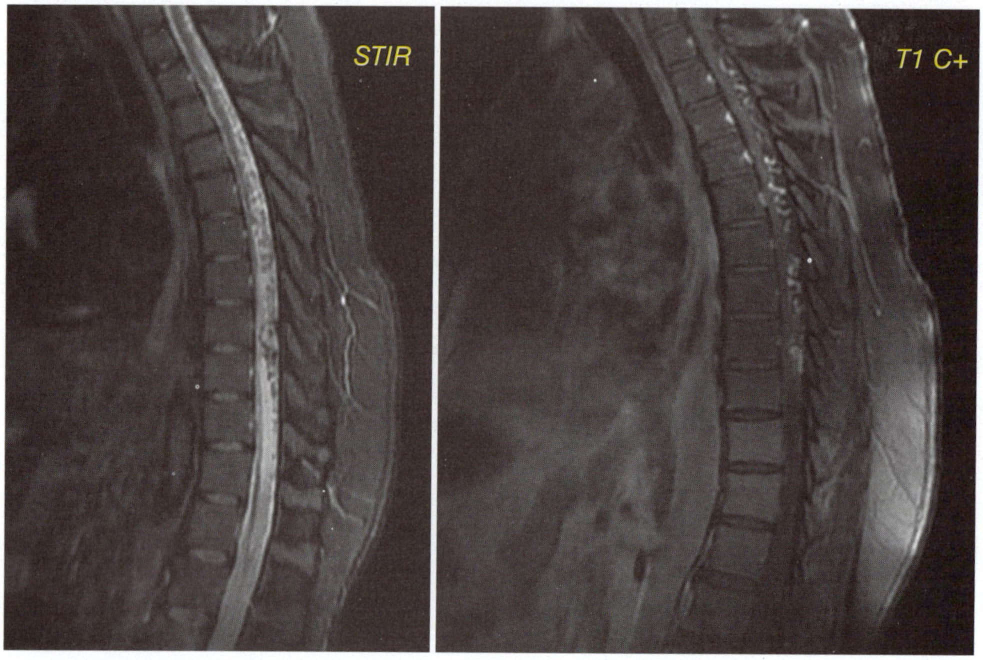

Clinical details: A 50-year-old lady with progressive weakness of bilateral lower limbs.

1. **Describe the findings in the images provided.**
2. **What is the most appropriate diagnosis?**
3. **Which is the gold standard investigation?**
4. **Enumerate one treatment option.**

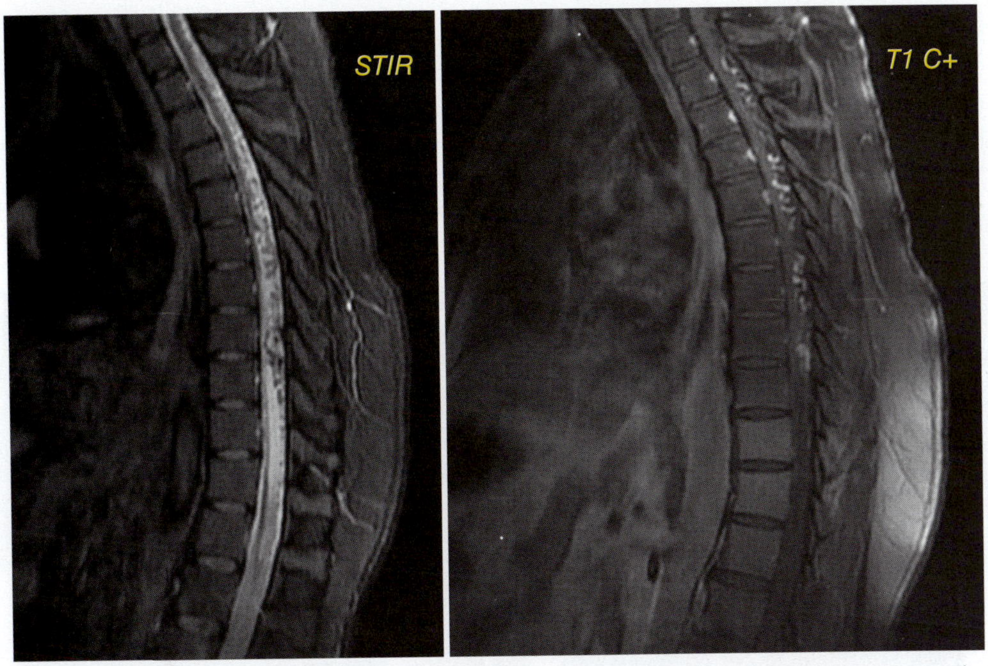

In a case of spinal dural arteriovenous fistulas (SDAVF), STIR: Numerous serpiginous hypointensities are seen in the thecal sac in the lower cervical and upper dorsal levels. Sagittal T1 post-contrast: Prominent enhancing veins and pial capillaries are seen from C4 to D9 level with scalloping of spinal cord.

Spinal Dural Arteriovenous Fistulas

- Spinal dural arteriovenous fistulas (SDAVF) is the most common spinal vascular malformation.
- Magnetic resonance imaging (MRI) features include cord oedema and dilated and tortuous appearing perimedullary veins. However, DSA (spinal angiography) is the gold standard investigation for confirming the diagnosis.
- Treatment options include endovascular embolization and surgical ligation of the SDAVF. Endovascular management is usually the management of choice (using cyanoacrylate glue or Onyx). Surgical ligation is considered if endovascular embolization fails.

OSCE 100

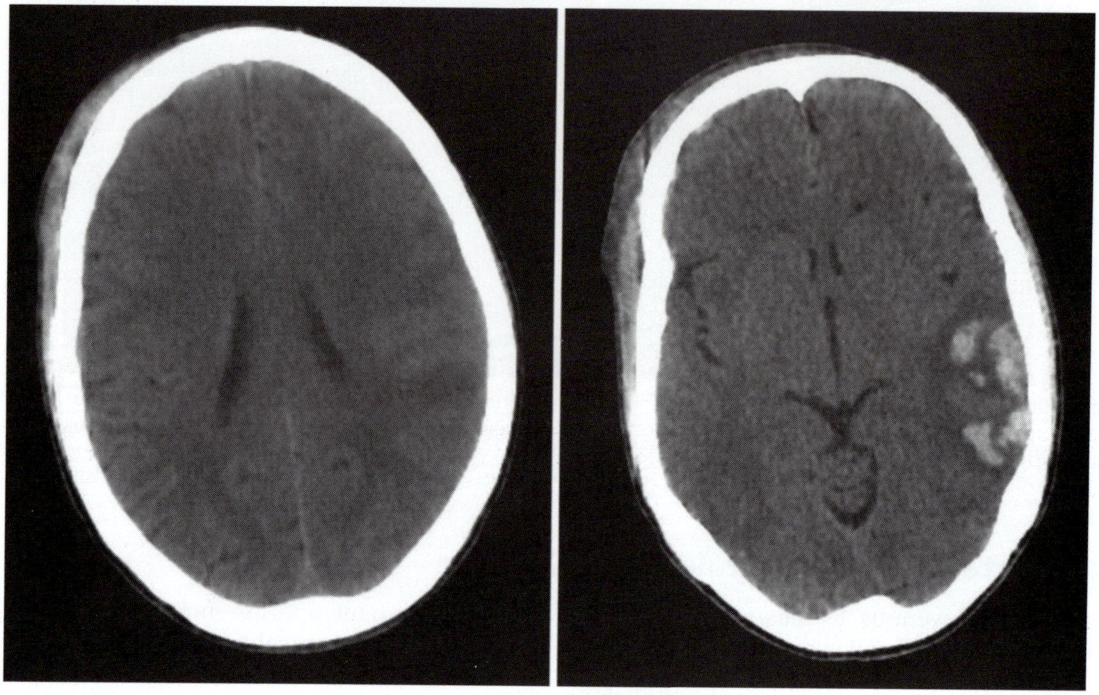

Clinical details: History withheld.

1. **Describe the imaging findings in the images provided.**
2. **What is the classical injury pattern observed in this case?**
3. **List two points to differentiate between extradural haematoma and subdural haematoma.**
4. **Enumerate four types of brain herniation syndromes.**

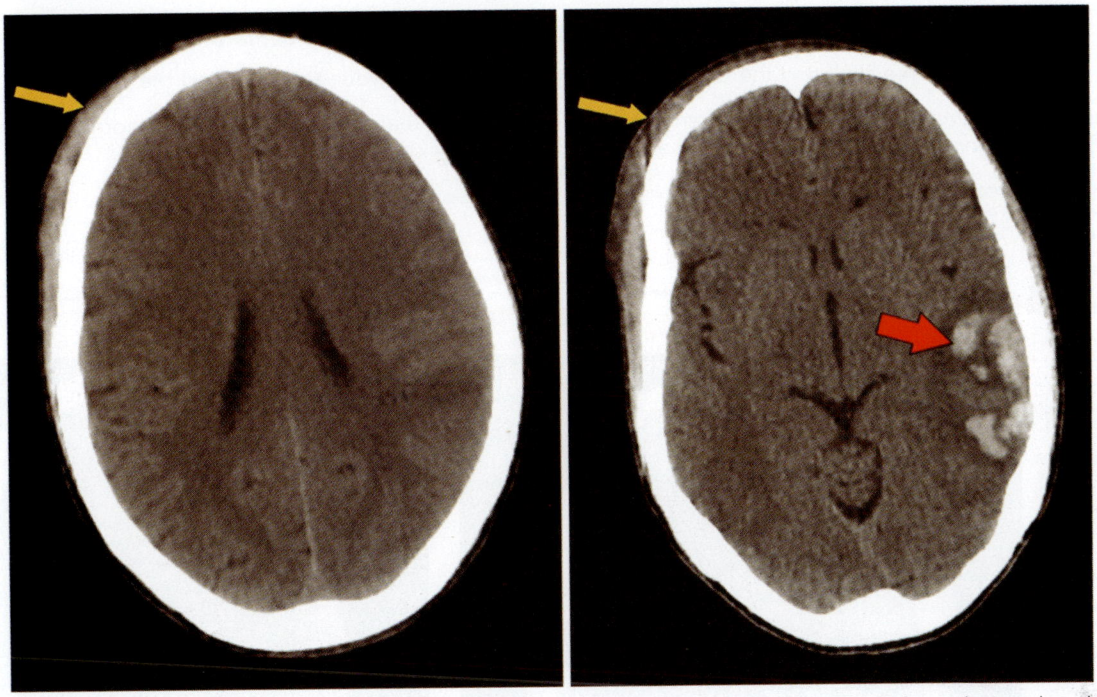

Axial non-contrast computed tomography (NCCT) brain images reveal haemorrhagic contusions with perilesional oedema (*red arrow*) in the left parietotemporal region. There is extracalvarial soft tissue swelling at the right frontal scalp (*yellow arrow*).

Coup-Contrecoup Injury (Brain)

- Coup-contrecoup injuries are a common type head injury pattern which involve damage at the impact site and the opposite side of the head. They commonly result in cerebral contusions and subarachnoid haemorrhage.

MECHANISM

- Skull acceleration causes coup injury at the impact site.
- Subsequent deceleration leads to contrecoup injury on the opposite side.
- Dual-sided pattern of damage due to the brain's interaction with the moving skull.

Feature	Extradural Haematoma (EDH)	Subdural Haematoma (SDH)
Location	Between the skull and the dura	Between the dura and the arachnoid
Involved vessel	Middle meningeal artery, a branch of the maxillary artery (from the external carotid artery (ECA))	Tear of subdural cortical bridging veins (drain to the dural sinuses)
Appearance	Biconvex or lens-shaped	Crescent-shaped or biconcave
Crossing sutures on CT	Often does not cross suture lines	May cross suture lines, spreading diffusely over the hemispheres
Treatment	Surgical evacuation	

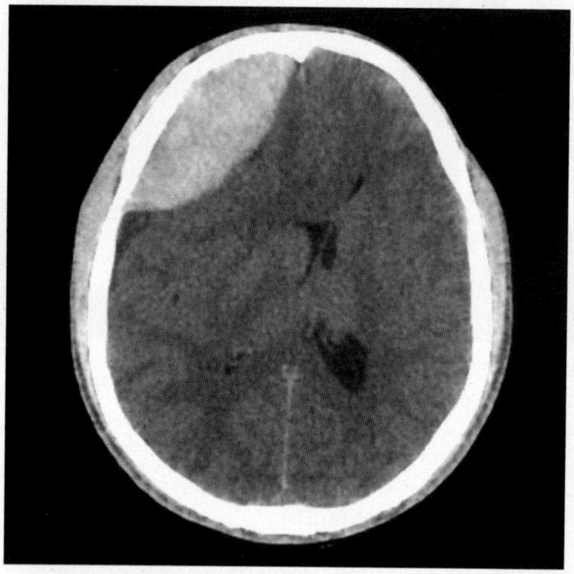

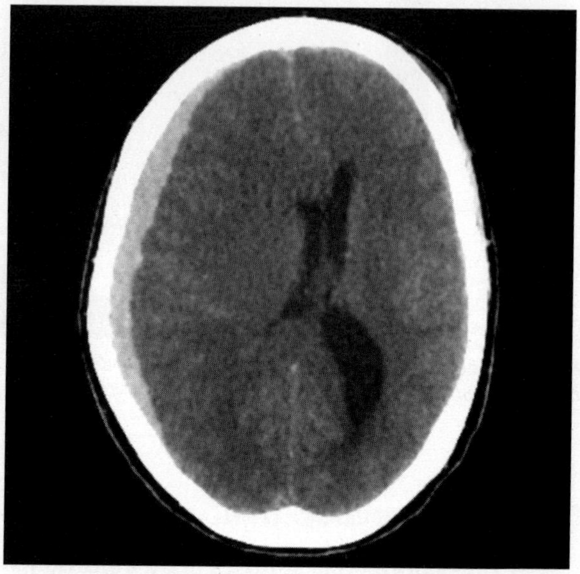

Brain herniation occurs when a brain structure herniates into an adjacent space due to mass effect caused by any expanding intracranial space occupying lesion like a large haematoma or a neoplasm.

Types of herniation syndromes include following:

1. Subfalcine herniation
2. Descending and ascending transtentorial herniations
3. Tonsillar herniation
4. Transalar herniation
5. Paradoxical brain herniation

OSCE

101

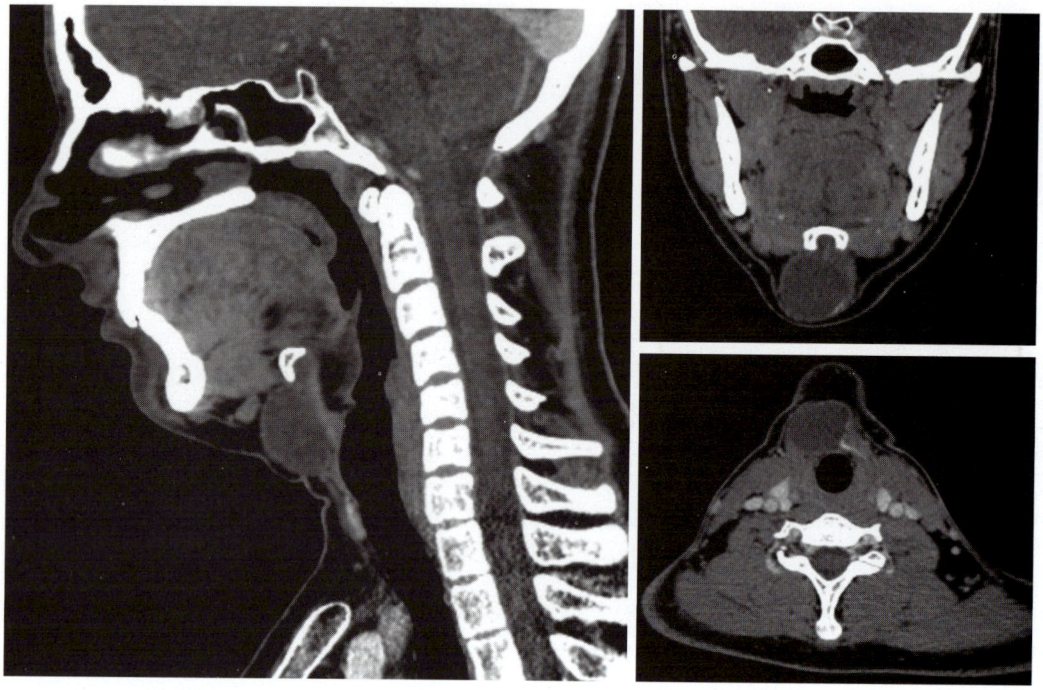

Clinical details: A 20-year-old presented with increasing neck swelling.

1. Describe the findings in the images provided.
2. What is the most appropriate diagnosis.
3. Which is the most common location?
4. Name one common association with respect to thyroid.

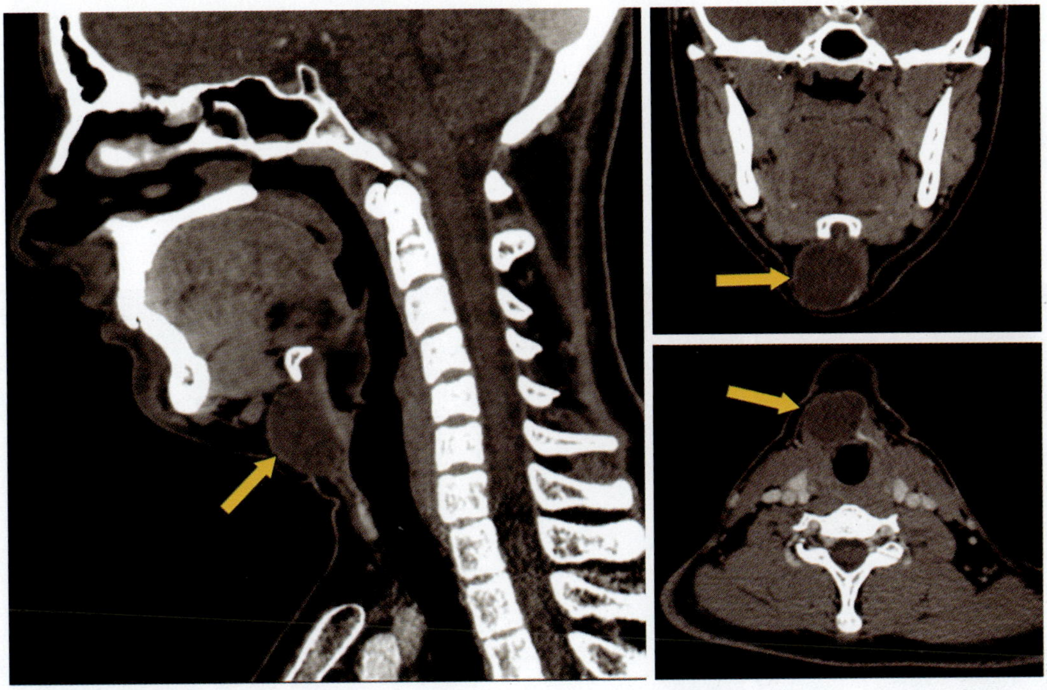

Sagittal, axial and coronal contrast-enhanced computed tomography (CECT) neck demonstrates a well-defined, midline thin-walled infrahyoid cystic lesion with rim of enhancement – thyroglossal duct cyst (TGDC).

Thyroglossal Duct Cyst

- Thyroglossal duct cysts (TGDCs) are one of the most common congenital midline neck cystic lesions. TGDC is a congenital lesion which occurs because of failure of regression of segments of thyroglossal duct.
- Most common location = infrahyoid midline neck (65%–70%).
- It characteristically shows movement with tongue movement. TGDC is usually seen within 2 cm of the midline.
- Association with ectopic thyroid is well known.

RADIOLOGICAL FEATURES

- Ultrasound is usually the first investigation and shows a well-defined anechoic to hypoechoic midline cystic lesion.
- Computed tomography (CT) features include a well-defined cyst with fluid density and rim enhancement.
- On neck magnetic resonance imaging (MRI), TGDC is hypointense (fluid contents) to hyperintense (protein contents) on T1. High signal intensity is seen on T2 WI. Thin rim of enhancement is seen on post-contrast MRI.

OSCE

102

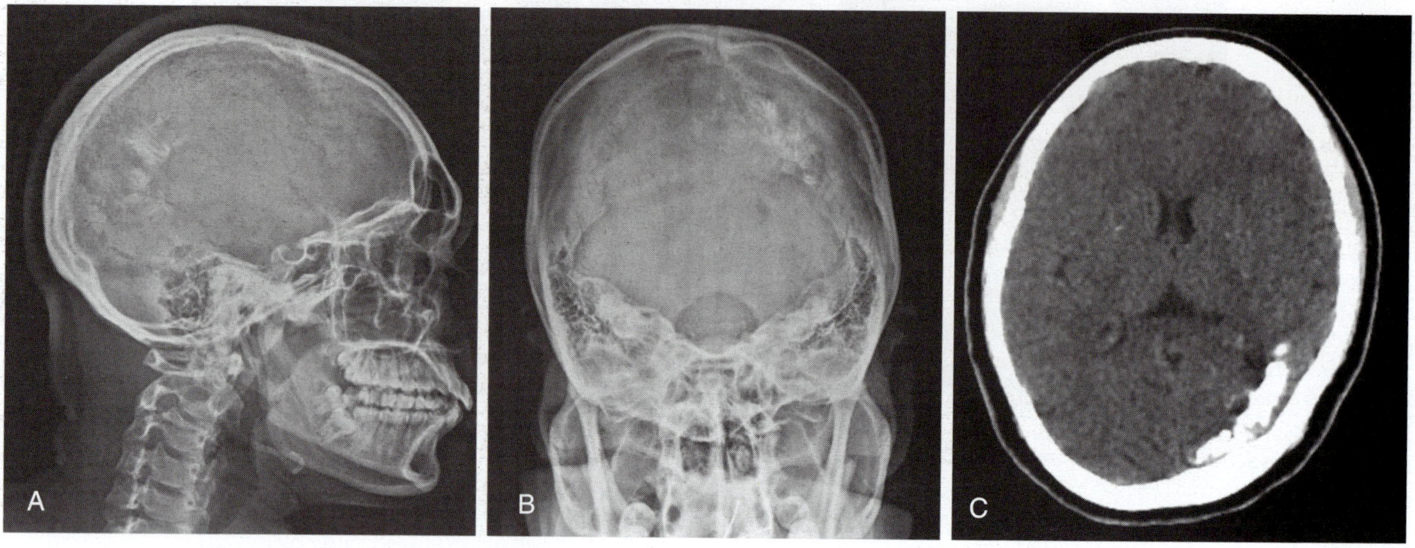

Clinical details: A young patient presented with a history of recurrent headaches and seizures.

1. **Describe the findings seen in images A, B and C.**
2. **What is the name of the characteristic skin involvement seen in this condition?**
3. **What is the most appropriate diagnosis?**
4. **What would you expect to see on post-contrast MRI brain images?**

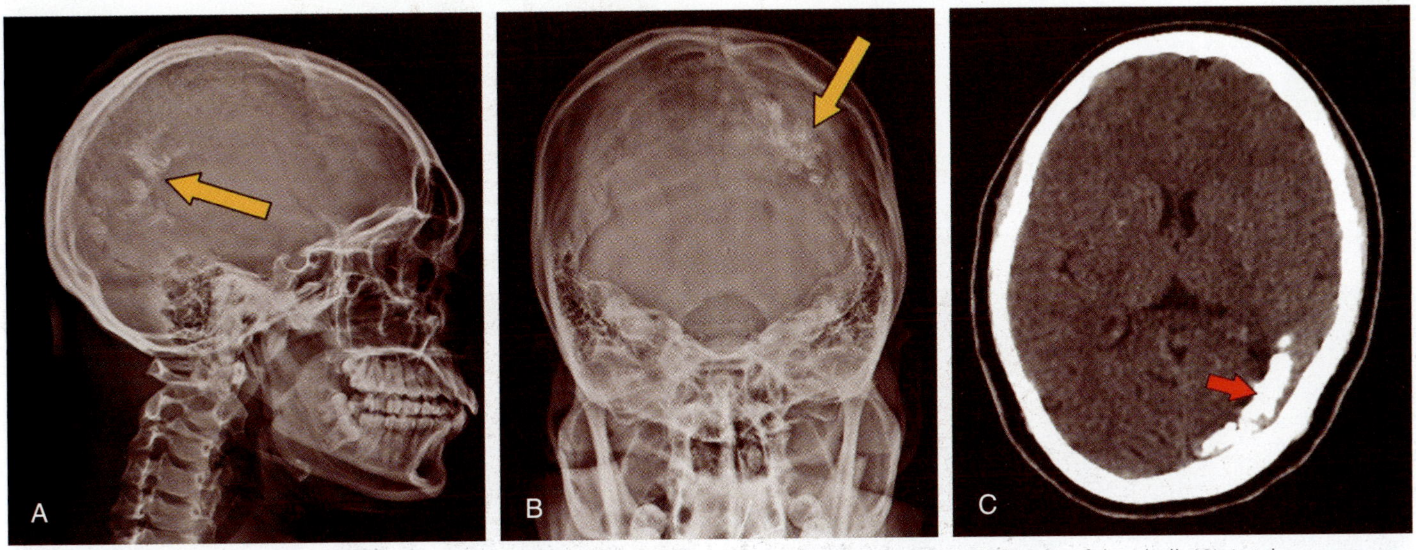

(A and B) Lateral and frontal skull radiographs demonstrate gyriform calcifications seen on the left side of the skull. (C) Axial non-contrast computed tomography (NCCT) brain reveals subcortical gyriform calcification in the left parieto-occipital region with associated parenchymal volume loss, with subtle adjacent calvarial thickening.

Sturge–Weber Syndrome

- Sturge–Weber syndrome (SWS) is a rare sporadic type of neurocutaneous syndrome or phacomatosis. It is also known as encephalotrigeminal angiomatosis. A gene mutation in GNAQ, located on chromosome 9q21, has been linked to Sturge–Weber syndrome. It is characterized by the presence of facial port wine stain, easily involving the ophthalmic division of the trigeminal nerve, leptomeningeal angioma and retinal choroidal angioma with or without glaucoma. In addition to the port wine stain, patients usually present with seizures (90% of cases by 1 year of age), migrainous headaches, hemiparesis or glaucoma.
- The port wine stain can be unilateral (two-thirds cases) or bilateral (one-third cases).
- Leptomeninges angiomas are most commonly located in the parieto-occipital region, followed by the frontal and temporal lobes. SWS is most commonly unilateral (80% of cases). However, bilateral involvement has been observed (20%).

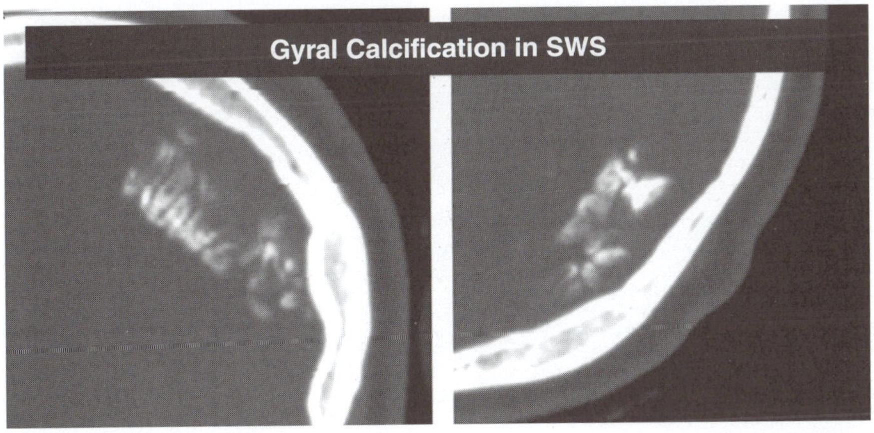

RADIOLOGICAL FEATURES

- Computed tomography (CT) typically demonstrates tram-track type of cortical/subcortical gyral calcifications, associated parenchymal volume loss, ipsilateral choroidal plexus enlargement, calvarial thickening and hyperpneumatization of the ipsilateral sinuses.
- In addition to the above features, post-contrast magnetic resonance imaging (MRI) reveals prominent leptomeningeal enhancement in the region of the gyral calcifications. The gyral calcifications demonstrate blooming on GRE/SWI sequences. Choroid plexus haemangioma may be seen.
- The primary goal of treatment for Sturge–Weber syndrome is to control seizures. Surgery is only considered in rare cases when other treatments have failed. Ophthalmological referral is often indicated for treatment of glaucoma.

OSCE

103

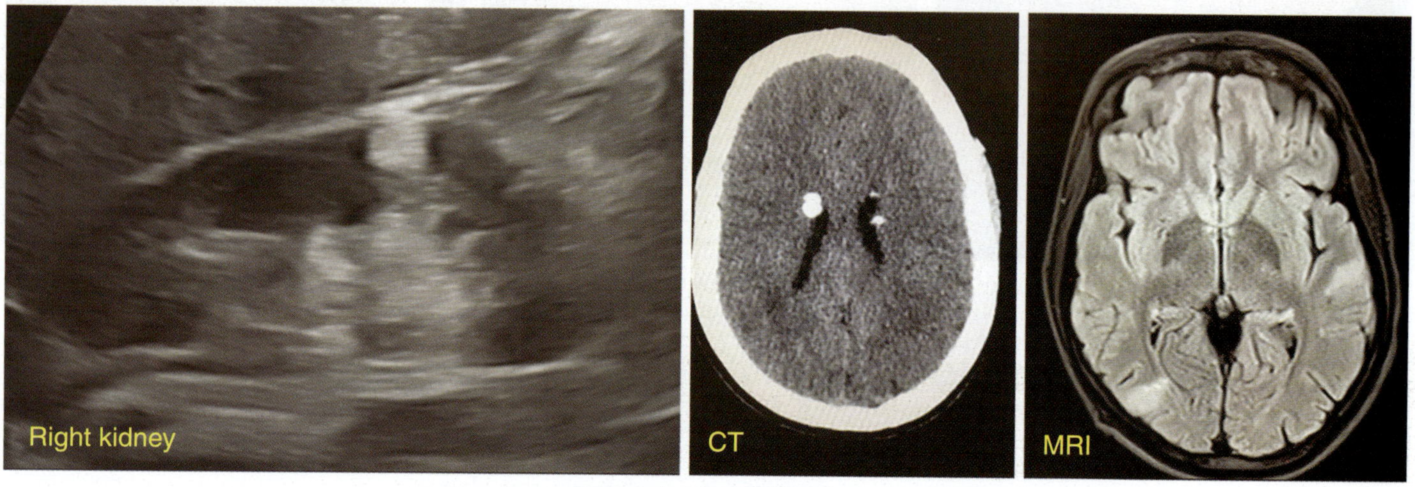

Clinical details: Withheld.

1. **Describe your findings in the provided images.**
2. **What is the most appropriate diagnosis?**
3. **Name the two genes associated with this pathology.**
4. **Name two thoracic abnormalities that can be associated with this.**

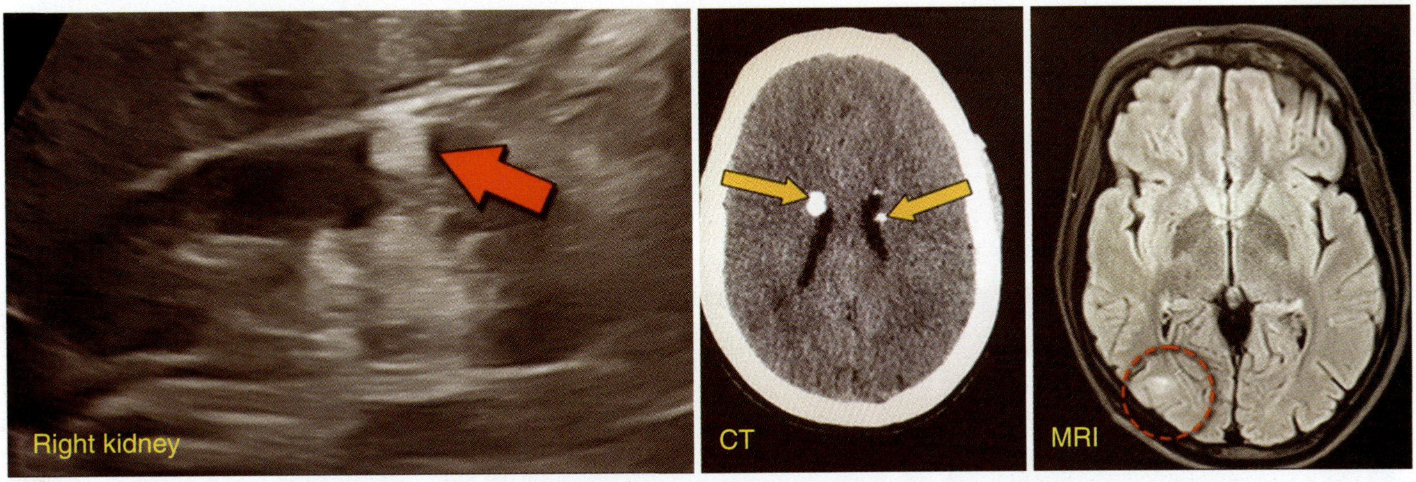

Ultrasonography (USG) right kidney demonstrates a hyperechoic lesion in the renal cortex, consistent with renal angiomyolipoma (*red arrow*). Axial computed tomography (CT) image shows bilateral periventricular calcified subependymal nodules (*yellow arrows*). Axial magnetic resonance imaging (MRI) FLAIR sequence demonstrates a hyperintense cortical tuber in the right parieto-occipital region.

Tuberous Sclerosis

- Tuberous sclerosis or Bourneville disease is a rare neurocutaneous disorder/phakomatosis. It is characterized by a classical clinical tried known as the Vogt triad (EPI-LOI-A): EPIlepsy (seizures), Low IQ (intellectual disability) and Adenoma sebaceum (facial angiofibroma). It is caused by mutations in either the TSC1 or TSC2 gene, which are involved in regulating cell growth and division.

Common manifestations of tuberous sclerosis:

Central nervous system (CNS) manifestations	Cortical tubers: • T1 hypointense and T2/FLAIR hyperintense. • Half of the cortical/subcortical tubers are in the frontal lobe. • One-tenth exhibit enhancement. Subependymal nodules (SEN): • Usually calcified and seen along the walls of the lateral ventricles. Subependymal giant cell astrocytoma (SEGCA): • Frequently found close to the foramen of Monro. • Larger with more avidly enhancement than SEN. • May result in obstructive hydrocephalus. Abnormalities in the white matter such as radial bands.
Thoracic manifestations	Lymphangioleiomyomatosis (LAM): • Bilateral tiny lung cysts with uniform distribution. Chylous effusion and pneumothorax Cardiac rhabdomyomas
Abdominal manifestations	Renal angiomyolipomas: • Multiple, bilateral and large fat containing masses. • Large size increases the risk of haemorrhage. Renal cysts Renal carcinoma and oncocytomas Hepatic angiomyolipomas
Musculoskeletal manifestations	Sclerotic bony lesions and bone cysts

OSCE

104

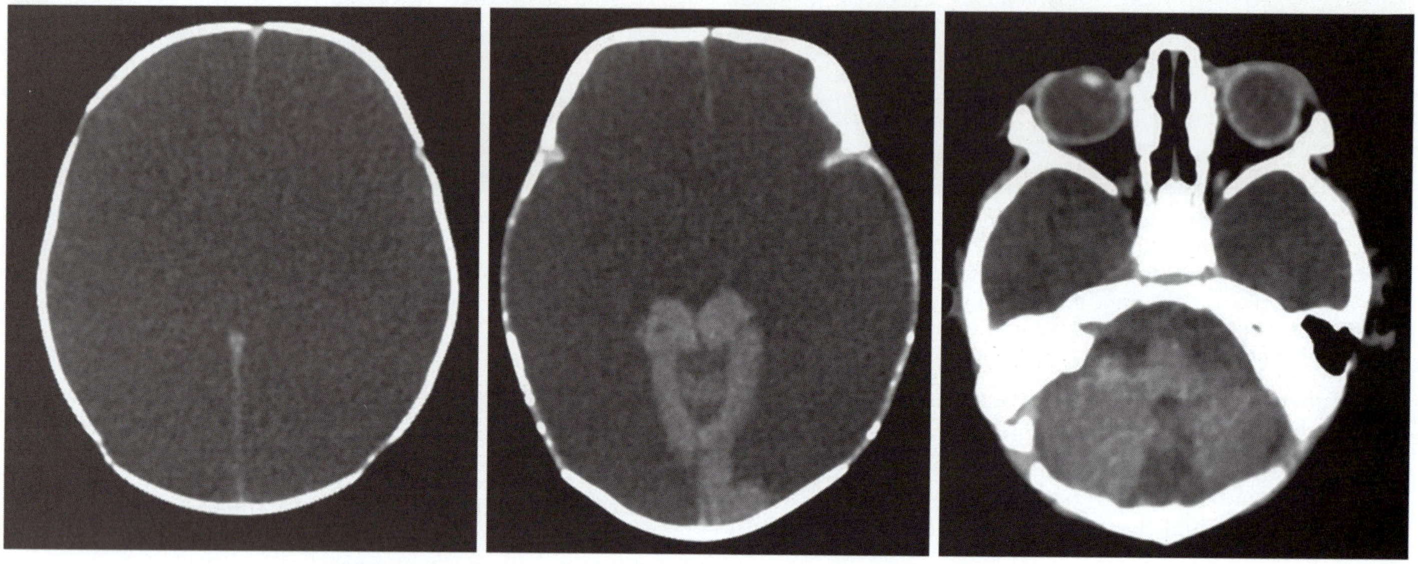

Clinical details: An infant with history of seizures and failure to thrive.

1. **Describe your findings in the given images.**
2. **What is the most appropriate diagnosis?**
3. **List two imaging differentials.**
4. **How would you differentiate this pathology from its differentials?**

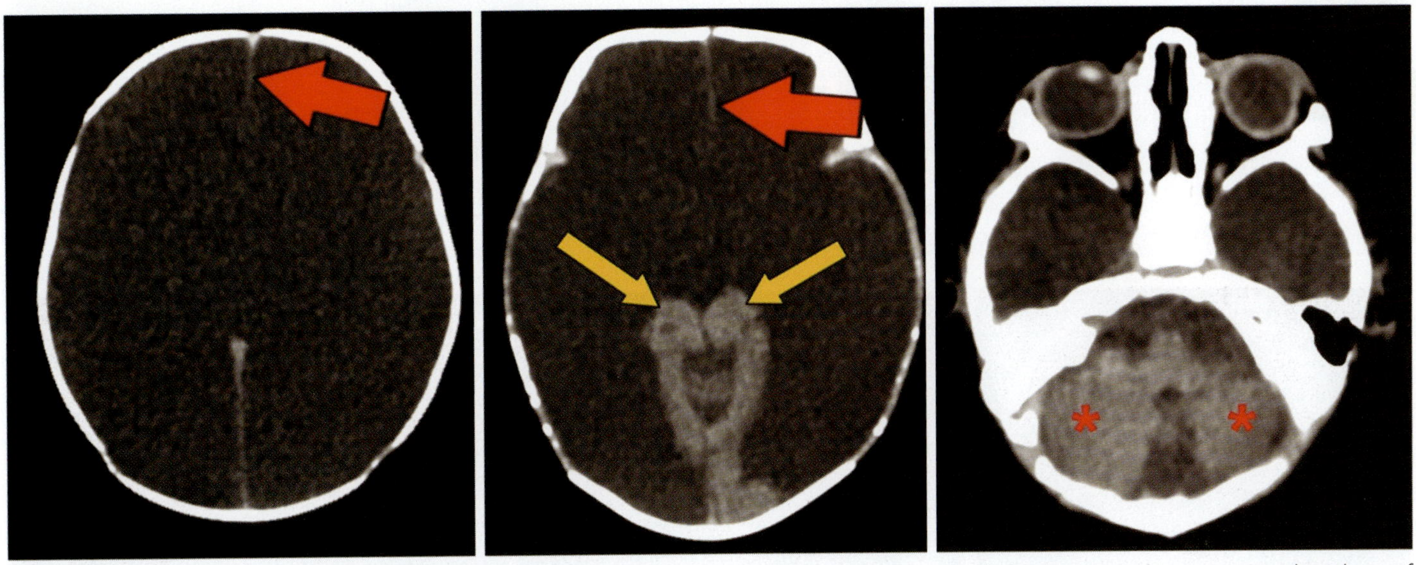

Axial non-contrast computed tomography (NCCT) brain images in a case of hydranencephaly demonstrate near-complete loss of the supratentorial brain parenchyma and replaced by cerebrospinal fluid (CSF) density fluid. The falx (*red arrows*), thalami (*yellow arrows*) and the posterior fossa structures (*) are preserved.

Hydranencephaly

- Hydranencephaly ('water-bag' brain) is a rare congenital neurodevelopmental abnormality characterized by the absence of cerebral hemispheres. It is thought to be caused by bilateral occlusion of the internal carotid arteries (ICAs) before 16 weeks of gestation. The falx, thalami, brainstem, cerebellum and meninges are usually preserved. Temporal and occipital lobe remnants are frequently observed. Macrocephaly is usually present. Prenatal ultrasound or vascular imaging reveals the absence of the middle cerebral arteries.
- Distinguishing hydranencephaly from other conditions is crucial for accurate diagnosis. The top differential diagnoses include severe hydrocephalus, alobar holoprosencephaly (HLE), severe bilateral open-lip schizencephaly and cystic encephalomalacia.

Feature	Hydranencephaly	Severe Hydrocephalus	Alobar Holoprosencephaly
Absent cerebral hemispheres	Yes (absent)	Thin, compressed cortex	No
Falx	Present	Present	Absent
Middle cerebral artery (MCA)	Absent	Preserved	Preserved
Thalami	Present (not fused)	Present (not fused)	Fused
Midline facial abnormalities	Not associated	Not associated	Associated with midline facial abnormalities

OSCE

105

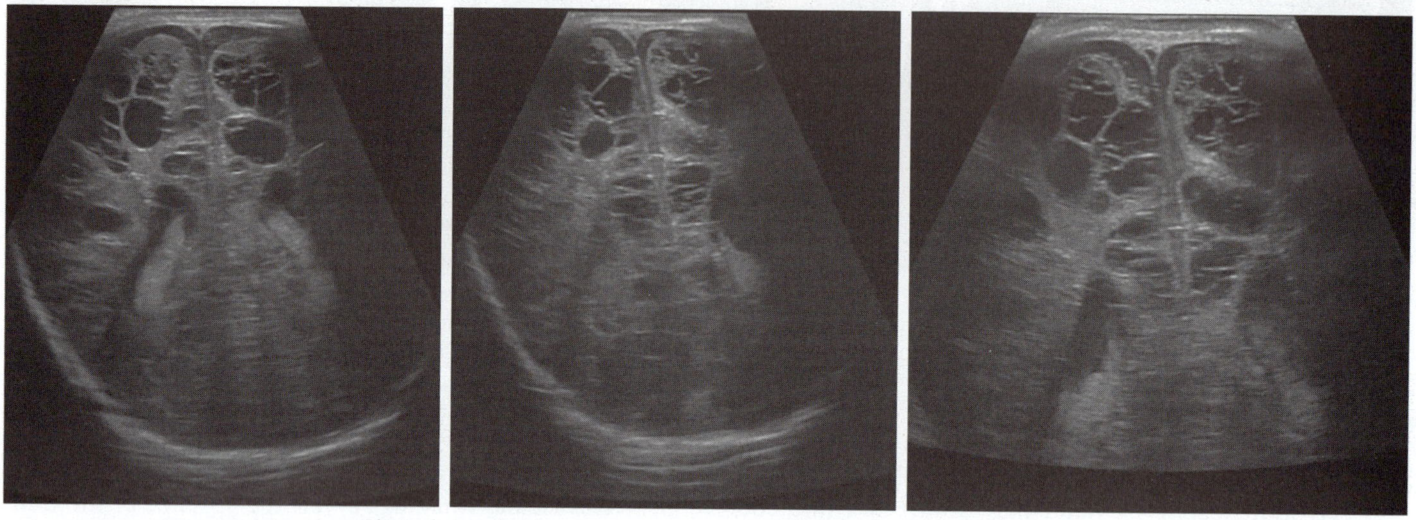

Clinical details: A premature neonate with lethargy and seizures.

1. **Identify the investigation performed.**
2. **Describe the findings observed in the provided images.**
3. **What is the most appropriate diagnosis?**
4. **What is the underlying aetiology?**

appear isointense to grey matter, while larger lesions exhibit heterogeneity due to cystic changes, necrosis or haemorrhage. T2-weighted images similarly show isointensity to grey matter, with larger lesions displaying heterogeneity and a frequent hypointense rim. Gadolinium-enhanced T1-weighted images reveal moderate to heterogenous enhancement in solid components. GRE/SWI are particularly sensitive to detecting haemorrhagic components.

- MRI provides detailed imaging of masses and surrounding structures (cavernous sinus and optic chiasm).
- On T1-weighted images, masses are typically isointense to grey matter. Larger lesions may show heterogeneity (cystic changes, necrosis and haemorrhage). On T1-weighted sagittal scans, the posterior pituitary 'bright spot' is either absent (20%) or displaced into the supradiaphragmatic cistern (80%).
- T2-weighted images exhibit isointensity, with larger lesions showing heterogeneity and a hypointense rim.
- Gadolinium-enhanced T1-weighted images reveal moderate to heterogeneous enhancement in solid components. GRE/SWI are sensitive to detecting haemorrhagic components.
- A macroadenoma extending above the pituitary fossa tends to compress the central part of the optic chiasm, housing fibres from the nasal retina, resulting in the common manifestation of bitemporal hemianopia.
- Pituitary macroadenomas may exhibit invasive growth, with a tendency to extend into the cavernous sinuses. Prolactin-secreting tumours often exhibit cavernous sinus extension, evident by a substantial increase in prolactin levels upon sinus invasion. Coronal MRI plane is the best for assessing the extent of cavernous sinus invasion.
- The Knosp classification is used to determine the extent of cavernous sinus invasion by pituitary macroadenoma.

Differential Diagnosis	Key Features
Pituitary macroadenoma	• Commonest pituitary region mass • Hormone-producing activity
Pituitary hyperplasia	• Physiological in young/pregnant/lactating females • End-organ failure such as hypothyroidism
Meningioma	• Separate identifiable pituitary • Hyperdense on non-contrast computed tomography (NCCT) • Dural tail sign • Avid enhancement
Craniopharyngioma (papillary type)	• More likely to be cystic with the presence of calcifications
Lymphocytic hypophysitis	• Seen in peripartum females
Saccular cerebral aneurysms	• Presence of flow void on MRI
Pituitary carcinoma	• Rare

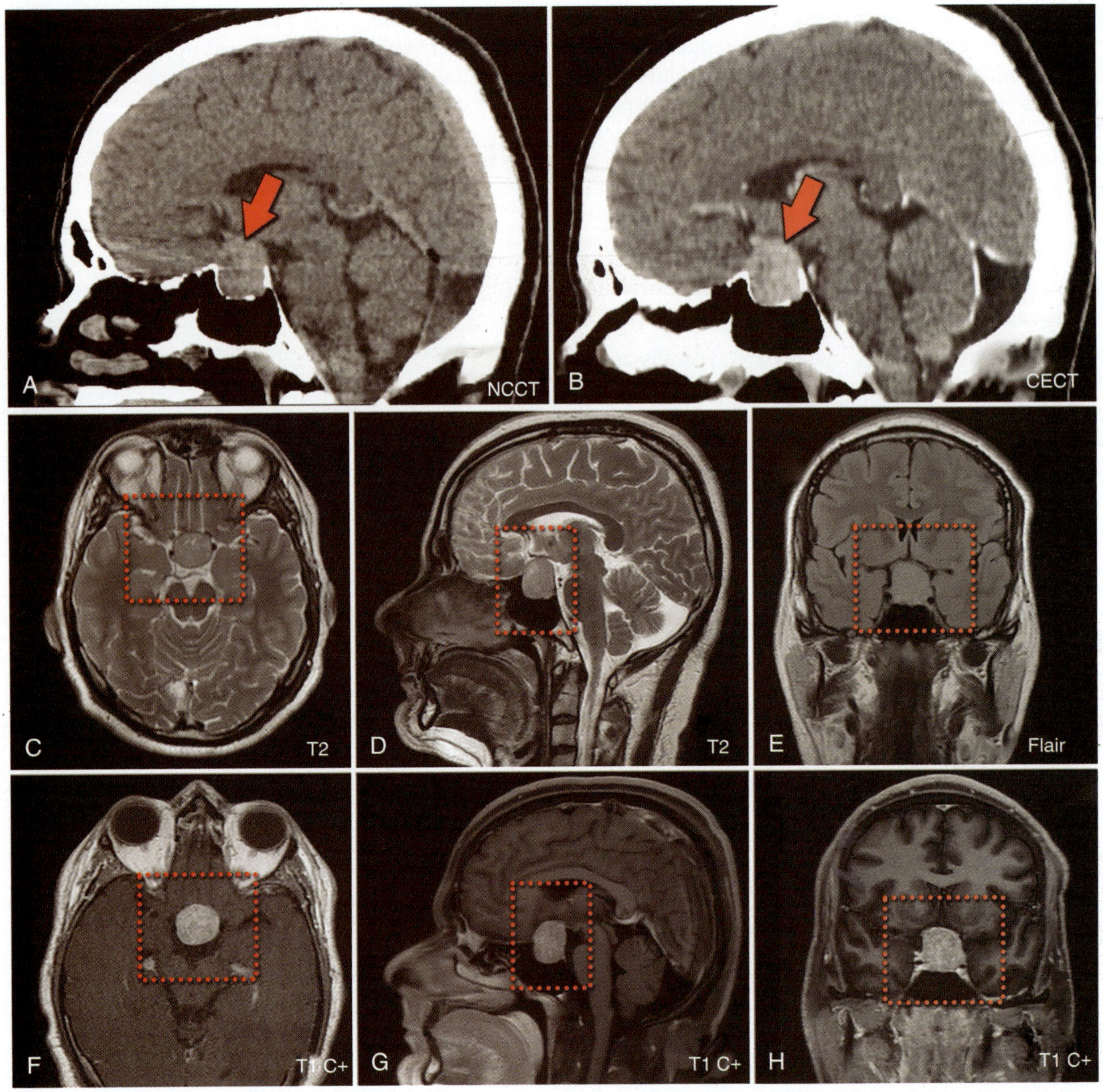

Sagittal non-contrast computed tomography (NCCT) and contrast-enhanced computed tomography (CECT) brain (A and B) show expansion of the sella with a mildly hyperdense lobulated sellar/suprasellar mass showing nearly homogeneous post-contrast enhancement. On magnetic resonance imaging (MRI), it appears isointense to mildly hyperintense on T2 (C and D) and hypointense on T1 with marked post-contrast enhancement (F–H). There is involvement of the bilateral cavernous sinuses with partial encasement of the bilateral cavernous internal carotid arteries. There is displacement of the bilateral supraclinoid internal carotid arteries and bilateral A1 anterior cerebral arteries along with compression of the optic chiasma superiorly. Findings are in keeping with pituitary macroadenoma.

Pituitary Macroadenoma

- Pituitary macroadenomas, defined as adenomas exceeding 10 mm, constitute the most common suprasellar masses in adults. They are roughly twice as prevalent as pituitary microadenomas. Most pituitary adenomas are secretory (~65%), with prolactinomas being the most common (~50%).

RADIOLOGICAL FEATURES

- On computed tomography (CT), the attenuation varies based on haemorrhagic, cystic or necrotic components, while solid adenomas without haemorrhage typically exhibit brain-like attenuation (30–40 HU). Moderate post-contrast enhancement is usually observed. Their slow growth leads to an enlarged pituitary fossa with thinned and remodelled bone. This may give a 'snowman' or a 'figure of 8' appearance.
- Magnetic resonance imaging (MRI) offers exquisite delineation of the mass and clear visualization of surrounding structures like cavernous sinus and optic chiasm. On T1-weighted images, they typically

OSCE

106

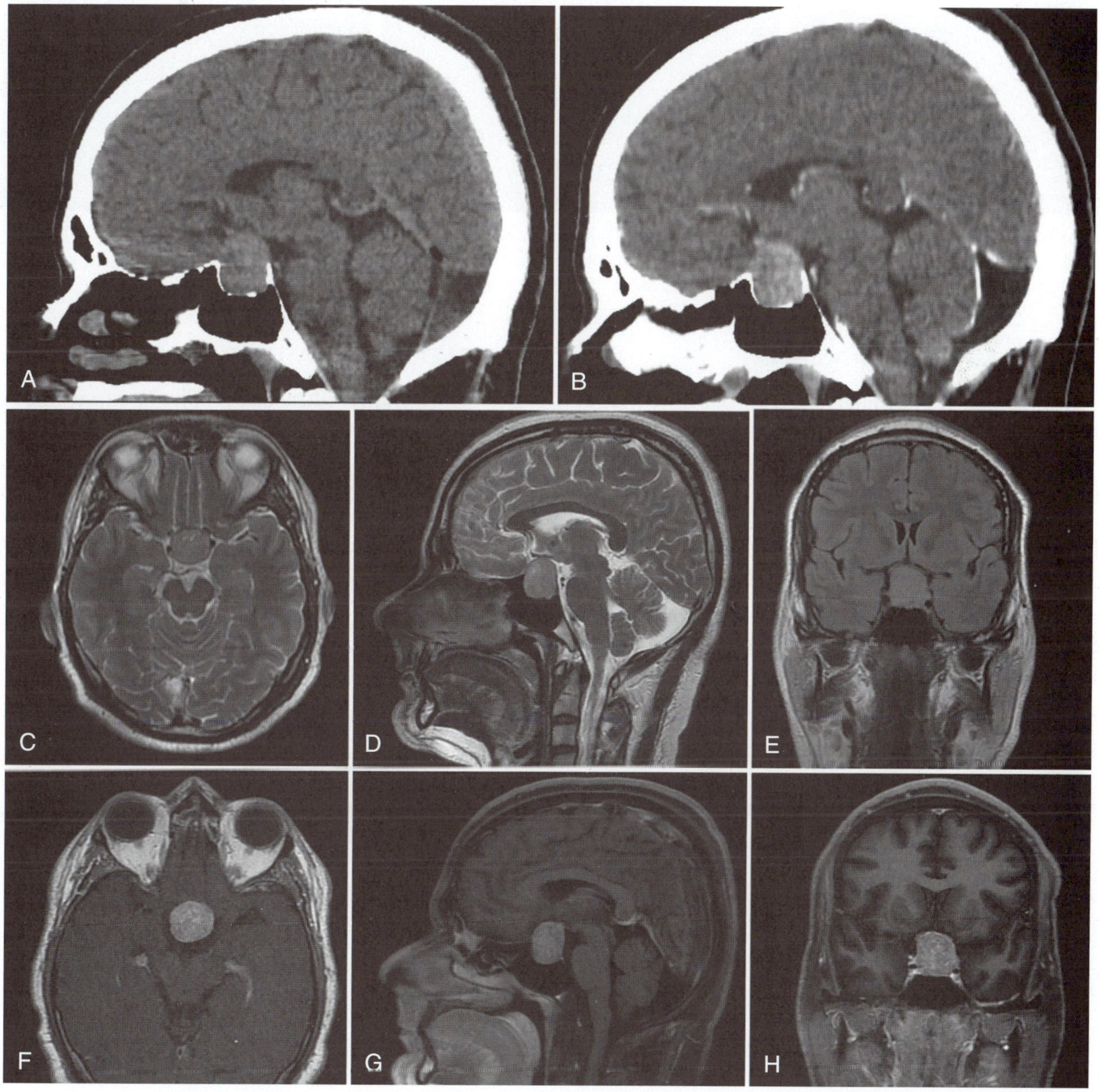

Clinical details: A 30-year-old male presented with headaches and visual disturbance.

1. **Describe the findings and the most appropriate diagnosis.**
2. **Which is the best magnetic resonance imaging (MRI) plane for assessment of cavernous sinus invasion by pituitary macroadenoma?**
3. **Name the classification used to determine the extent of cavernous sinus invasion by pituitary macroadenoma.**
4. **Which hormone is most likely to be secreted by a secretory pituitary macroadenoma?**

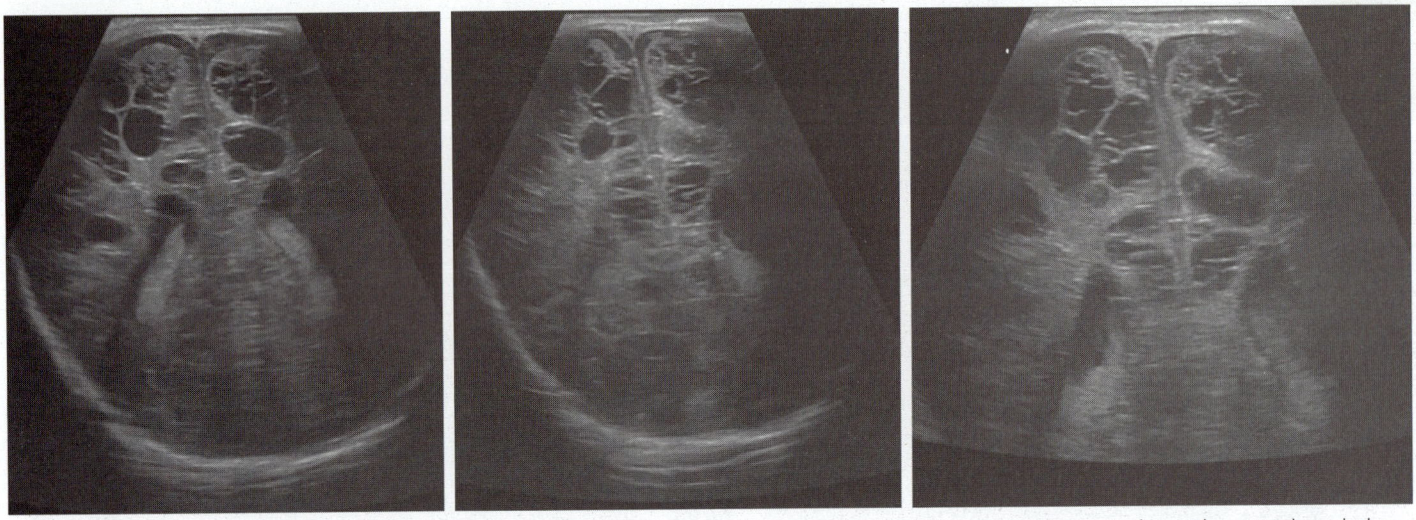

Transcranial ultrasonography demonstrates bilateral extensive cystic lesions in the bilateral periventricular, subcortical and deep white matter, consistent with grade IV periventricular leukomalacia. (PVL).

Periventricular Leukomalacia

- Periventricular leukomalacia (PVL) or white matter injury of prematurity is caused by perinatal hypoxic-ischaemic insult. It typically involves periventricular parenchyma with development of widespread cystic lesions in advanced cases. It most commonly occurs in premature neonates and neonates with low birth weight (<1500–2000 g).
- Patients may present with spastic cerebral palsy, seizures, mental retardation or visual/hearing impairment.

RADIOLOGICAL FEATURES

- Transcranial ultrasonography is a first line of investigation in suspected PVL.

Grading of Periventricular Leukomalacia (PVL)	
Grade 1	Increased periventricular echogenicity persisting more than 7 days
Grade 2	Development of small periventricular cysts
Grade 3	Development of extensive periventricular cysts, particularly in the fronto-parietal and occipital regions
Grade 4	Extensive subcortical cysts

PART H

Thorax

OSCE

109

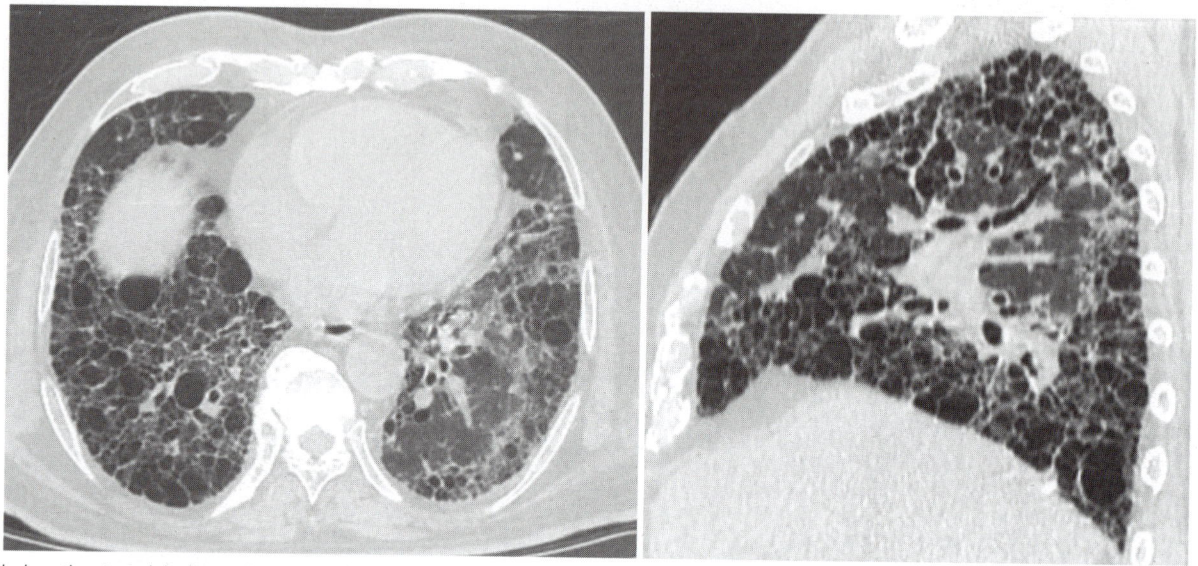

Clinical details: An elderly male presented with progressive shortness of breath. There is no history of fever or expectoration.

1. **Describe the imaging findings.**
2. **What is the most appropriate radiologic pattern of interstitial lung disease (ILD) seen here?**
3. **Enumerate two systemic diseases which can cause this pattern.**
4. **What hallmark imaging feature of this pathology is seen in this particular case?**

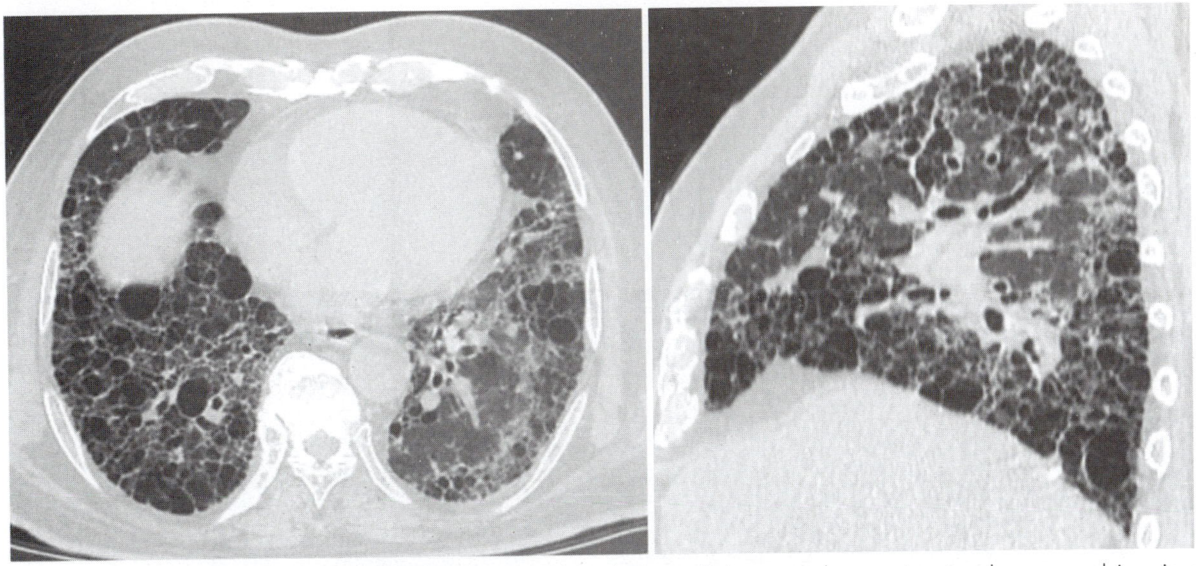

High-resolution computed tomography (HRCT) thorax (axial and sagittal) images show extensive honeycombing in subpleural location, associated with traction bronchiectasis, ground-glass opacification and reticulation.

Interstitial Lung Disease (Usual Interstitial Pneumonia Pattern)

- Usual interstitial pneumonia (UIP) is a subtype of interstitial lung disease (ILD) characterized by the presence of honeycombing in subpleural location and basilar predominance. Honeycombing is more predominant than ground-glass opacification. Traction bronchiectasis is seen in advanced disease.

RADIOLOGICAL FEATURES

- Honeycombing is considered to be the hallmark imaging finding of UIP. If more than 5% of the lung parenchyma is involved by honeycombing, this is considered highly specific for UIP.
- Most common differential is non-specific interstitial pneumonia (NSIP) in which ground-glass opacification is more predominant than honeycombing and immediate subpleural sparing is seen. Contrary to UIP, NSIP shows good response to steroids.
- Other differentials include fibrotic hypersensitivity pneumonitis (involving the mid and upper zones with centrilobular nodules and air trapping) and amiodarone lung fibrosis (presence of hyperdense liver on a non-contrast computed tomography [NCCT]).

UIP	NSIP
• Honeycombing is the hallmark feature	• Honeycombing is minimal to absent
• Ground-glass opacities are not prominent	• Ground-glass opacities are common
• Involvement of the subpleural lung parenchyma	• Immediate subpleural sparing
• Apico-basilar gradient	• No apico-basilar gradient
• Heterogeneous involvement of the lung	• Homogeneous involvement
• Traction bronchiectasis is more common	• Traction bronchiectasis is less common

OSCE

110

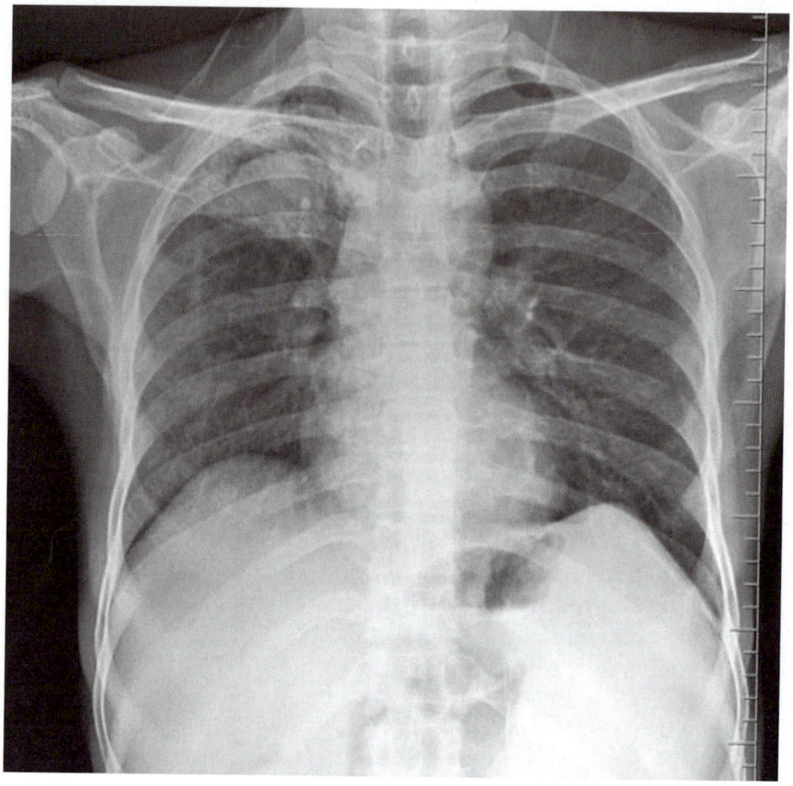

Clinical details: A middle-aged patient presented with history of evening rise of temperature, cough and sputum for the past 7 months.

1. **Describe the findings seen in the provided images.**
2. **What is the most appropriate diagnosis?**
3. **What could be the underlying aetiology for cavity formation?**
4. **What is 'Monod sign'?**

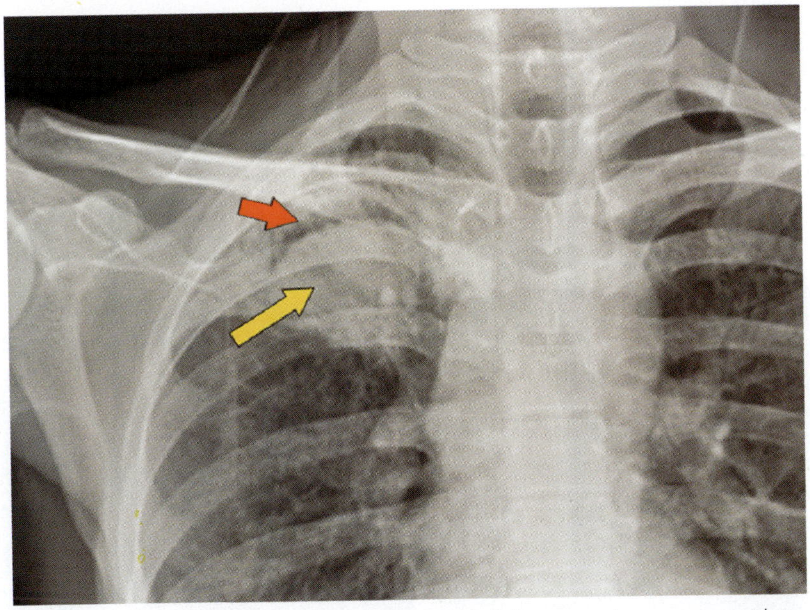

Zoomed image of frontal chest radiograph demonstrates a cavity in the right upper lungs zone with a mycetoma (*yellow arrow*) in a case of aspergilloma. A crescent-shaped lucency seen in the superior aspect of the cavity – Monod sign.

Aspergilloma

- Infection of *Aspergillus fumigatus* in a pre-existing cavity in lung may cause aspergilloma or a fungal ball in an immunocompetent patient. The pre-existing cavity may be due to cavity pulmonary tuberculosis, sarcoidosis or cystic bronchiectasis – pulmonary tuberculosis being the most common. Patients may present with haemoptysis.

RADIOLOGICAL FEATURES

- Chest radiograph and high-resolution computed tomography (HRCT) thorax reveal a nodular opacity/mass within the lung cavity. Prone HRCT may be used to demonstrate that the fungal ball/mycetoma within the cavity is mobile. A thin crescent of air usually surrounds the mycetoma and is known as the Monod sign.

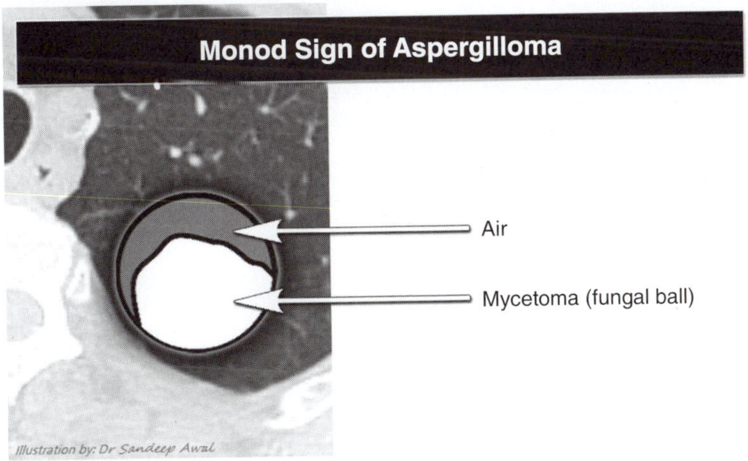

OSCE

111

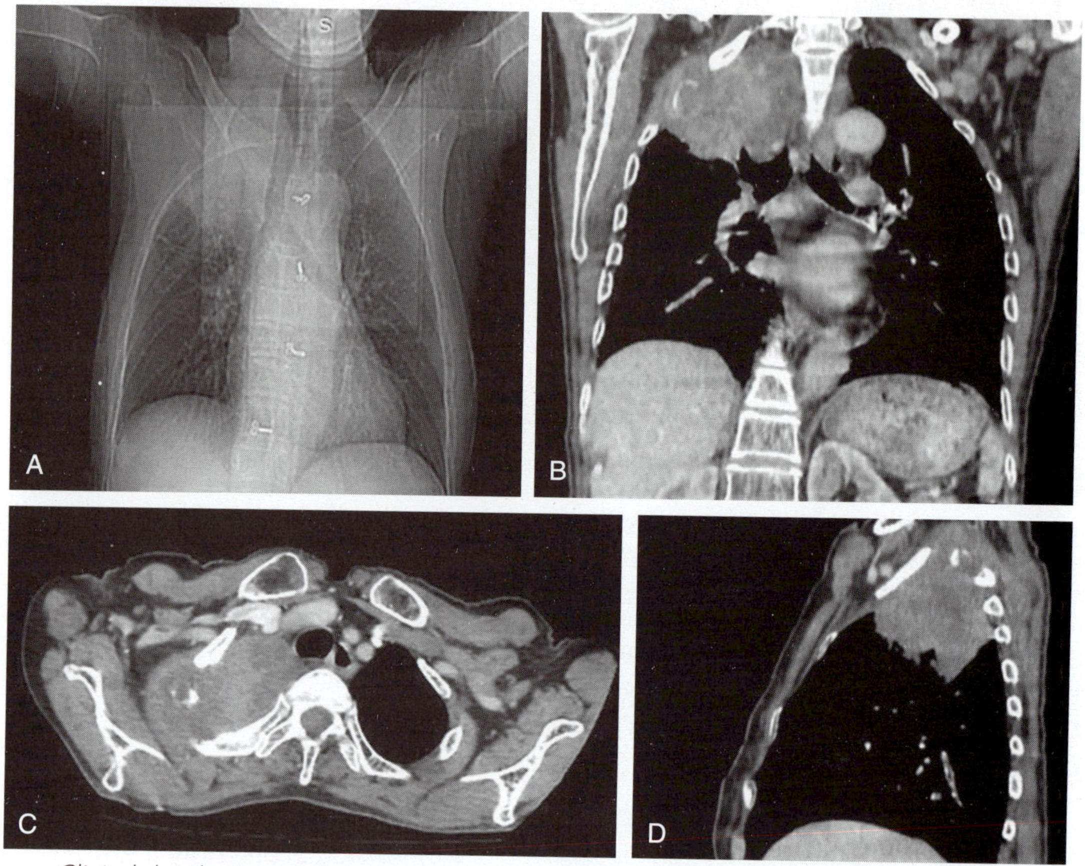

Clinical details: An elderly male patient presented with longstanding right shoulder pain.

1. **Describe the imaging findings.**
2. **Provide the most appropriate diagnosis.**
3. **What should be the next appropriate imaging?**
4. **What is Horner syndrome?**

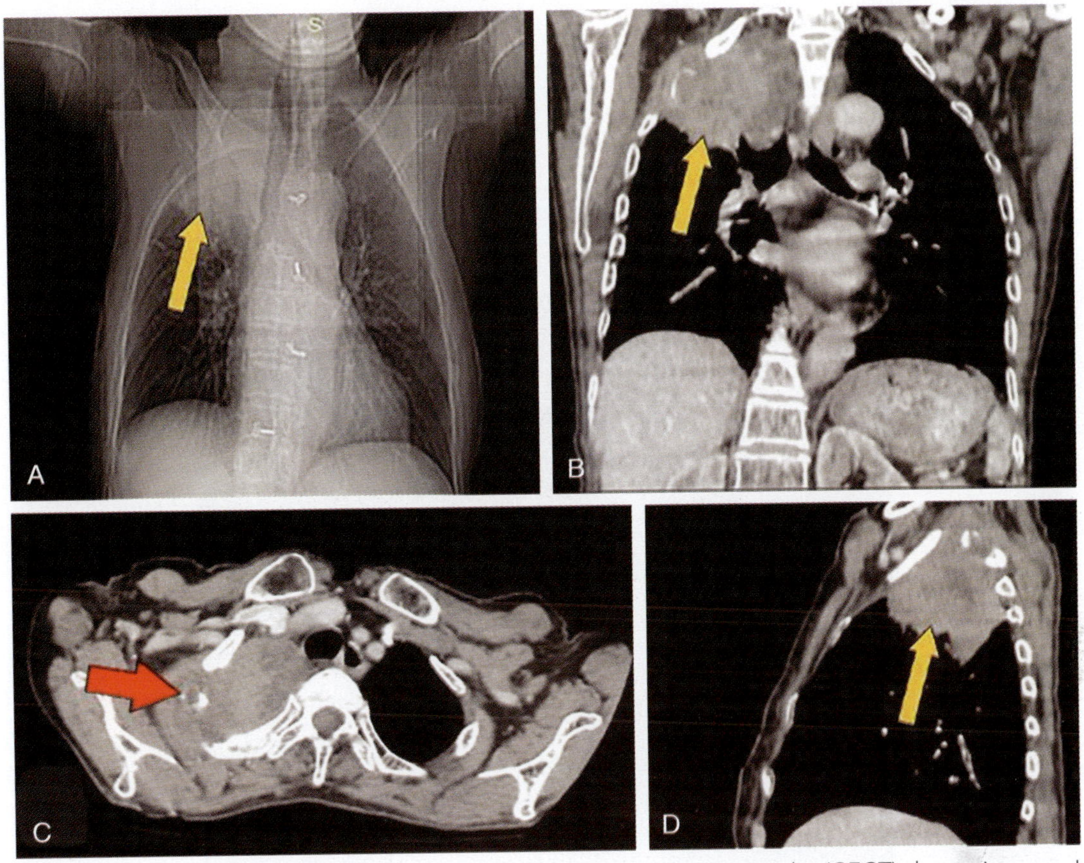

(A–D) Scout image, coronal, axial and sagittal contrast-enhanced computed tomography (CECT) thorax images: Large heterogeneously enhancing irregular mass involving right lung apex (*yellow arrows*). It invades and erodes the right second rib (*red arrow*) and right apical chest wall

Pancoast Tumour (Superior Sulcus Tumour)

- A Pancoast tumour (superior sulcus tumour) comprises a variety of tumours located in apical lung and invading the apical chest wall. It comprises approximately 3%–5% of bronchogenic carcinomas.
- Common symptoms include shoulder pain, muscle weakness/atrophy and paraesthesia. Horner syndrome may be seen and includes ptosis, miosis, enophthalmos and anhidrosis of the ipsilateral face. Majority of superior sulcus tumours are non-small cell carcinomas.

RADIOLOGICAL FEATURES

- Plain chest radiograph demonstrates a homogenous soft tissue opacity at lung apex with or without rib involvement. Ultrasound may aid in guided biopsy.
- Computed tomography (CT) is excellent at delineating the extent of rib/bony involvement. Magnetic resonance imaging (MRI) is more sensitive and specific than CT for demonstrating the soft tissue and brachial plexus involvement. Positron emission tomography (PET) CT can be used for evaluating the status of nodal and distal metastasis.

OSCE

112

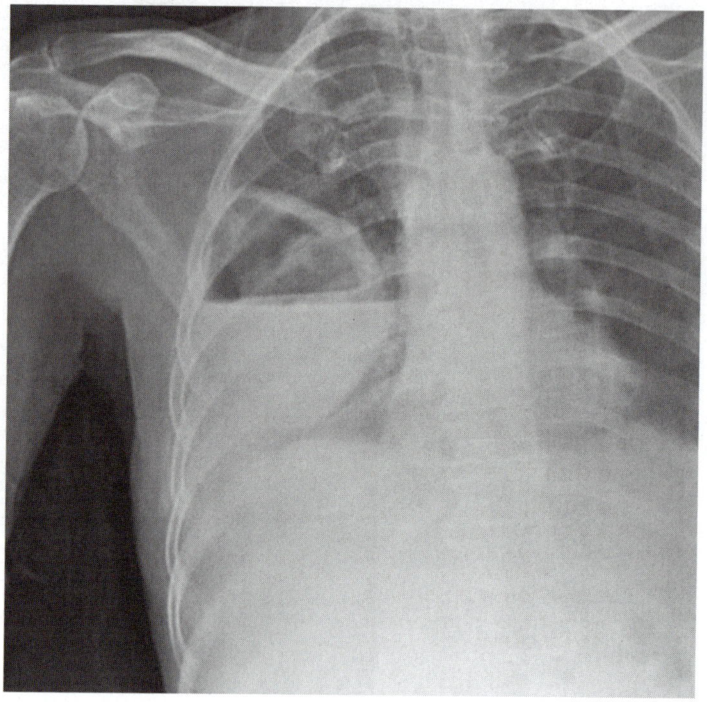

Clinical details: A middle-aged male patient presented with fever, chills and cough of 2 weeks' duration.

1. **Describe your findings.**
2. **What is the most appropriate diagnosis?**
3. **What is the next imaging modality recommended?**
4. **Give two appropriate differentials.**

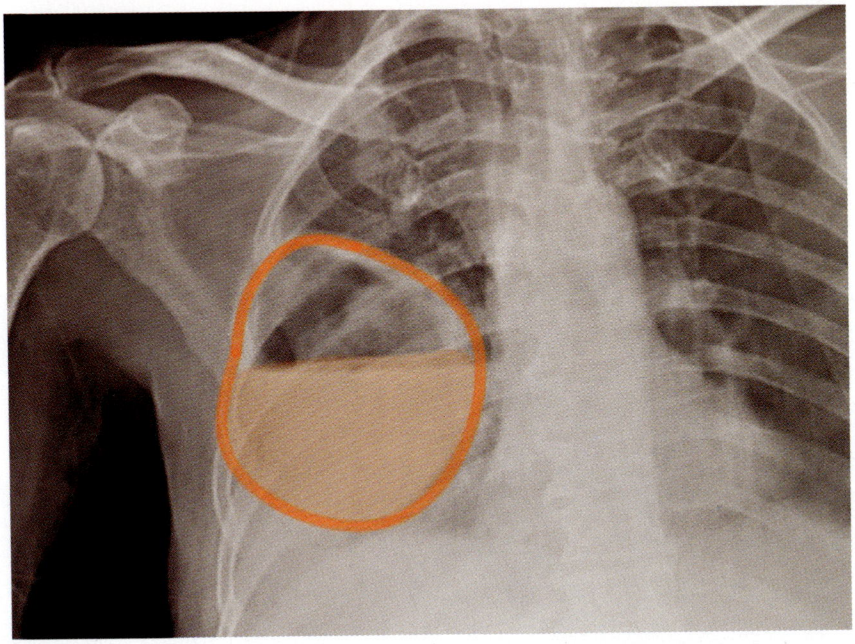

Frontal chest radiograph demonstrates a thick-walled cavitary lesion in the right middle and lower lung zones with an air–fluid level.

Lung Abscess

- Lung abscess is an infected cavitary lesion within the lung. A wide range of organisms can produce a lung abscess, but the common ones include *Staphylococcus*, *Streptococcus* and *Klebsiella*.

RADIOLOGICAL FEATURES

- On X-ray and computed tomography (CT) thorax, lung abscess is seen as a cavity with an air–fluid level. There may be features of surrounding consolidation in some cases, making it difficult to evaluate. CT is superior to chest radiograph in differentiating lung abscess from empyema.
- Other differential diagnosis includes cavitating metastasis with necrosis and lung cancer.

Lung Abscess	Empyema
Spherical or round shaped	Lens shaped/lenticular
Thickened, irregular abscess walls	Split pleura sign: Enhancing, regular thickening of pleura with separation of its visceral and parietal layers
Acute angle with the chest wall	Obtuse angle with the chest wall

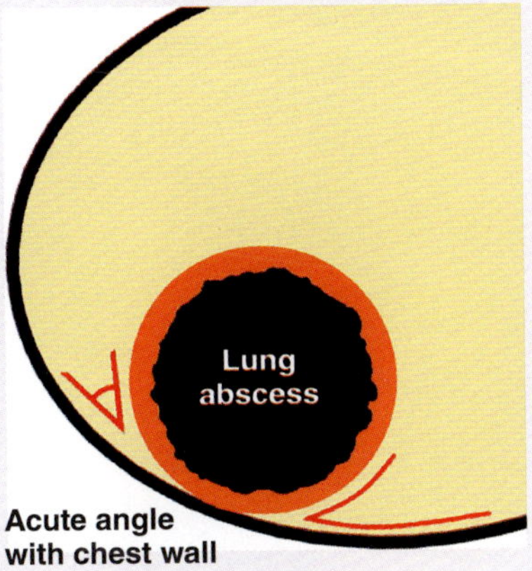

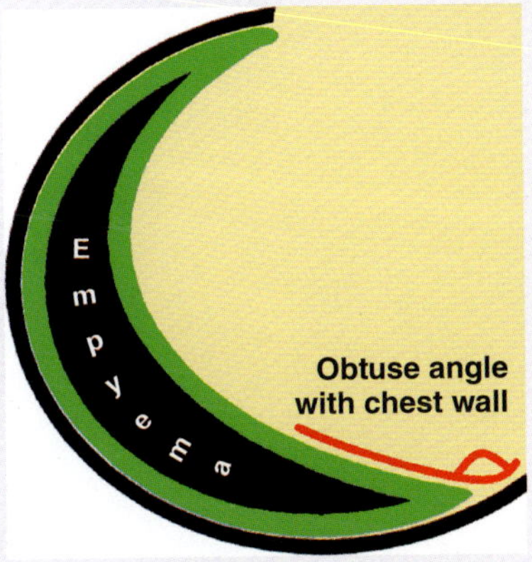

OSCE

113

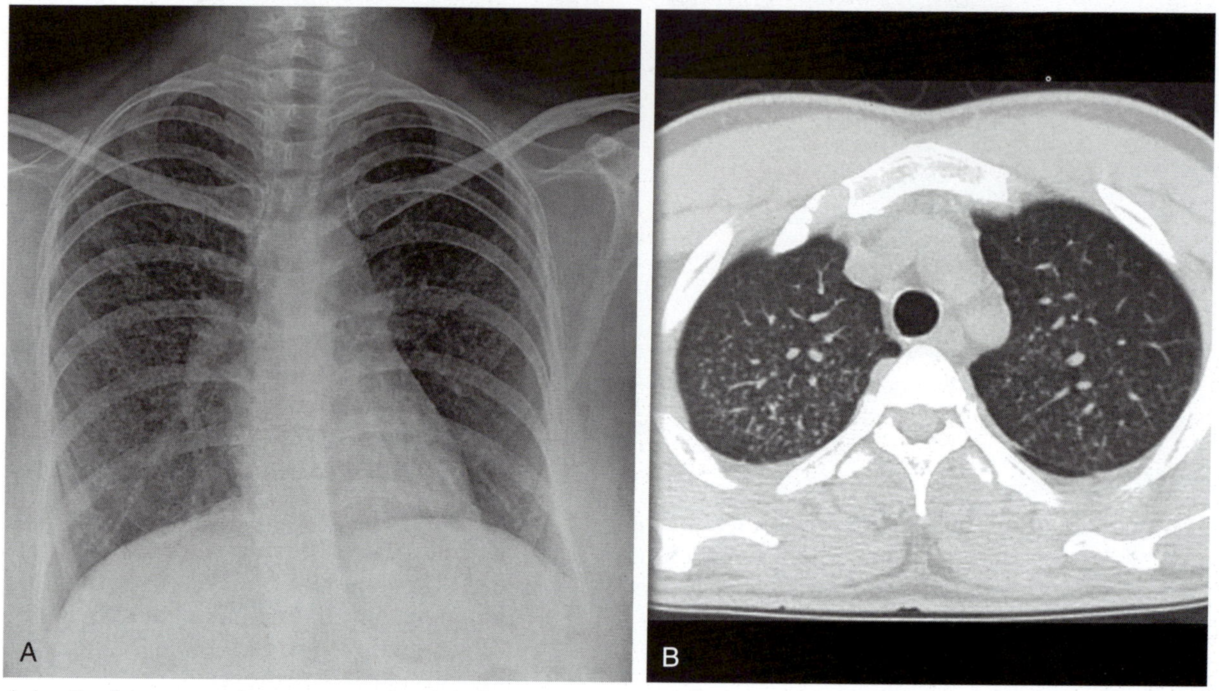

Clinical details: A young patient presented with lethargy, night sweats, fever and raised erythrocyte sedimentation rate (ESR).

1. **Describe the features seen on the (A) radiograph and in the (B) computed tomography (CT) images.**
2. **What is the most appropriate diagnosis?**
3. **List three causes of miliary metastasis in the lungs.**
4. **List two differences between primary and re-activation tuberculosis (TB).**

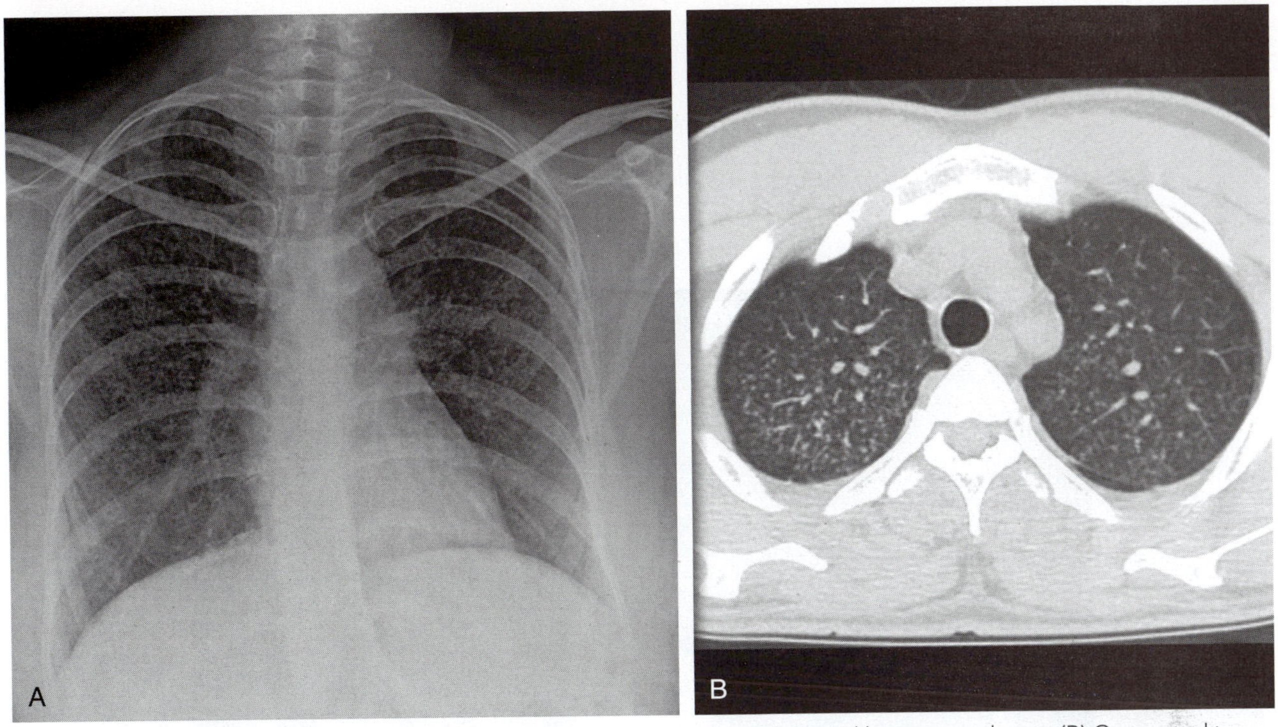

(A) Frontal chest radiograph reveals innumerable tiny nodules scattered in the bilateral lung parenchyma. (B) Computed tomography (CT) scan of the lungs shows multiple tiny nodules scattered in bilateral upper lobes of lung.

Miliary Tuberculosis

Miliary tuberculosis is a rare manifestation of tuberculosis, characterized by multiple tiny 'millet-seed' like nodular opacities (1–3 mm), scattered randomly and uniformly in bilateral lung parenchyma. Miliary tuberculosis represents a haematogenous spread of tuberculosis infection. If untreated, it has a poor prognosis.

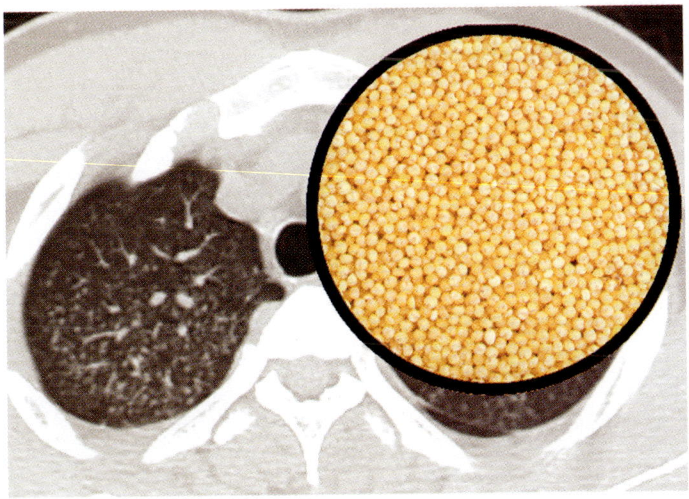

RADIOLOGICAL FEATURES

It can be seen in both primary and post-primary (reactivation) tuberculoses. Both radiographs and computed tomography (CT) scan reveal the presence of innumerable tiny nodular opacities scattered in the bilateral lungs. Usually, there is no associated cavitation and no significant lymph nodal enlargement.

Causes of miliary metastasis include thyroid carcinoma, renal cell carcinoma, breast carcinoma, malignant melanoma and osteosarcoma.

Primary Tuberculosis	Reactivation Tuberculosis
• Usually involves lung bases	• Upper lobes are more commonly involved
• Lymphadenopathy is common	• Lymphadenopathy is rare
• Pleural effusion is common	• Pleural effusion is uncommon
• Cavity formation is uncommon	• Cavitation is common in active disease

Note: Miliary pattern can be seen in both primary and post primary (reactivation) tuberculoses

OSCE

114

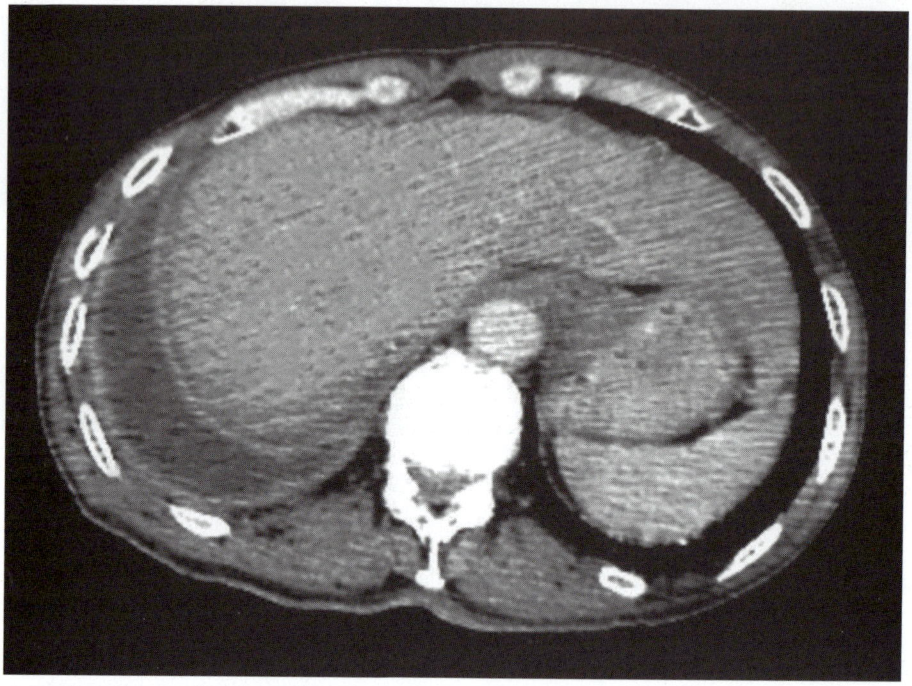

Clinical details: An elderly male presented with history of chronic cough, fever and weight loss. Frontal chest radiograph showed the presence of right costophrenic angle blunting. Contrast-enhanced computed tomography (CT) of the thorax was subsequently performed.

1. **What is 'split pleura sign'?**
2. **Provide two differentiating points between an empyema and a peripherally located pulmonary abscess.**
3. **What is the management of choice in a case of empyema?**
4. **What is empyema necessitans and its most common causative organism?**

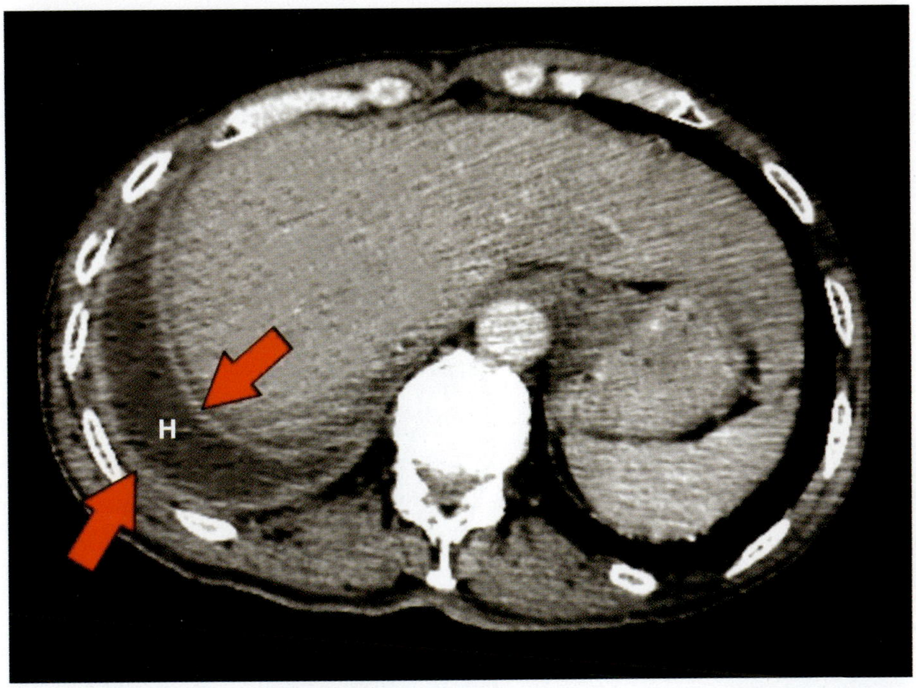

Selected axial section of the basal lungs in a contrast-enhanced computed tomography (CT) scan of the thorax reveals a right-sided hypodense pleural collection (*H*) with enhancing parietal and visceral pleural layers (*red arrows*), demonstrating the split pleura sign of pleural empyema.

Pleural Empyema

- A pleural empyema is referred to purulent collection within the pleural cavity, usually unilateral. It is also called pyothorax and commonly occurs following pneumonia with an associated parapneumonic effusion.
- The majority of the empyemas are due to *Staphylococcus* or *Streptococcus* infections, but it can also be seen in the setting of mycobacterial infection (tuberculosis).

RADIOLOGICAL FEATURES

- On a radiograph, it usually resembles a pleural effusion but, in some cases, it can also mimic a peripherally located pulmonary abscess. Computed tomography (CT) scan is considered superior to a chest radiograph in differentiating between a lung abscess and an empyema. On contrast-enhanced CT of the thorax, pleural empyema is seen as a hypodense fluid collection within the pleural cavity with thickened and enhancing layers of parietal and visceral pleurae. This is termed the 'split pleura sign', and it is the most reliable indicator for distinguishing pleural empyema from peripheral pulmonary abscess.
- A pleural empyema is considered an emergency and requires prompt drainage of the infected purulent collection along with antibiotic support.

Lung Abscess	Empyema
Spherical or round shaped	Lens shaped/lenticular
Thickened, irregular abscess walls	Split pleura sign: Enhancing, regular thickening of pleura with separation of its visceral and parietal layers
Acute angle with the chest wall	Obtuse angle with the chest wall

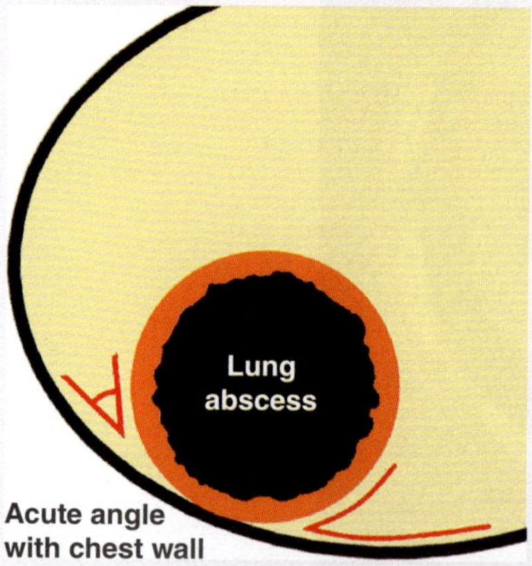

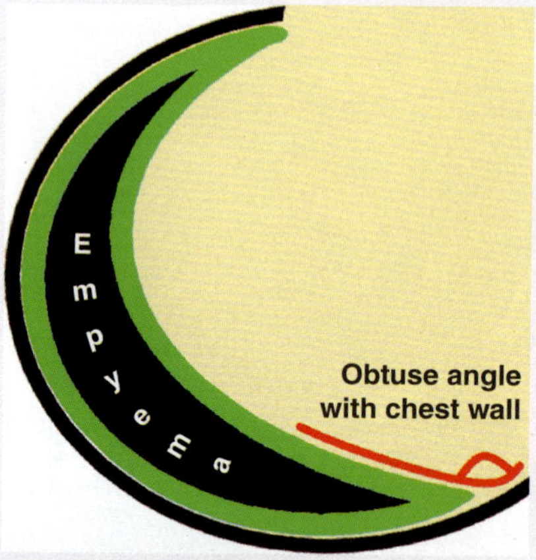

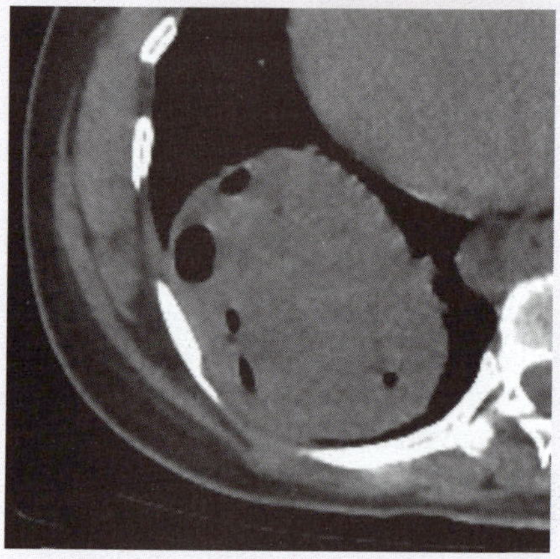

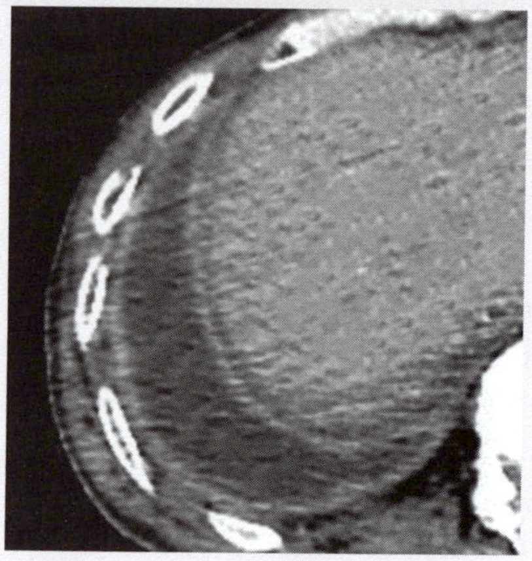

- Empyema necessitans denotes the extension of pleural empyema beyond the confines of the pleural cavity, into the chest wall and adjacent soft tissues. The most common cause of empyema necessitans is *Mycobacterium tuberculosis* followed by adenomyosis. CT thorax is the best modality for the evaluation of empyema necessitans, and typically reveals the presence of an empyema which extends beyond the pleural cavity infiltrating into the chest wall. Management can be done by both open and closed drainage procedures along with appropriate antibiotic cover.

OSCE

115

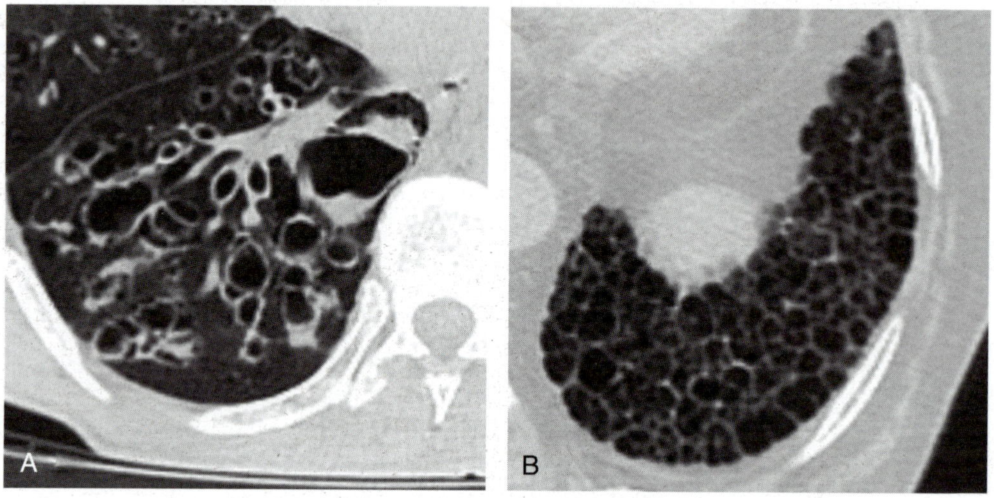

Clinical details: History withheld.

1. **Describe the computed tomography (CT) findings seen in both patients A and B.**
2. **List two CT features that are helpful in diagnosing bronchiectasis.**
3. **Enumerate two causes of central bronchiectasis.**
4. **Which interstitial lung disease (ILD) is characterized by the findings seen in patient B?**

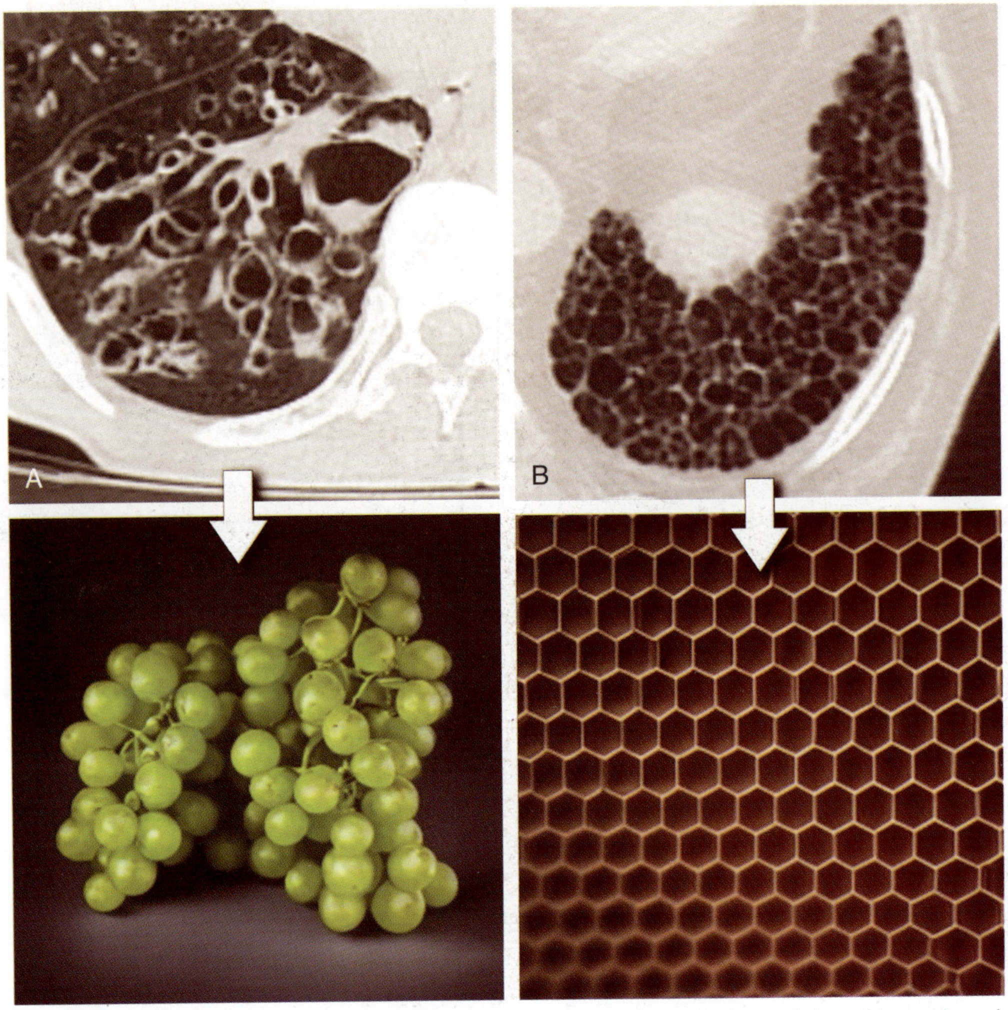

Axial computed tomography (CT) thorax images: (A) Cystic bronchiectasis in the right lower lobe of lung ('bunch of grapes appearance') and (B) extensive honeycombing in the left lower lobe of lung.

Bronchiectasis

Bronchiectasis is defined as the irreversible dilatation of the airways. It originates predominantly from chronic inflammation, with mechanisms encompassing bronchial obstruction and wall damage due to mucous plugging.

Patient usually presents with recurrent respiratory infections, longstanding cough with expectoration and haemoptysis.

COMMON CAUSES OF BRONCHIECTASIS

- Idiopathic bronchiectasis (most common cause)
- Cystic fibrosis, primary ciliary dyskinesias as like Kartagener syndrome and Young syndrome
- Post-pneumonia or bronchitis
- Pulmonary tuberculosis
- Allergic bronchopulmonary aspergillosis
- Parenchymal fibrosis due to interstitial lung diseases (ILD; usual interstitial pneumonia [UIP]) causing traction bronchiectasis
- Mounier-Kuhn syndrome and Williams–Campbell syndrome

Macroscopically there are three types of bronchiectasis:

1. Cylindrical bronchiectasis – commonest type
2. Varicoid bronchiectasis
3. Cystic bronchiectasis (+/– air–fluid levels)

Central bronchiectasis is seen in allergic bronchopulmonary aspergillosis (ABPA), cystic fibrosis and Mounier-Kuhn syndrome.

RADIOLOGICAL FEATURES

COMMON CT FEATURES OF BRONCHIECTASIS

- Visualization of bronchus in the peripheral lung within 1 cm of the pleura
- Lack of bronchial tapering in the peripheral lung
- Increased bronchial arterial ratio: Ratio of the diameter of bronchus and its accompanying artery greater than 1.5.

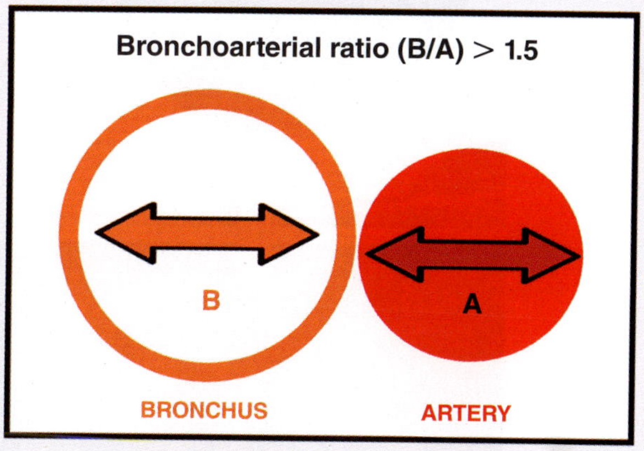

- Bronchial wall thickening and air trapping

SIGNS

- Signet ring sign
- Tram track sign – cylindrical bronchiectasis
- String of pearls sign – varicose bronchiectasis
- Cluster of grapes sign – cystic bronchiectasis

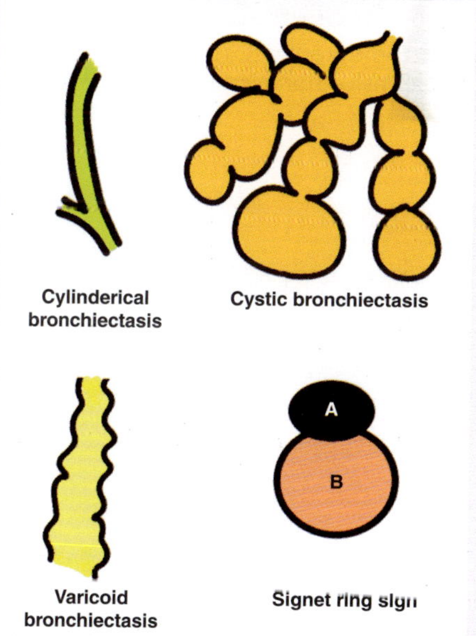

OSCE

116

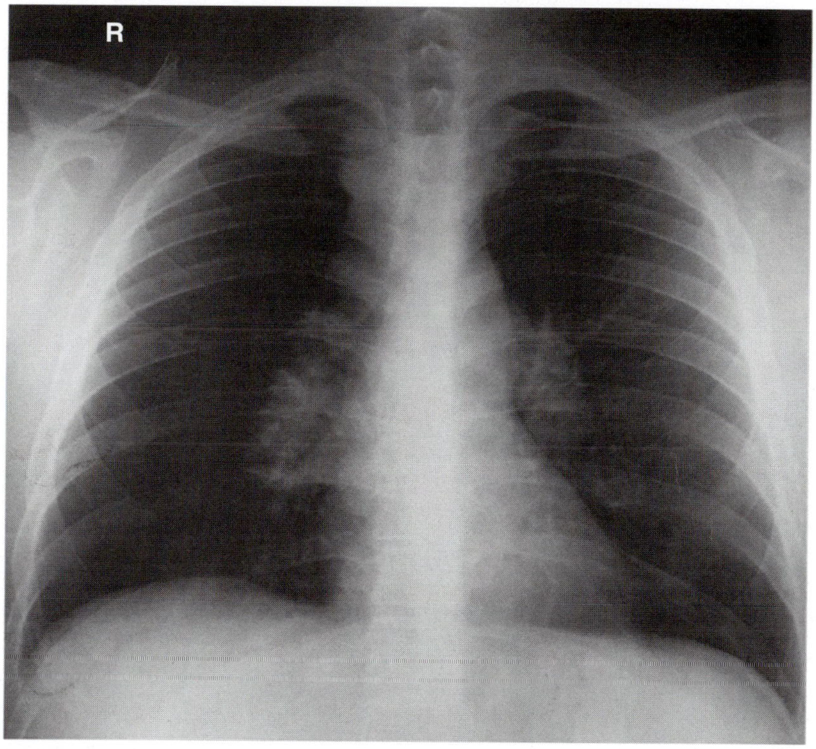

Clinical details: A middle-aged patient presented with a history of dyspnoea for 3 months and a painful rash over the shins.

1. **Described findings seen in the above radiograph.**
2. **What is the most appropriate diagnosis?**
3. **What is the classification for staging?**
4. **What is the role of scintigraphy of this pathology?**

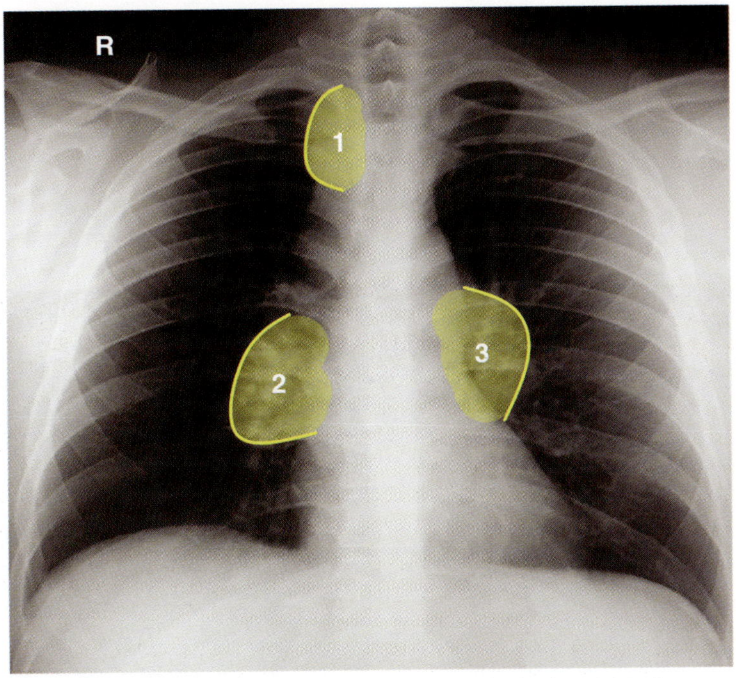

Frontal chest radiograph reveals bilateral hilar lymphadenopathy along with thickened right paratracheal stripe indicative of enlarged right paratracheal lymph nodes (1-2-3 sign or Garland triad).

Sarcoidosis

- Thoracic involvement is common in sarcoidosis, with over 90% of patients presenting with pulmonary and/or mediastinal involvement. Erythema nodosum, a painful red nodular rash, can be a symptom seen in patients diagnosed with sarcoidosis.

RADIOLOGICAL FEATURES

- Mediastinal involvement is usually in the form of lymph nodal enlargement, whereas parenchymal involvement can range from reticulonodular opacities, airspace opacities, lung nodules and coalescing ill-defined nodules. End-stage lung disease in sarcoidosis is characterized by pulmonary fibrosis, commonly seen in the upper and mid lung zones.
- On high-resolution computed tomography (HRCT) thorax, two nodules are usually seen in the perilymphatic distribution. The enlarged tube mediastinal lymph nodes may show egg-shell calcifications. End-stage pulmonary fibrosis can be associated with tractional bronchiectasis.

THE CLASSIC RADIOLOGICAL SIGNS SEEN IN THORACIC SARCOIDOSIS

Garland triad (1-2-3 sign or pawnbroker's sign)	Lymph node enlargement on chest radiographs involving (1) right paratracheal lymph nodes, (2) right hilar lymph nodes and (3) left hilar lymph nodes
Galaxy sign	Coalescent mass-like region formed due to coalescing granulomas/ nodules, surrounded by tiny nodules, showing a galaxy-like appearance

Pulmonary sarcoidosis on a frontal chest radiograph is classified into five stages (Siltzbach classification/ Scadding criteria):

SILTZBACH CLASSIFICATION/SCADDING CRITERIA

Stage 0	Normal chest radiograph
Stage I	Hilar or mediastinal lymphadenopathy only
Stage II	Parenchymal involvement + lymphadenopathy
Stage III	Parenchymal involvement only
Stage IV	End-stage pulmonary fibrosis

- Gallium-67 scintigraphy is a scan that can be used to assess sarcoidosis activity, treatment response and extrathoracic involvement. It is not specific for sarcoidosis, but it can also be used to see inflammation in other conditions. The gallium equivalent of the 1-2-3 sign is known as the lambda sign.

OSCE

117

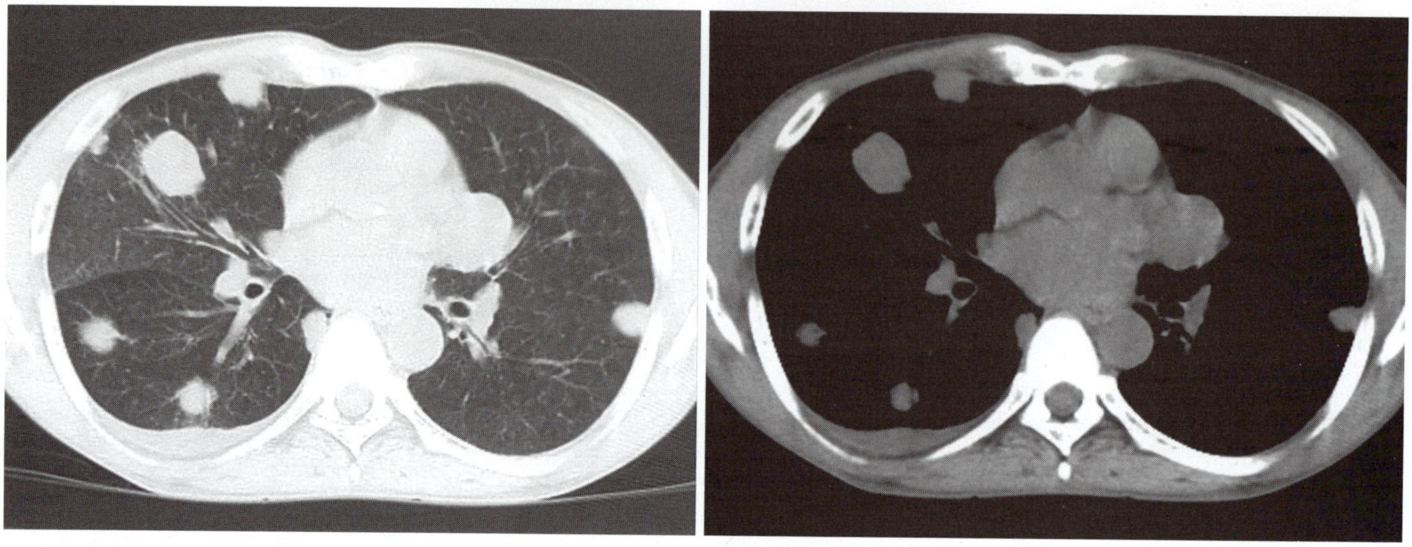

Clinical details: History withheld.

1. **Enumerate three causes of cannonball metastasis in the lungs.**
2. **Pulmonary metastasis from which primary cancer can lead to the development of pneumothorax?**
3. **What is 'feeding vessel sign'?**
4. **List two causes of miliary metastasis.**

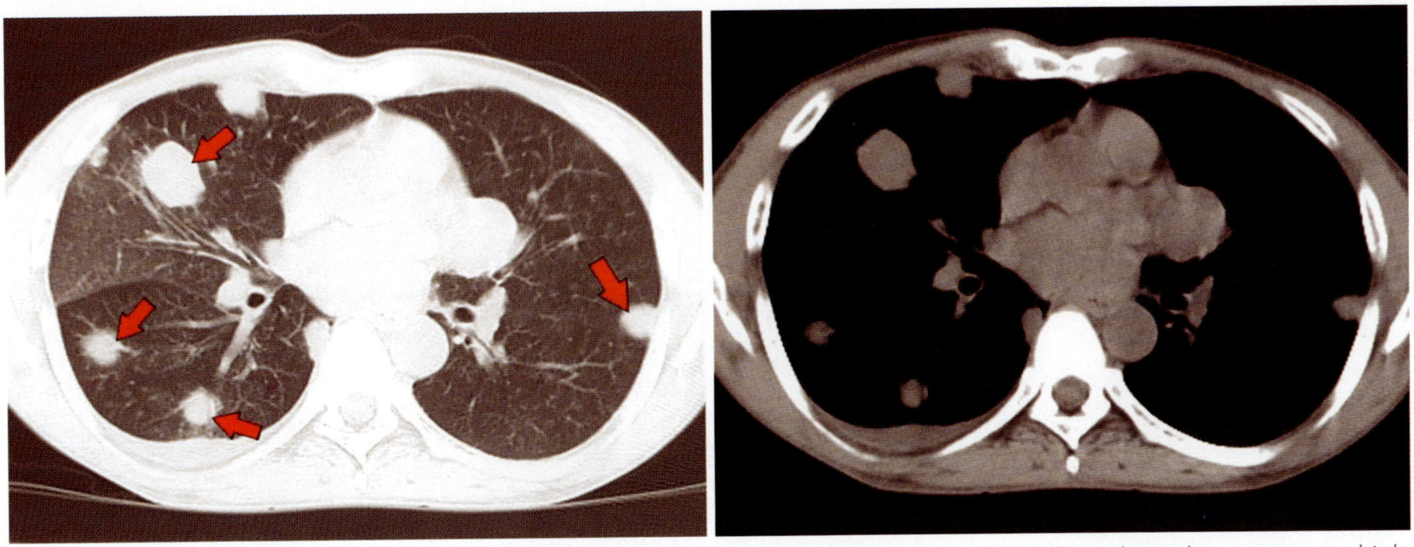

Selected axial section of a computed tomography (CT) thorax study with lung and mediastinal windows demonstrate multiple rounded nodules of varying sizes, scattered in the bilateral lung parenchyma.

Lung Metastasis

- **Cannonball metastases** are characterized by the presence of multiple rounded, well-defined, lung metastases. While various types of primary tumours can exhibit this pattern, certain primary tumours tend to specifically manifest as cannonball metastases (mnemonic = CREPS):

CANNONBALL METASTASES

C: Choriocarcinoma or colorectal carcinoma

R: Renal cell carcinoma (RCC)

E: Endometrial cancer

P: Prostate cancer

S: Synovial sarcoma

- Necrotic tumours near the pleura can cause pneumothorax, with **osteosarcoma** being a classic culprit for pulmonary metastases causing pneumothorax. Pneumothorax can also result from cystic/cavitary lung metastases.
- Cavitation of metastasis is seen in 5% of cases. Causes of cavitating metastasis to the lung consist of (1) squamous cell carcinoma (most common), (2) transitional cell tumours, (3) colon cancer and (4) sarcoma.
- Miliary metastasis can be attributed to various primary cancers, including thyroid carcinoma, renal cell carcinoma, breast carcinoma, malignant melanoma and osteosarcoma.
- The occurrence of calcification in metastatic lesions is most frequently associated with osteogenic sarcoma, synovial sarcoma, chondrosarcoma, thyroid carcinoma and mucinous adenocarcinoma.
- The 'feeding vessel sign' can be seen when a small pulmonary artery has a direct connection to a nodule. It can be seen in metastases, infarcts, vascular lesions such as arteriovenous malformations (AVMs) and septic emboli.

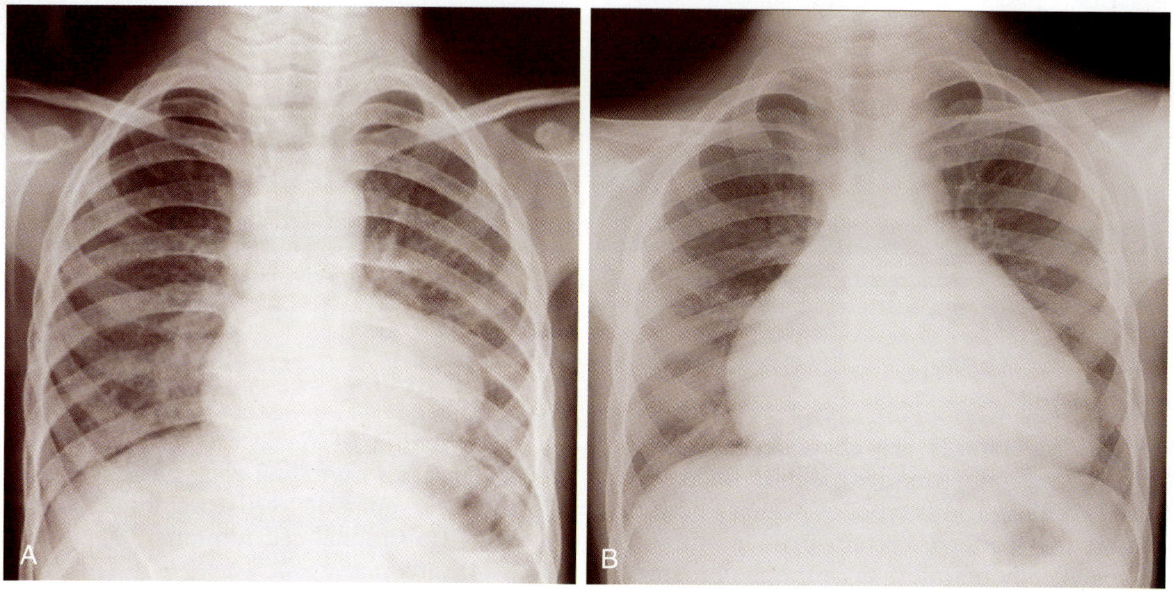

Clinical details: History withheld.

1. **Name the classical sign and the appropriate diagnosis in case A.**
2. **What is the most commonly associated cardiovascular anomaly seen in A?**
3. **Name the classical sign and the appropriate diagnosis in case B.**
4. **Maternal lithium intake is associated with which congenital cardiac anomaly?**

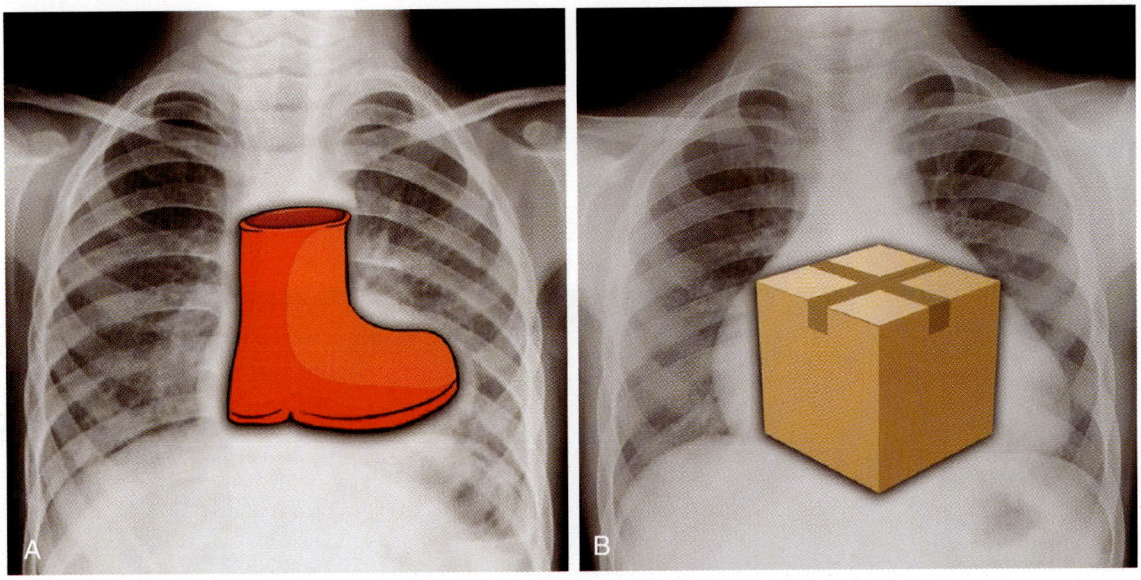

(A) Boot-shaped heart in a case of tetralogy of Fallot with upwards prominence of the cardiac apex (due to right ventricular enlargement) and (B) box-shaped heart in a case of Ebstein anomaly with marked cardiac enlargement.

Tetralogy of Fallot

Tetralogy of Fallot (TOF) is a congenital heart defect characterized by four anatomical abnormalities:

- Ventricular septal defect (VSD)
- Pulmonary stenosis (right ventricular outflow tract obstruction)
- Overriding aorta
- Right ventricular hypertrophy

TOF is the most common cyanotic congenital cardiac anomaly. The boot-shaped heart appearance is a common finding in TOF. It is caused by a combination of two factors:

I. Right ventricular hypertrophy: This causes the apex of the heart to turn upwards, giving it a boot-like appearance.

II. Concave pulmonary arterial segment.

TOF is commonly associated with right-sided aortic arch (25% of cases), atrial septal defect (ASD) and extracardiac associations such as foetal rubella syndrome, DiGeorge syndrome and congenital lobar emphysema.

Ebstein Anomaly

Ebstein anomaly is a rare congenital cardiac anomaly characterized by the apical displacement of the tricuspid valve into the right ventricle. This results in atrialization of the right ventricle's inlet portion as well as adhesion of the septal and posterior leaflets to the myocardium.

The characteristic appearance of Ebstein anomaly on the chest radiograph is known as box-shaped heart. It is usually associated with ASD, with a right to left shunt causing cyanosis. It is known to be associated with chromosomal anomalies, such as trisomy 13, trisomy 21, and Turner syndrome, Wolff–Parkinson–White syndrome and maternal intake of lithium carbonate.

OSCE

119

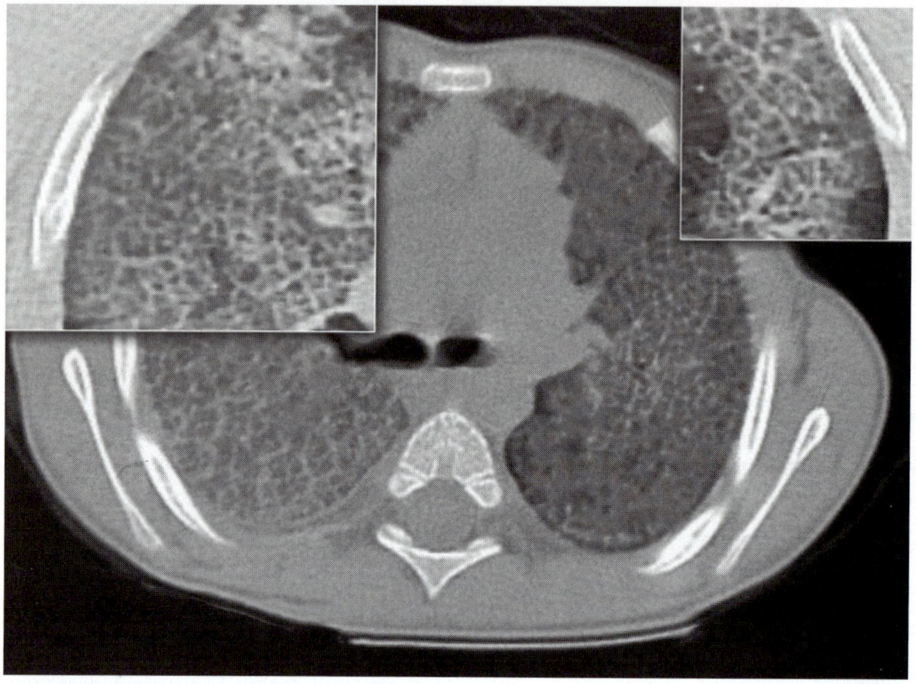

Clinical details: A middle-aged smoker presented with exertional dyspnoea and non-productive cough.

1. **Describe the findings seen in the provided image.**
2. **What is crazy paving appearance?**
3. **List three common causes of crazy paving appearance.**
4. **What is the standard treatment of pulmonary alveolar proteinosis (PAP)?**

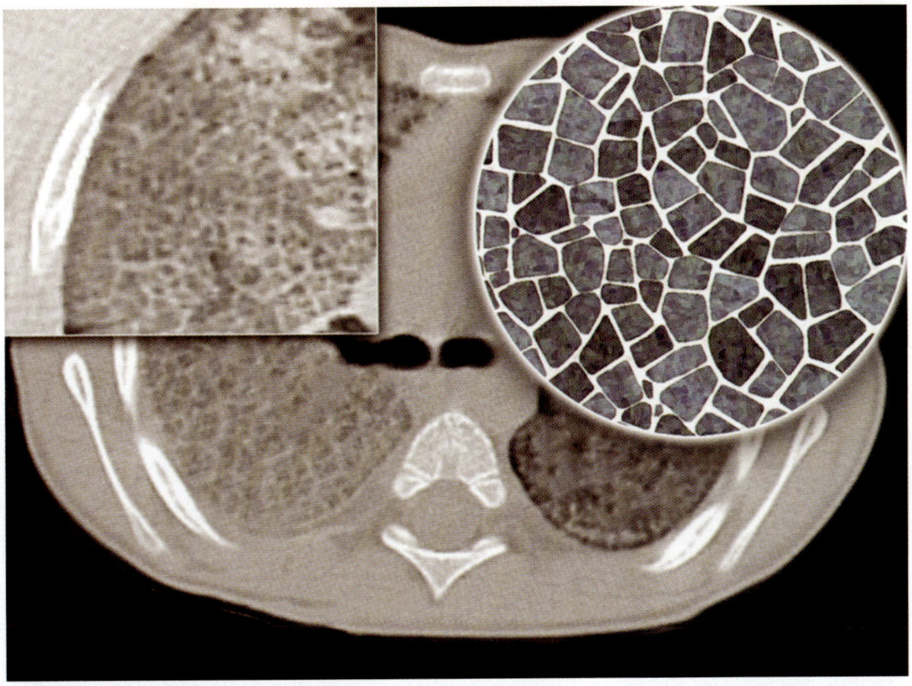

Axial high-resolution computed tomography (HRCT) lung reveals diffuse ground-glass opacities in the bilateral lung parenchyma, with interlobular septal thickening, giving it a crazy paving appearance.

Crazy Paving and Pulmonary Alveolar Proteinosis

Crazy paving is a radiological pattern that can be seen on chest computed tomography (CT) scans, characterized by ground-glass opacities with thickening of the interlobular and intralobular septa. This pattern is non-specific and can be caused by a variety of pathologies:

CRAZY PAVING APPEARANCE

Idiopathic	• Pulmonary alveolar proteinosis (PAP)
	• Organising pneumonia (OP)
	• Non-specific interstitial pneumonia (NSIP)
Infectious	• Pneumocystis carinii pneumonia (PCP)
Cancer	• Mucinous bronchoalveolar carcinoma (BAC)
Inhalational	• Lipoid pneumonia
Miscellaneous	• Acute respiratory distress syndrome (ARDS)
	• Pulmonary oedema
	• pulmonary haemorrhage

PAP is an uncommon disease caused due to abnormal surfactant accumulation in the lungs. Majority of the patients are young to middle-aged adults. PAP is strongly associated with smoking. There is an increased risk of *Nocardia* infection, which could result in brain abscesses. One-third of the cases may lead to pulmonary fibrosis.

Most cases of this condition necessitate therapeutic saline bronchoalveolar lavage, though spontaneous resolution can occasionally occur. GM-CSF supplementation shows varying levels of effectiveness.

OSCE

120

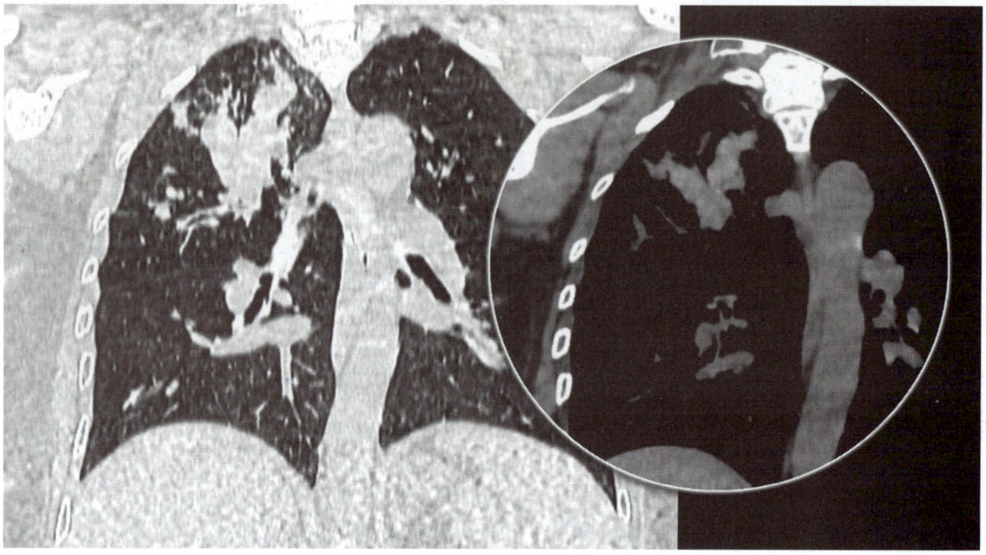

Clinical details: A 30-year-old male patient presenting with long history of chronic cough and wheeze.

1. **Describe the imaging findings seen in the given images.**
2. **What are ASPER criteria?**
3. **What is the characteristic radiological sign seen in the above case?**
4. **What is the distribution of bronchiectasis seen in this pathology?**

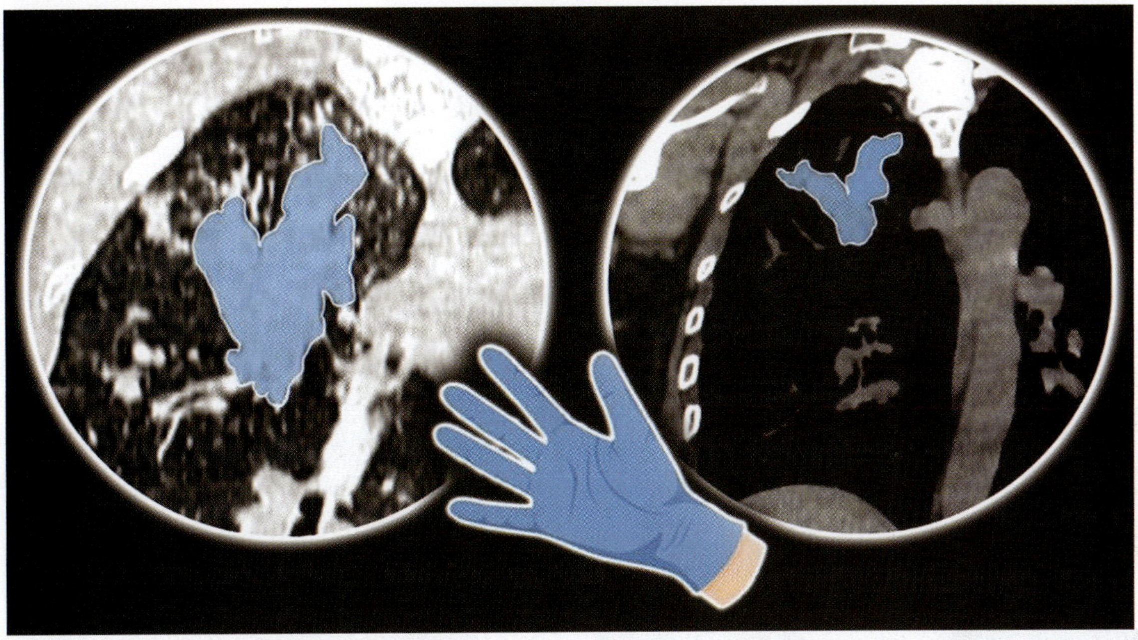

Selected coronal sections of computed tomography (CT) lung with lung window and mediastinal window reveal tubular branching opacities involving the right upper lung, along with surrounding tiny nodules in a case of allergic bronchopulmonary aspergillosis showing the typical finger-in-glove appearance.

Allergic Bronchopulmonary Aspergillosis

Allergic bronchopulmonary aspergillosis (ABPA) is a fungal infection of the lungs that results from an allergic response to *Aspergillus* antigens. It is commonly seen in patients with underlying bronchial asthma or cystic fibrosis.

ASPER criteria include following:

A: Asthma/atopy

S: Serum IgG/IgE against *Aspergillus*

P: Proximal bronchiectasis or central bronchiectasis

E: Elevated levels of IgE (IgE $>$ 1000 ng/mL)

R: Reactive skin test

RADIOLOGICAL FEATURES

- Fleeting lung opacities
- Centrilobular nodules, may show tree in bud appearance
- Bronchiectasis which is characteristically apex the central, upper lobes of lung
- Mucoid impaction may be seen in the form of bronchoceles. This may give rise to the typical finger-in-glove appearance in which the bronchoceles appear as thick tubular branching structures pointing towards the lung hilum.
- Late sequelae are represented by upper lobe predominant fibrotic changes.

OSCE

121

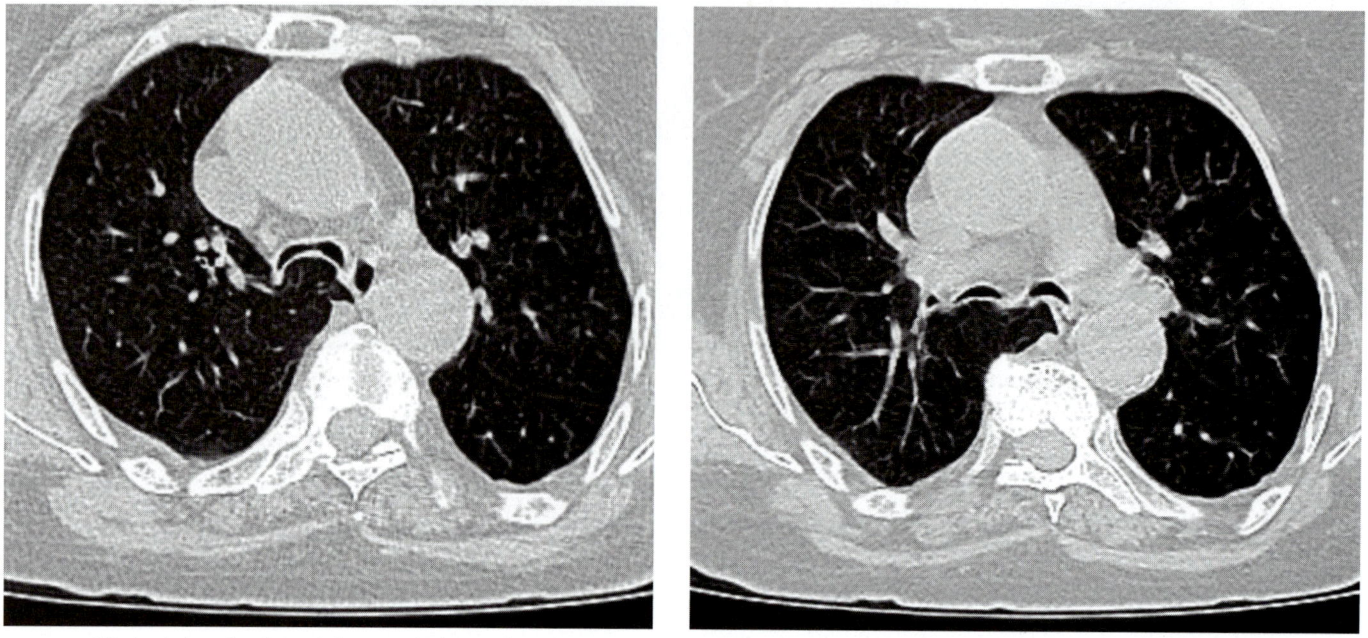

Clinical details: A middle-aged obese female patient presented with a history of chronic dyspnoea and cough.

1. **Describe the findings seen in the provided images.**
2. **What should be the computed tomography (CT) protocol to diagnose this entity?**
3. **Enumerate two causes of tracheomalacia?**
4. **What is the radiation-free alternative that can be used in effacement of the central airway dynamics?**

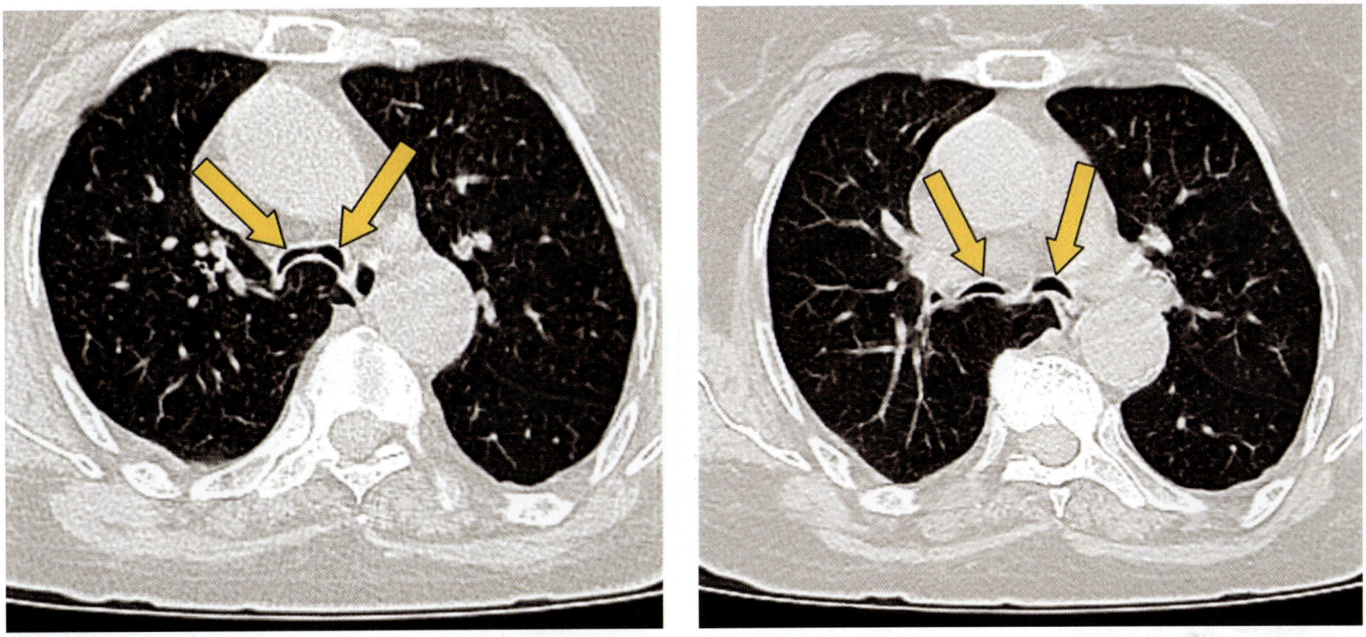

Expiratory axial high-resolution computed tomography (HRCT) thorax images at two different levels demonstrate marked collapse of the trachea and bronchi.

Tracheobronchomalacia

- Tracheobronchomalacia is defined as excessive compressibility of the airways secondary to weakness the tracheal and bronchial walls. If only the trachea is involved, it is known as tracheomalacia.
- Common causes in adults include (1) ageing, (2) chronic airway diseases like asthma and chronic obstructive pulmonary disease (COPD), (3) prolonged intubation like tracheostomy and (4) recurrent or chronic lung infections.
- Causes of congenital tracheomalacia include (1) cystic fibrosis, (2) Mounier-Kuhn syndrome, (3) Marfan syndrome, (4) Ehlers–Danlos syndrome, etc.
- As per recent RadioGraphics article, the exaggerated narrowing of the trachea and bronchial walls is termed as **expiratory central airway collapse (ECAC)**, and it comprises two separate entities, namely **excessive dynamic airway collapse (EDAC)** and **tracheobronchomalacia.**
- There is a cartilaginous weakening of the airway wall in tracheobronchomalacia. In EDAC, there is membranous malacia.

RADIOLOGICAL FEATURES

- Computed tomography (CT) of the lungs in suspected tracheobronchomalacia is ideally performed using a multidetector helical CT scanner. It should include both inspiratory and expiatory phases. During the expiratory phase, there is usually a bowing of the posterior membranous portion of the trachea or bronchial walls forming a crescent-like shape in axial images. During expiration, there should be a decrease in the anterior to posterior diameter of the involved airways by more than 50%. Dynamic CT is considered to be more accurate than a conventional expiratory CT. Images acquired only during inspiration may be totally normal or may reveal of semilunar configuration with mild tracheomegaly.
- Cine magnetic resonance imaging (MRI) is a newer radiation-free alternative that can be used in the assessment of central airways in cases of EDAC and tracheobronchomalacia.

OSCE

122

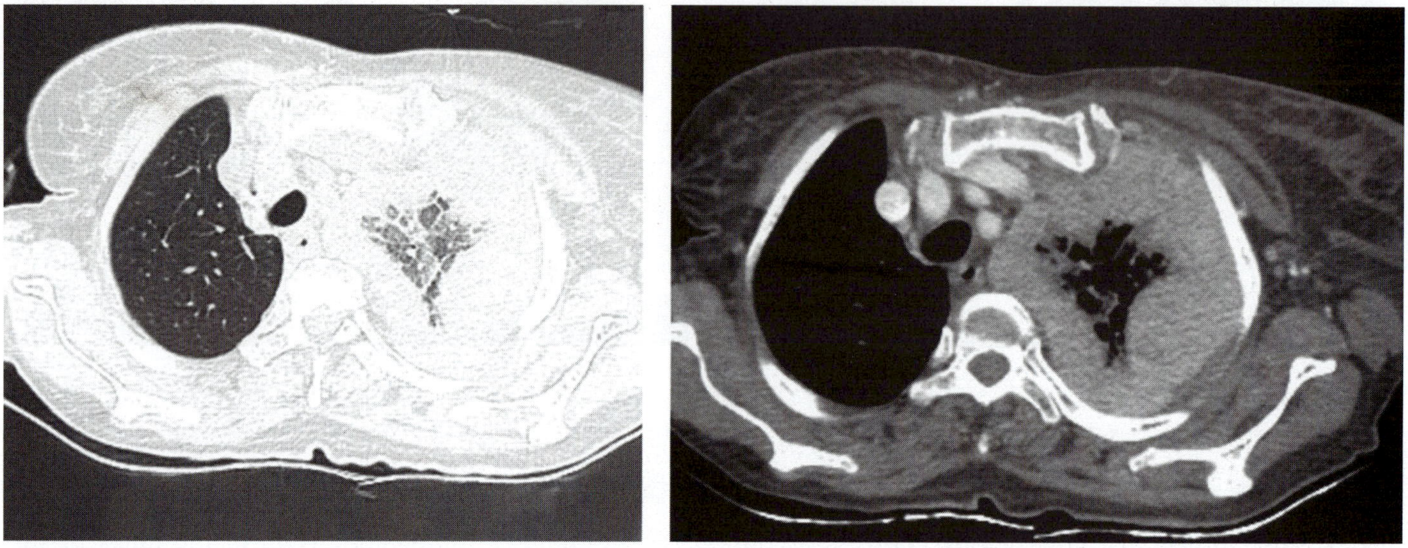

Clinical details: A 60-year-old female presented with chronic dyspnoea, left-sided chest pain and a history of asbestos exposure.

1. **Describe the findings seen in the provided images.**
2. **What is frozen mediastinum sign?**
3. **Which occupational exposure is closely associated with this pathology?**
4. **Apart from the pleura, name one more organ which can be affected by this entity.**

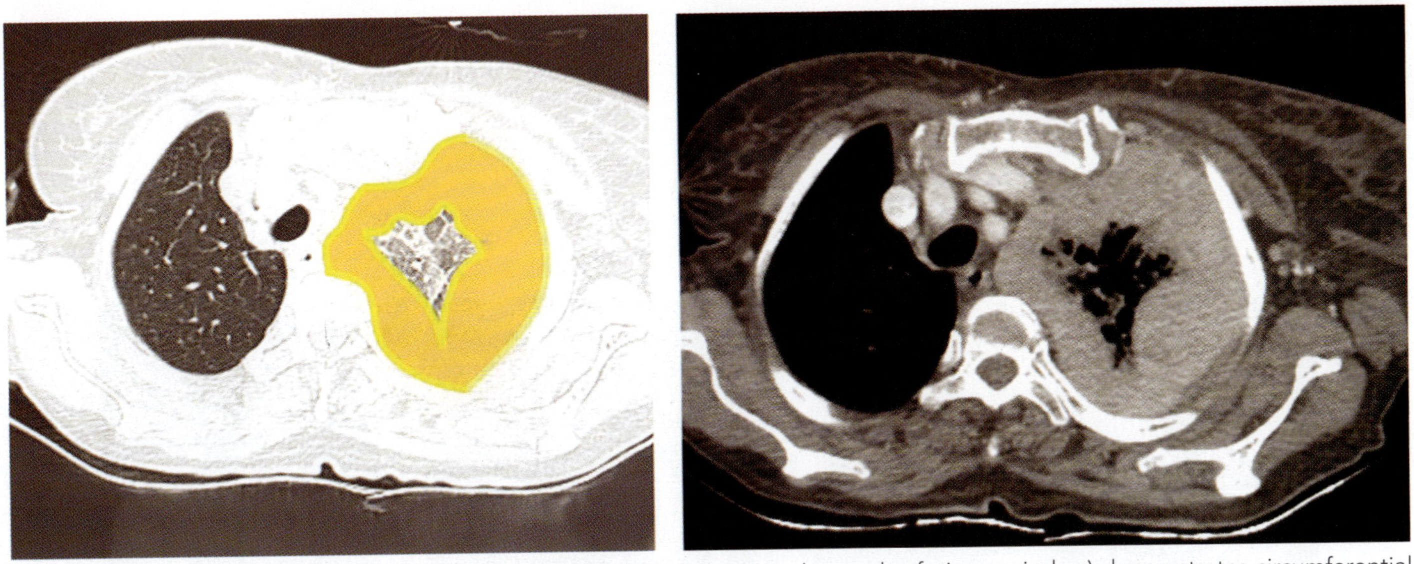

Axial contrast-enhanced computed tomography (CECT) thorax (lung window and soft tissue window) demonstrates circumferential left-sided pleural thickening with a lobulated appearance. The right side appears to be comparatively normal.

Mesothelioma

- Mesothelioma, also called malignant mesothelioma, is the most common primary neoplasm of the pleura. It is a highly malignant neoplasm which most commonly arises from the mesothelial cells. It arises in relation to parietal pleura. It can also be rarely seen in the peritoneum, pericardium or tunica vaginalis of the testis.
- Unilateral pleural thickening in a patient with a significant history of asbestos exposure is indicative of mesothelioma. However, not all types of asbestos fibres are associated with mesothelioma. The crocidolite type of asbestos fibres is the most common culprit. Even the family members of those working in the asbestos industry have an increased risk of developing mesotheliomas. There is usually a 20–40-year latency period between the exposure of asbestos and the development of mesothelioma. Women are more likely to develop non-asbestos-related peritoneal mesothelioma. Persistent pleural irritation, prior radiation, simian virus 40 and erionite exposure are the other risk factors.
- Histologically, three types are identified: Epithelioid type (60%–80%), sarcomatous type (10%–15%) and the mixed type (10%–25%).

RADIOLOGICAL FEATURES

- Radiographs may show concentric unilateral pleural thickening with pleural effusion. Computed tomography (CT) commonly reveals unilateral nodular concentric pleural thickening, which can involve the fissures as well. Calcifications may be seen in 20% of the cases. Despite the presence of significant pleural thickening/effusion, the affected hemithorax may be normal in volume without any definite mediastinal shift. This frozen appearance of the mediastinum/hemithorax is termed as the 'frozen mediastinum sign' or the 'frozen hemithorax sign'.
- Metastatic adenocarcinoma of the pleura is a differential which cannot be differentiated from mesothelioma on imaging alone.

OSCE

123

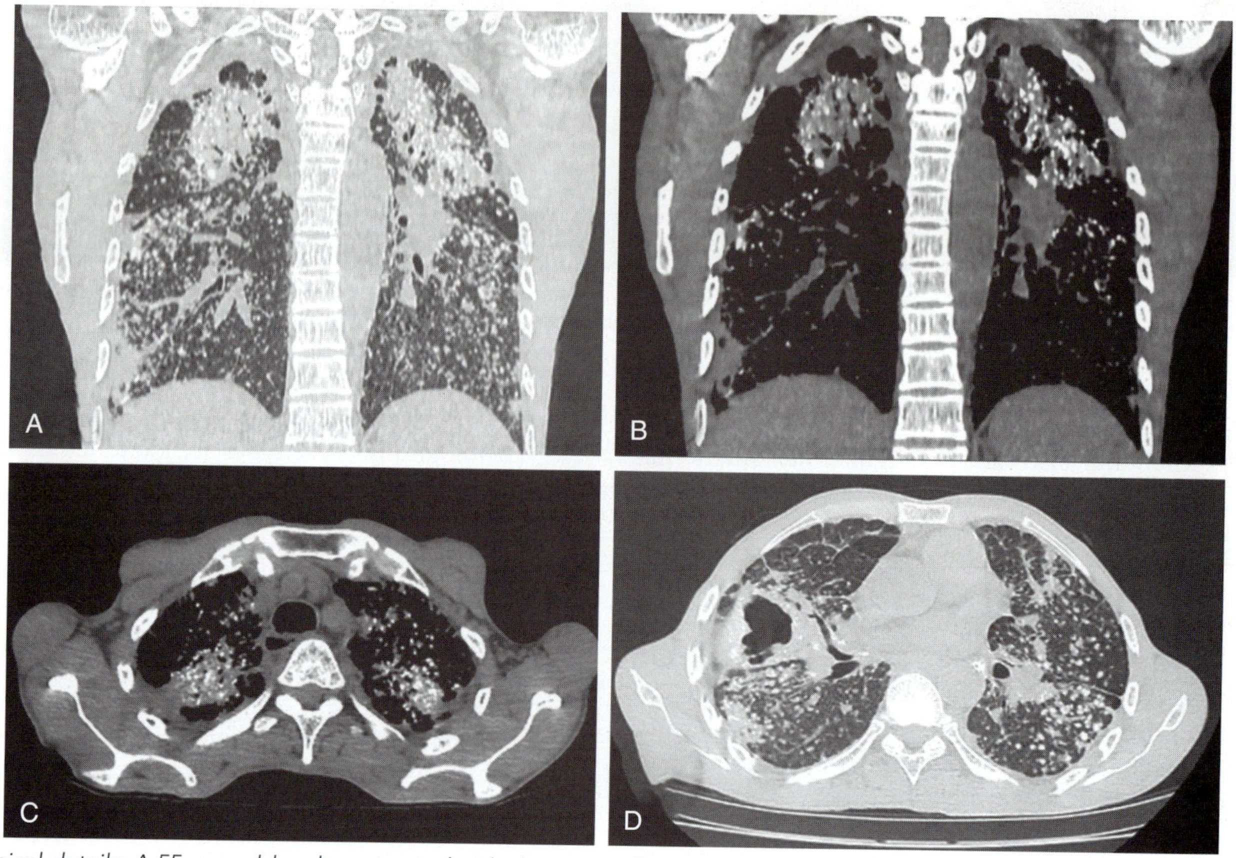

Clinical details: A 55-year-old male presented with shortness of breath and chronic fever with a long history of quarrying.

1. **Describe the imaging findings observed in the provided images.**
2. **What is the most appropriate diagnosis?**
3. **List three causes of egg-shell calcifications in lymph nodes.**
4. **What is Caplan's syndrome?**

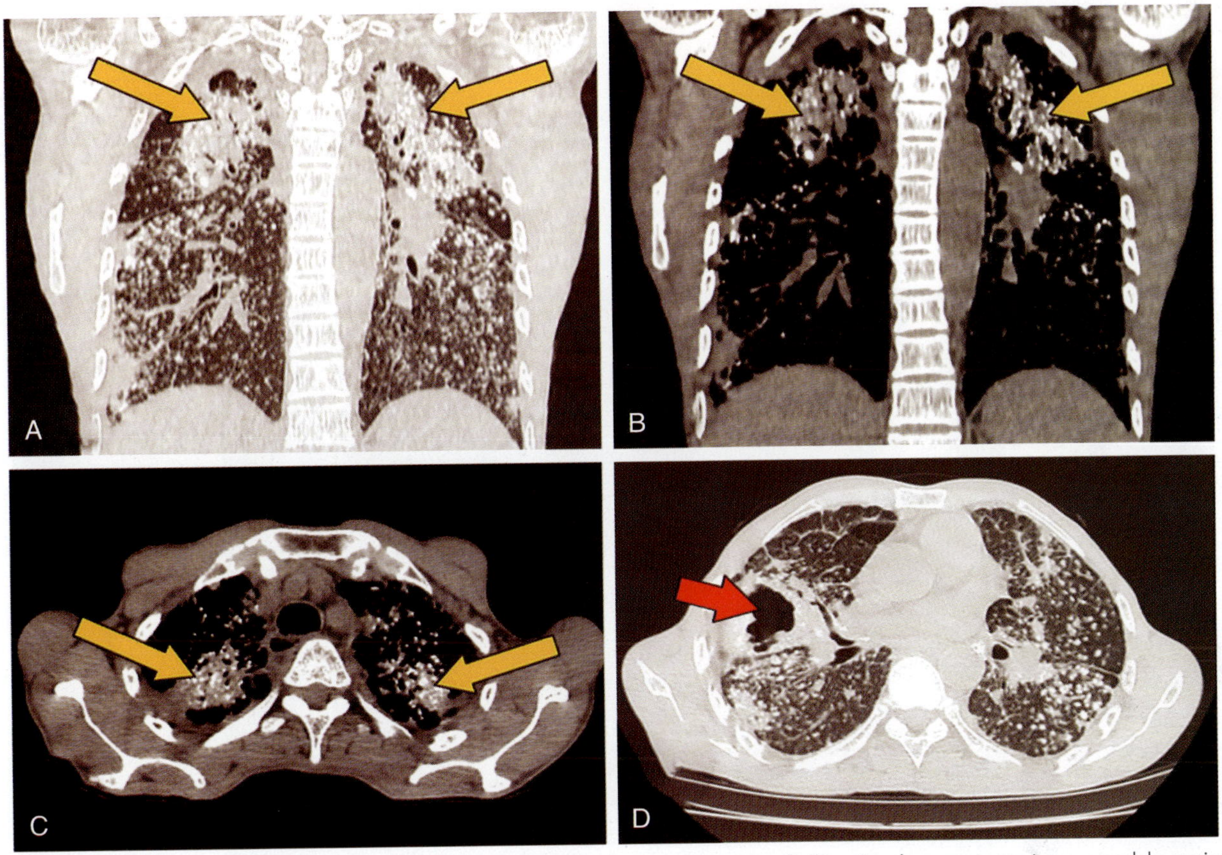

(A–D) Coronal and axial sections of computed tomography (CT) thorax in a case of silicosis, demonstrate innumerable variable-sized nodules with tiny calcifications scattered in the bilateral lungs, with mass-like patchy opacities in the bilateral upper lobes. Additionally, (D) there is a lung cavity in the right upper lobe, indicating concomitant tuberculosis.

Silicotuberculosis and Progressive Massive Fibrosis

- Pneumoconiosis is defined as a spectrum of lung diseases which are caused due to the inhalation of dust particles. Examples include asbestosis, silicosis, coal workers pneumoconiosis, siderosis, berylliosis, baritosis, stannosis and talcosis.
- Silicosis is a fibrotic type of pneumoconiosis which results from inhalation of fine particles of silica, specifically in individuals working in mines, quarries, tunnelling or the sandblasting industry.

RADIOLOGICAL FEATURES

- Typical findings of classic silicosis include multiple bilateral perilymphatic nodular opacities and multifocal patchy consolidations. There is a predilection of the upper two-thirds of the lungs. With advancing disease, the nodules may increase in size and may coalesce to form mass-like opacities. Egg-shell type of calcification is seen in the hilar and mediastinal lymph nodes.

PROGRESSIVE MASSIVE FIBROSIS

- Progressive massive fibrosis (PMF) refers to the mass-like conglomeration of nodules seen in the upper lobes of lung, in cases of silicosis and coal workers pneumoconiosis. These mass-like areas are commonly located in the posterior aspects of the upper lobes and contain calcifications. There may be progressive shrinkage and migration towards the hila overtime.
- Silicosis patients have a higher risk of developing pulmonary tuberculosis.
- Silicosis may be associated with connective tissue diseases:

Caplan's syndrome	Rheumatoid arthritis (RA) + necrobiotic nodules + silicosis
Erasmus syndrome	Systemic sclerosis (SSc) + silicosis

- Egg-shell type of calcifications is seen: Silicosis, coal workers pneumoconiosis, sarcoidosis, treated lymphoma and rarely amyloidosis, blastomycosis and histoplasmosis.

OSCE

124

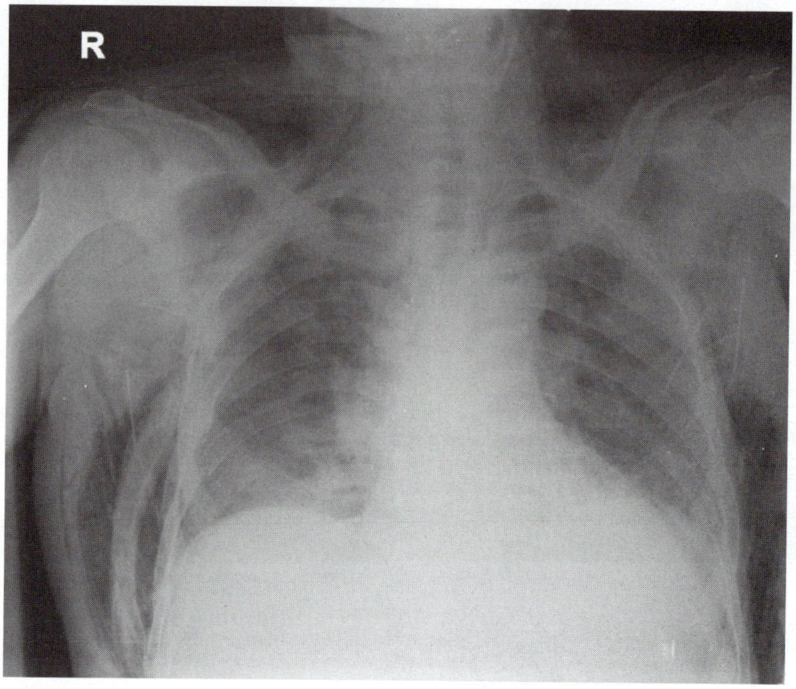

Clinical details: A middle-aged patient presented to the accident and emergency department.

1. **Describe the findings seen in the above radiograph.**
2. **What is 'ginkgo leaf sign'?**
3. **Define flail chest.**
4. **Name one infective cause of subcutaneous emphysema.**

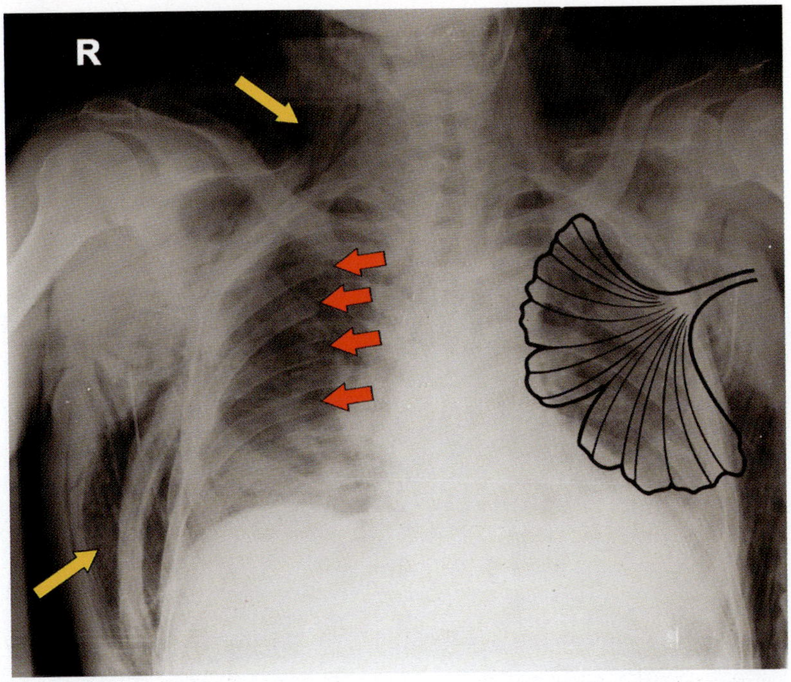

Frontal chest radiograph demonstrates multiple right-sided rib fractures (*red arrows*) and marked subcutaneous oedema from neck to visualized thorax (*yellow arrows*). On the left side, the classic ginkgo-leaf sign of subcutaneous emphysema is demonstrated.

Subcutaneous Emphysema

- Subcutaneous emphysema (surgical emphysema) is defined as the presence of air within the subcutaneous soft tissues.
- It can be secondary to significant penetrating trauma, infection by gas forming organisms (necrotizing fasciitis), iatrogenic causes such as insertion of chest drainage tube and internal causes such as pneumothorax and pneumomediastinum.

RADIOLOGICAL FEATURES

- On a plain radiograph, it is visualized as linear streaky lucencies involving the subcutaneous soft tissues. The ginkgo leaf sign in chest is a radiographic finding that is seen in extensive subcutaneous emphysema of the chest wall. Air infiltrates the fibres of the pectoralis major muscle, creating a branching pattern of lucency that resembles the ginkgo leaf. On the computed tomography (CT) scan, the lung window is much better than soft tissue windows in visualizing subcutaneous air. CT can also reveal a small pneumothorax or pneumomediastinum, which might have been missed on the radiograph.
- Flail chest is characterized by the fracture of three or more consecutive ribs at two or more locations. It may be associated with underlying pulmonary contusions or lacerations, pneumothorax and subcutaneous emphysema.

[Note: Not to be confused with the Ginkgo leaf sign of spinal meningioma.]

OSCE

125

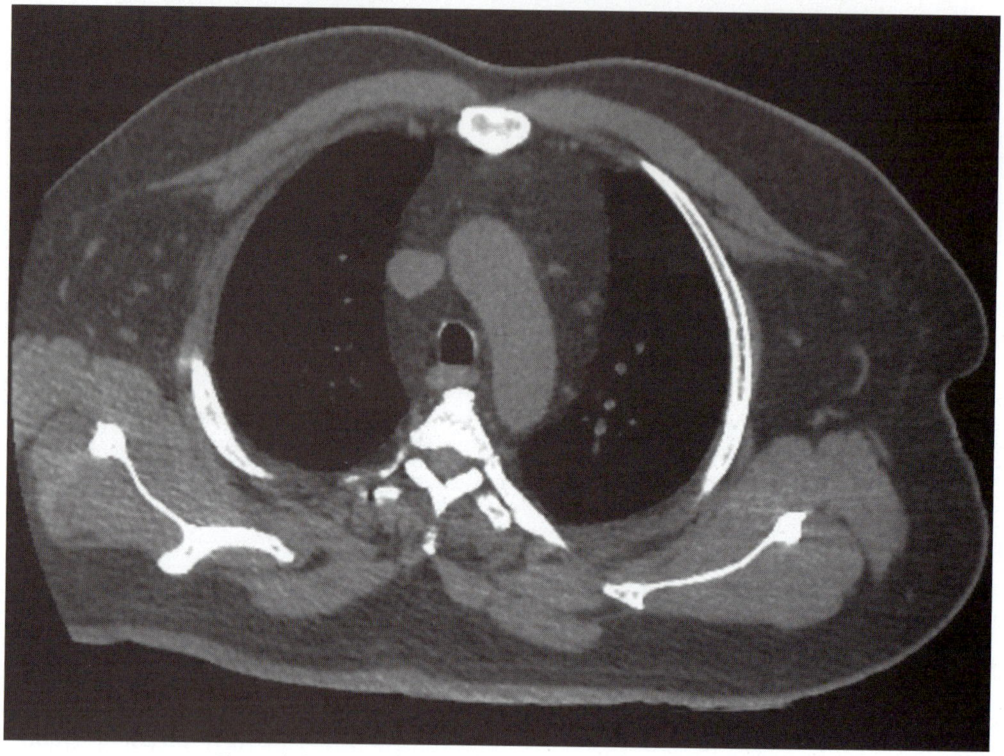

Clinical details: Incidental finding in an obese patient.

1. **Describe the findings seen in the provided image.**
2. **What is the most appropriate diagnosis?**
3. **Other than obesity, list two more associations with this entity.**
4. **What is Madelung disease?**

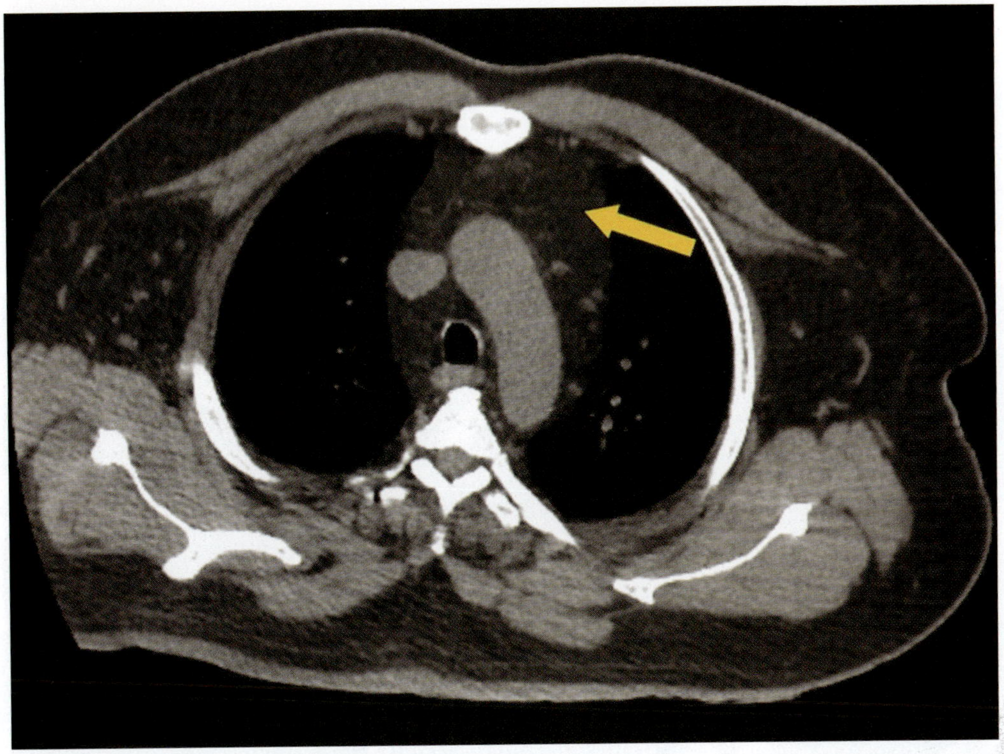

Axial computed tomography (CT) thorax demonstrates an excessive amount of unencapsulated fat involving the upper mediastinum, sharply outlining the mediastinal vascular structures.

Mediastinal Lipomatosis

- Mediastinal lipomatosis is a benign condition characterized by the deposition of excessive amount of unencapsulated fat in the mediastinum. The upper mediastinum is more commonly involved.
- The common associations include obesity, Cushing's syndrome, diabetes, hyperlipidaemia and usage of steroids. Mediastinal lipomatosis is usually asymptomatic, but in some cases, it may cause respiratory distress.

RADIOLOGICAL FEATURES

- On the plain frontal chest radiograph, it is seen as bilateral asymmetrical mediastinal widening. On the computed tomography (CT) scan, it is depicted as diffuse and homogeneous unencapsulated fat deposition in the mediastinum.
- Madelung disease, also known as lipomatosis of the neck, is a benign condition characterized by the presence of multiple areas of increased fat deposition involving the neck. It should not be confused with Madelung deformity, in which there is a radial bowing and shortening of the distal radius, with increased intraosseous space.

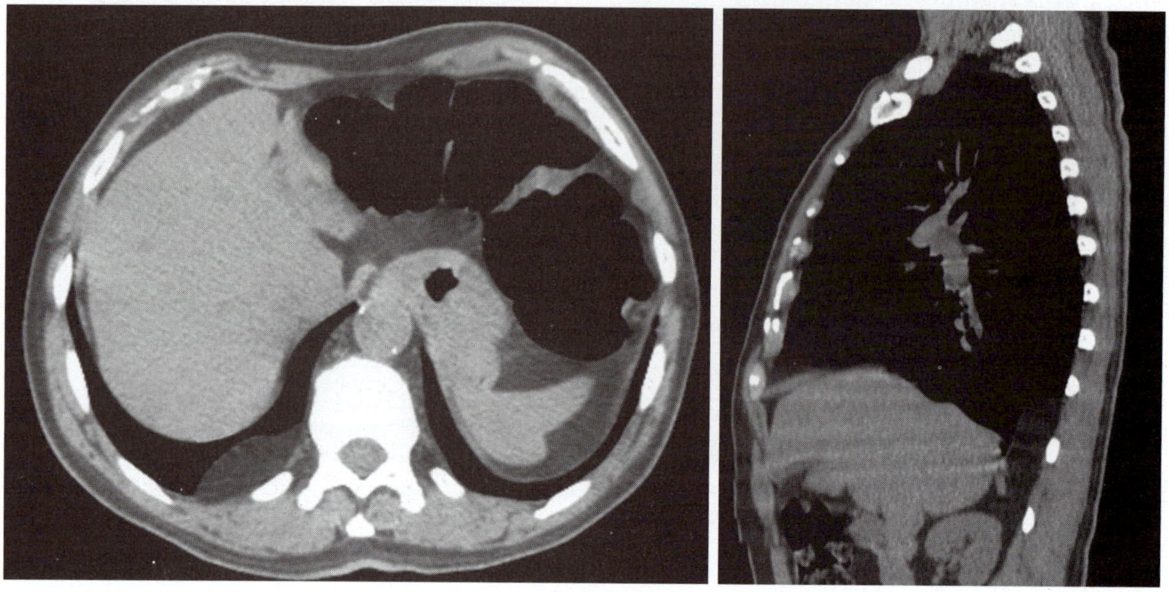

Clinical details: Incidental finding in an adult male patient.

1. **Describe the imaging findings.**
2. **What is the most appropriate diagnosis?**
3. **What are the types of congenital diaphragmatic hernias (CDHs) based on location?**
4. **Enumerate two differences between these types.**

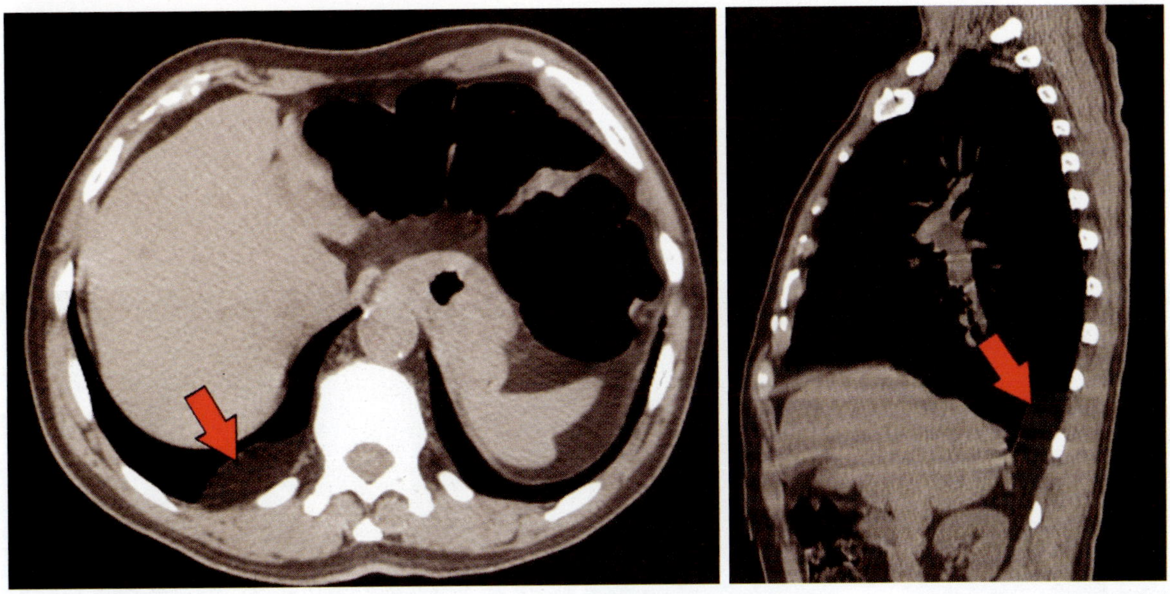

Axial and sagittal computed tomography (CT) thorax demonstrates herniation of peritoneal fat through a congenital defect in the posterior aspect of the right hemidiaphragm.

Bochdalek and Morgagni Hernia

- Congenital diaphragmatic hernias (CDHs) can be classified based on location into two types, namely Bochdalek hernia and Morgagni hernia.
- Bochdalek hernias are the most common type of CDH, usually occurring on the left side. They develop through the pleuroperitoneal canals, which are situated just lateral to the spine on either side of the body.
- Morgagni hernia is a type of retrosternal or parasternal hernia, representing approximately 2% of CDHs. It occurs when there is a protrusion through the Morgagni foramen, which is located adjacent to the xiphoid process.

Bochdalek Hernia	Morgagni Hernia
• Commonly posterolateral in location	• Commonly anterior in location
• More common on the left side	• More prominent on the right side
• Usually presents earlier in life	• Presents later in life
• Overall, more common than Morgagni hernia	• Less common than Bochdalek hernia
• Can be associated with ipsilateral pulmonary hypoplasia and congenital heart disease	• Can be associated with congenital heart disease

OSCE

127

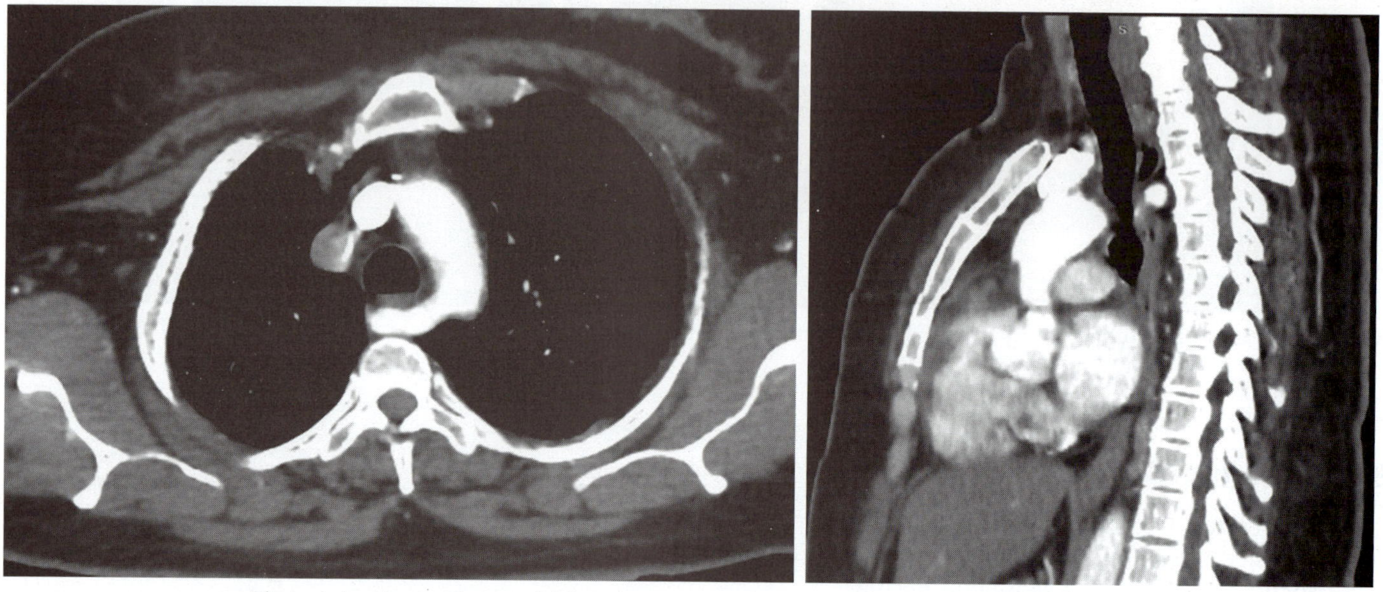

Clinical details: A 48-year-old female presented with longstanding mild dysphagia.

1. **Describe your findings in the provided images.**
2. **What is the most appropriate diagnosis?**
3. **What is diverticulum of Kommerell?**
4. **What is dysphagia lusoria?**

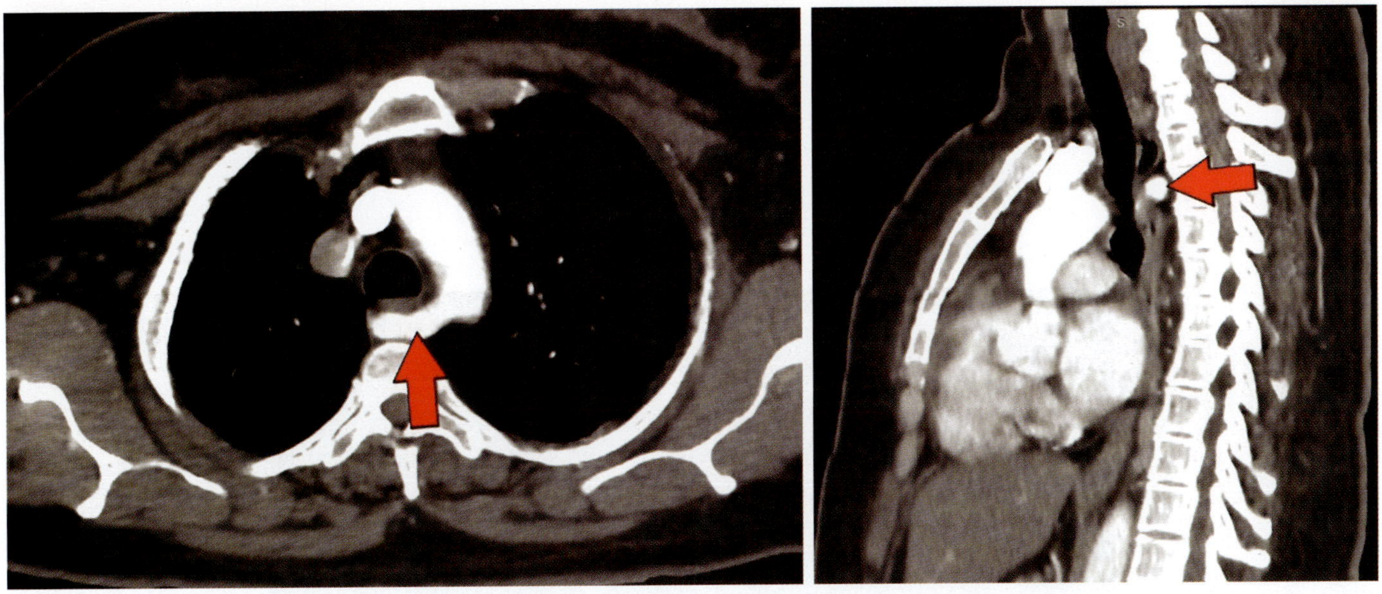

Axial and coronal post-contrast computed tomography (CT) images demonstrate the aberrant origin and course of the right subclavian artery from the distal left aortic arch and courses towards the right side and posterior to the oesophagus.

Aberrant Right Subclavian Artery

- Aberrant right subclavian artery (ARSA) is an aortic arch anomaly, in which there is an anomalous origin and course of the right subclavian artery. The ARSA arises from the distal left aortic arch, as the last branch of the aorta, and passes towards the right side.
- It passes posterior to the oesophagus in the majority of cases and may cause dysphagia in some cases, known as dysphagia lusoria. Diverticulum of Kommerell is the dilatation of the proximal ARSA seen in some cases of ARSA. Barium swallow (upper gastrointestinal [GI] contrast study) may show narrowing of the oesophagus at the level of the aortic arch without any mucosal irregularity.

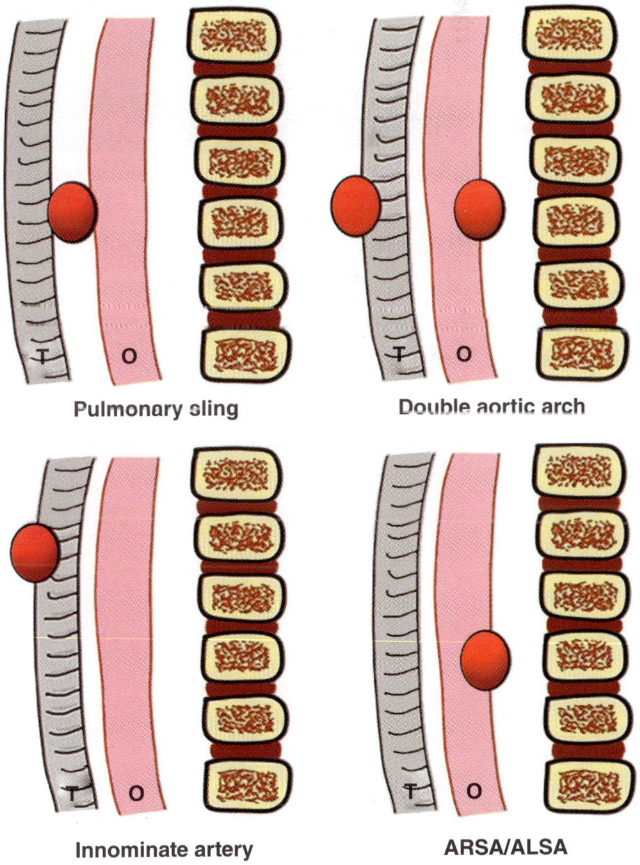

Vascular impressions

OSCE

128

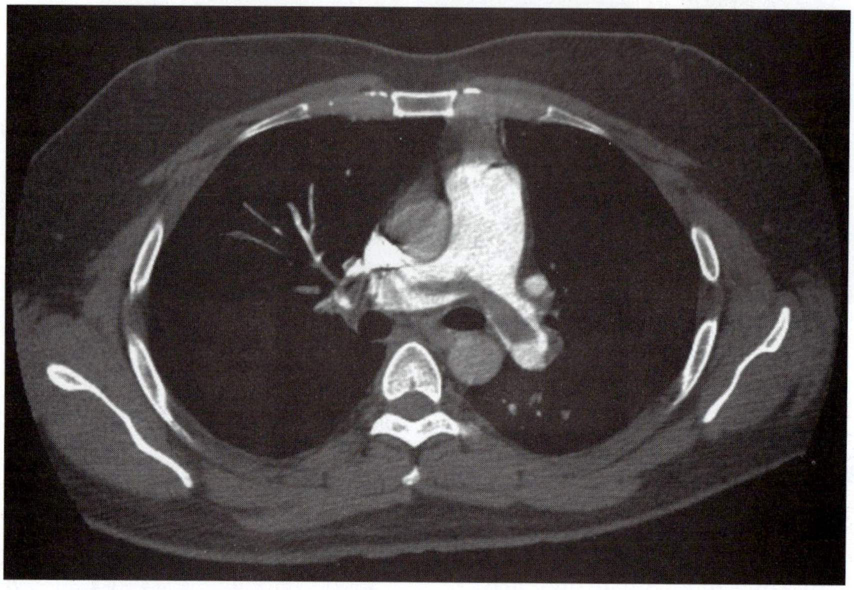

Clinical details: A middle-aged patient presented with acute dyspnoea, chest pain and palpitations.

1. **Identify the investigation performed.**
2. **Describe the findings seen in the image provided.**
3. **What is the most appropriate diagnosis?**
4. **What is 'Polo mint sign'?**

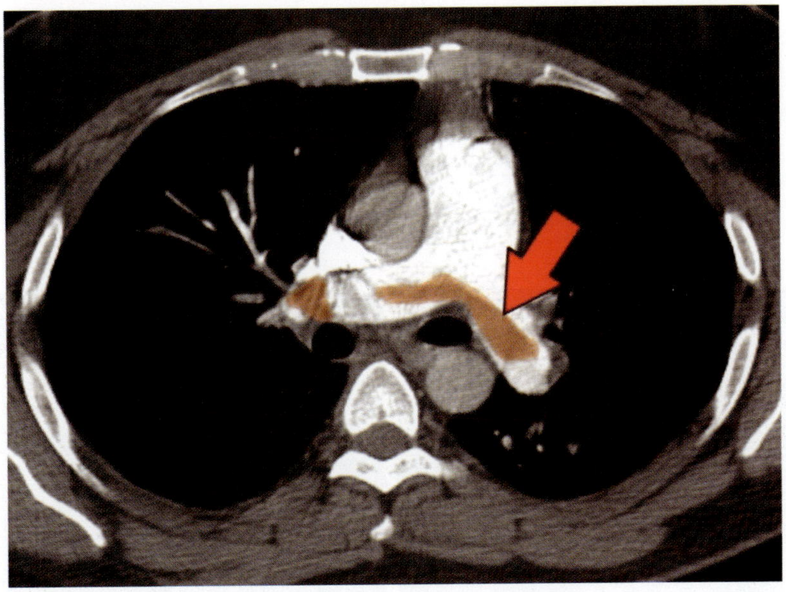

Axial computed tomography (CT) pulmonary angiography reveals saddle-shaped pulmonary embolism involving the pulmonary artery bifurcation and the bilateral main pulmonary arteries.

Pulmonary Embolism

- Pulmonary embolism (PE) is a clinical emergency in which characterized by the occlusion of the pulmonary artery or its branches by an embolus. This may be acute or chronic.
- Acute pulmonary emboli can be detected on computed tomography pulmonary angiography (CTPA), which reveals filling defects in the pulmonary arteries. A narrow ring of contrast, called the Polo mint sign, surrounds the central filling defect (thrombus) when the artery is seen in its axial plane on CTPA.
- A large PE that spans the pulmonary trunk's bifurcation and extends into the left and right pulmonary arteries is frequently referred to as a saddle PE. It can block both the left and right pulmonary arteries if it is large enough, causing right heart failure.

RADIOLOGICAL FEATURES

CHEST RADIOGRAPH SIGNS

Westermark sign: Focal area of hyperlucency (due to oligaemia) distal to the occluded artery.

Fleischner sign: Pulmonary artery enlargement due to the thrombus.

Hampton hump: Peripheral wedge-shaped lung opacity signifying lung infarct.

Chang sign: Dilatation of right descending pulmonary artery with an abrupt cut-off.

Palla's sign: Enlargement of the right descending pulmonary artery.

Acute PE	Chronic PE
Central filling defect (Polo mint sign and tram-track sign)	Eccentric filling defect
Hypodense thrombus (mean attenuation value lower 33 HU ±15)	Hyperdense thrombus (mean attenuation value higher 87 HU +30)
Increased diameter of the involved pulmonary artery	Reduced diameter of the involved pulmonary artery
–	Intraluminal webs or bands
–	Bronchial artery collateral formation
Pulmonary parenchyma shows infarct	Mosaic attenuation

- Although D-dimer is highly sensitive for the evaluation of PE and has a high negative predictive value, it has a high false positive rate.

OSCE

129

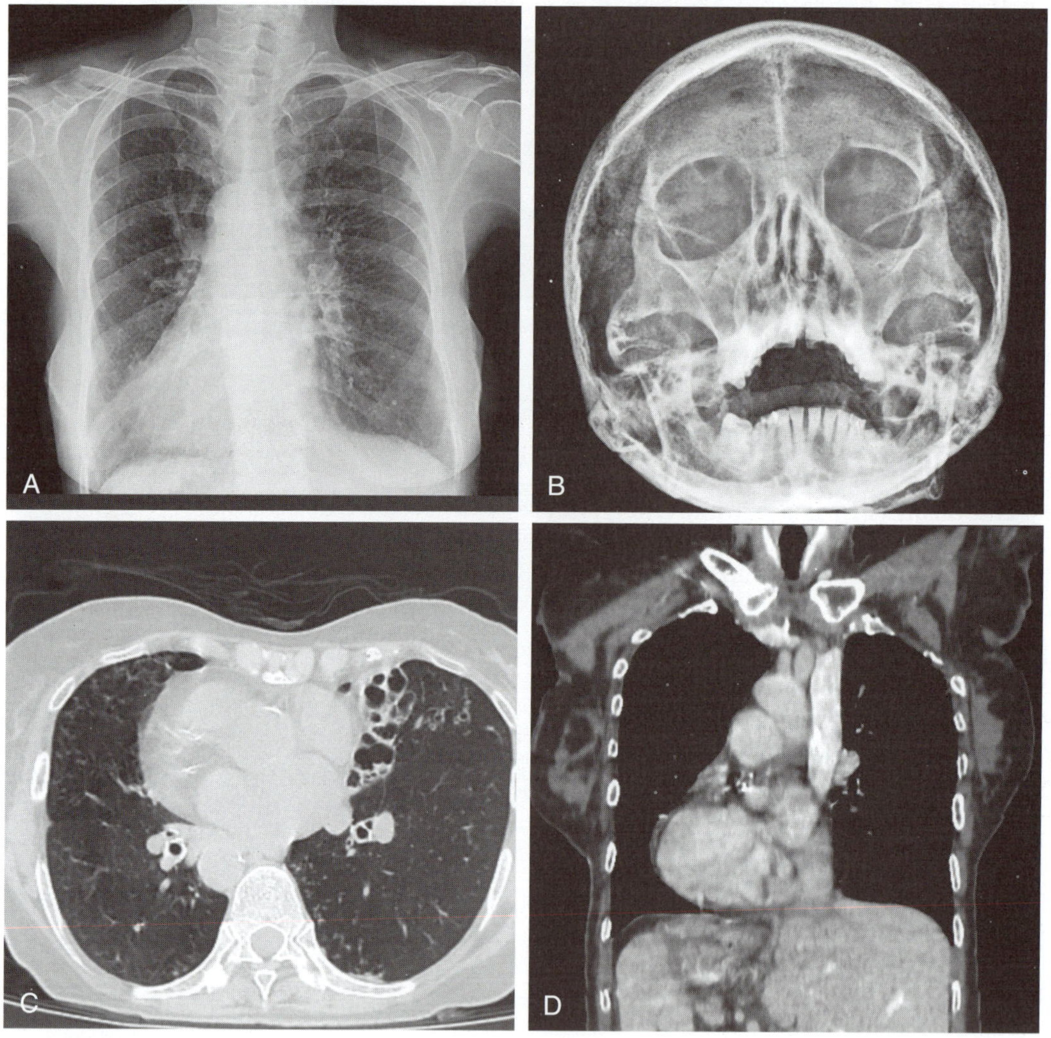

Clinical details: A middle-aged woman presented with a history of recurrent upper and lower respiratory tract infections.

1. **Describe the findings in the provided images.**
2. **What is the most appropriate diagnosis?**
3. **What is the inheritance pattern?**
4. **List two causes of upper lobe bronchiectasis and two causes of lower lobe bronchiectasis.**

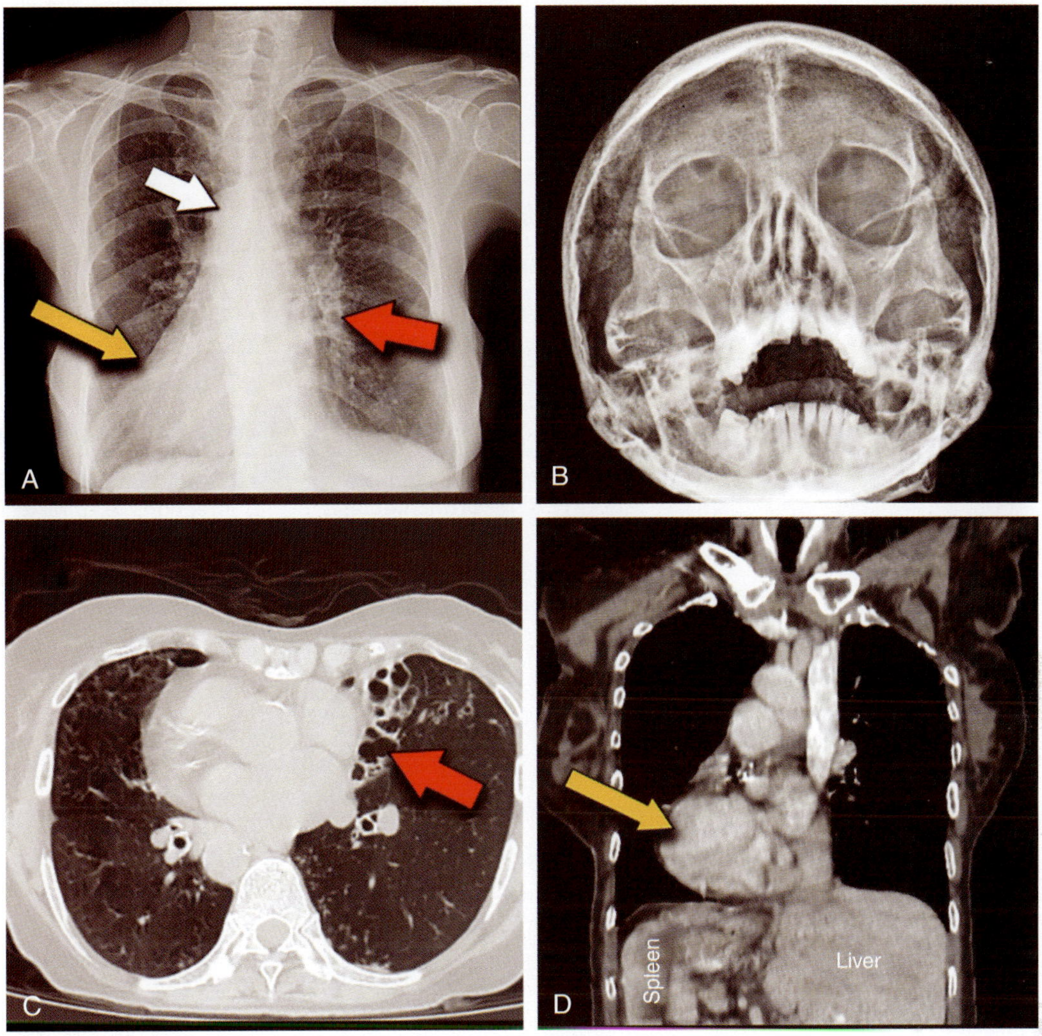

(A) Frontal chest radiograph shows dextrocardia (*yellow arrow*), right aortic arch (*white arrow*) and bronchiectasis (*red arrow*). Additionally, multiple small nodular opacities are present in bilateral lung fields.
(B) Frontal skull radiograph (Waters view) reveals bilateral opacified maxillary sinuses. Frontal and maxillary sinuses appear opacified/hypoplastic.
(C) Axial computed tomography (CT) thorax in lung window demonstrates bronchiectasis involving the lingula (*red arrow*). Tiny nodular opacities are also seen. Note the right-sided descending thoracic aorta.
(D) Coronal CT thorax in mediastinal window shows dextrocardia (*yellow arrow*), left-sided liver and right-sided spleen (total situs inversus).

Kartagener Syndrome

Kartagener syndrome, a subset of primary ciliary dyskinesia, manifests as an autosomal recessive disorder characterized by abnormal ciliary structure/function, resulting in compromised mucociliary clearance.

Kartagener syndrome is distinguished by a clinical triad of:

1. Situs inversus
2. Bronchiectasis
3. Chronic sinusitis with or without nasal polyps

Infertility is observed in males, while females have subfertility. Notably, there is no discernible gender predilection.

RADIOLOGICAL FEATURES

X-ray features:

- Situs inversus
- Bronchiectasis and bronchial wall thickening, mucous plugging with 'finger in glove sign' may be seen
- Predilection for right middle, lingular segment of left upper lobe and lower lobes
- Areas of consolidation
- X-ray paranasal sinuses (PNS) may show sinus opacification

Computed tomography features:

- Situs inversus
- Bronchiectasis
- Areas of consolidation
- Mucous plugging with mucoceles, tree-in-bud pattern/centrilobular nodules indicating mucous impaction and infection
- Mosaic perfusion may be seen
- Computed tomography (CT) PNS may show chronic sinusitis

BRONCHIECTASIS

Upper lobe bronchiectasis	• Cystic fibrosis • Tuberculosis
Lower lobe bronchiectasis	• Post infective bronchiectasis • Pulmonary aspiration diseases • Primary ciliary dyskinesia/Kartagener syndrome
Central bronchiectasis	• Allergic bronchopulmonary aspergillosis (ABPA) • Cystic fibrosis • Mounier-Kuhn syndrome
Middle lobe bronchiectasis	• Non-tuberculous mycobacterial infections (e.g. MAC infection)

OSCE

130

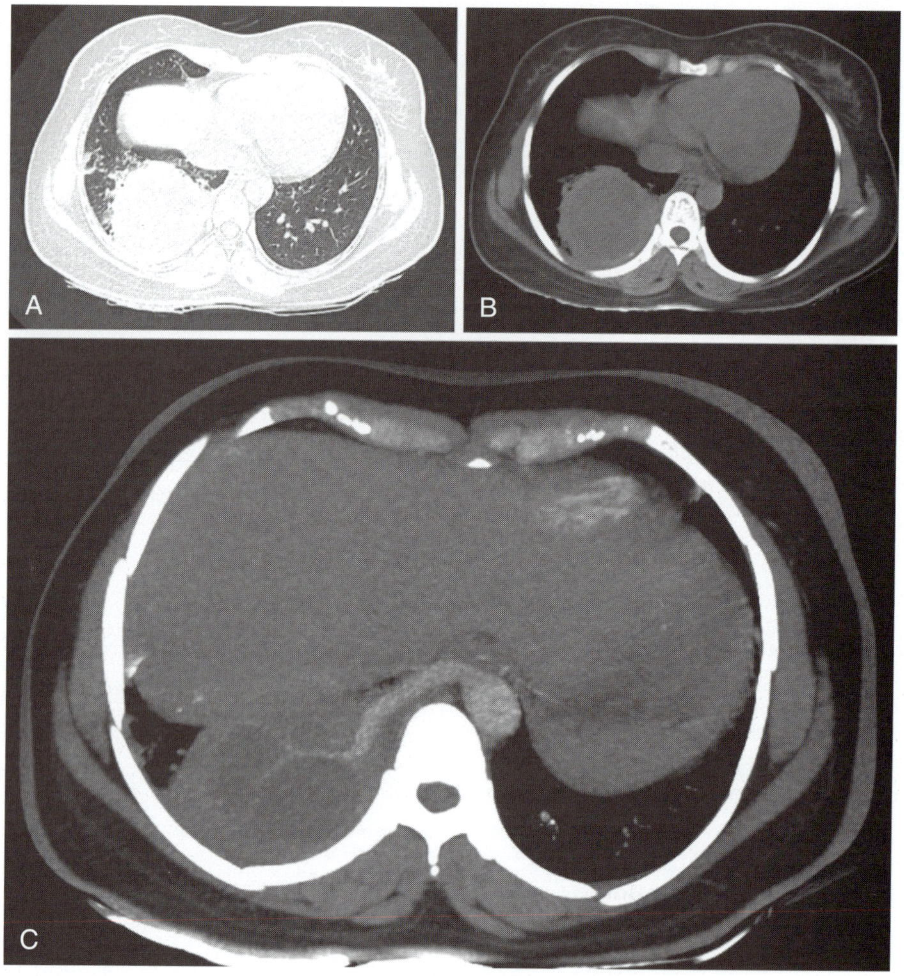

Clinical details: A female patient presented with recurrent chest infections since childhood.

1. **Describe the findings and the most appropriate diagnosis.**
2. **List three differentiating points between intralobar and extralobar sequestration.**
3. **What is 'hybrid lesion'?**
4. **What is the treatment? What is the scope of interventional radiology?**

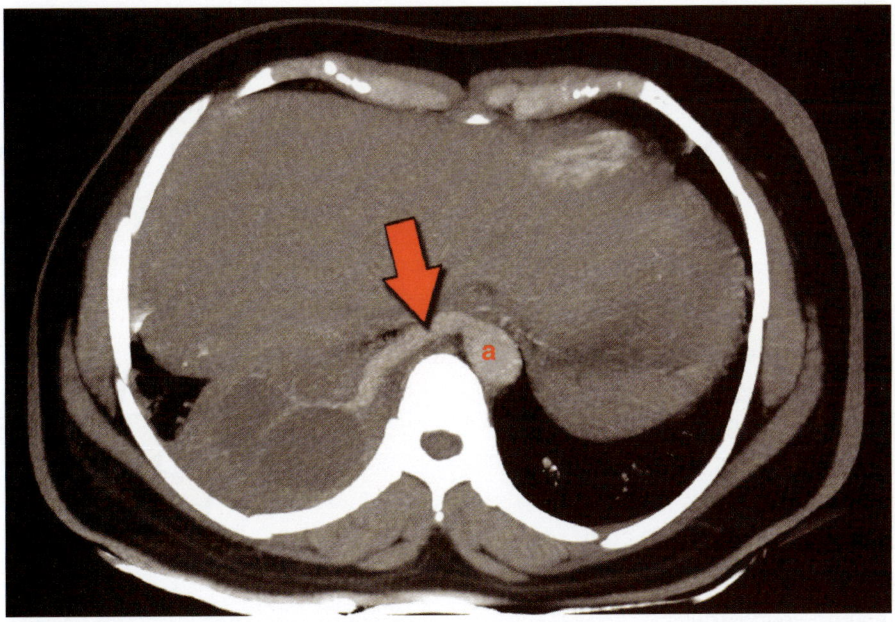

Axial contrast-enhanced computed tomography (CECT) thorax shows a rounded abscess with an aberrant feeding artery (*red arrow*) from the descending thoracic aorta. No bronchial supply observed. The venous drainage was from the right inferior pulmonary vein (not shown). Features are consistent with intralobar type of lung sequestration.

Bronchopulmonary Sequestration (Lung Sequestration)

- Bronchopulmonary sequestration is a congenital anomaly characterized by aberrant pulmonary tissue devoid of normal connections with the bronchial tree or pulmonary arteries. It can be categorized as intralobar or extralobar, with arterial supply originating from either the thoracic or abdominal aorta, and venous drainage either via the pulmonary or systemic veins.
- Clinical presentations vary, encompassing recurrent chest infections, bronchiectasis, haemoptysis or presenting as an asymptomatic lung mass.

RADIOLOGICAL FEATURES

- On antenatal ultrasound, it can be seen as an echogenic mass. Colour Doppler may help in identifying the feeding artery from the aorta.
- Chest X-ray (CXR) reveals a persistent lower lung opacity, frequently situated on the left side. Air bronchograms may be present.
- Computed tomography (CT) with contrast (contrast-enhanced CT [CECT]) or angiography (CTA) provides an optimal delineation of the arterial and venous vascular anatomy. It also helps differentiate between intralobar and extralobar sequestration.
- Traditionally, bronchopulmonary sequestration has been treated with surgical resection. Recent advances include successful trials of coil embolization as a minimally invasive alternative. Spontaneous involution, though rare, has been reported.

Intralobar Sequestration	Extralobar Sequestration
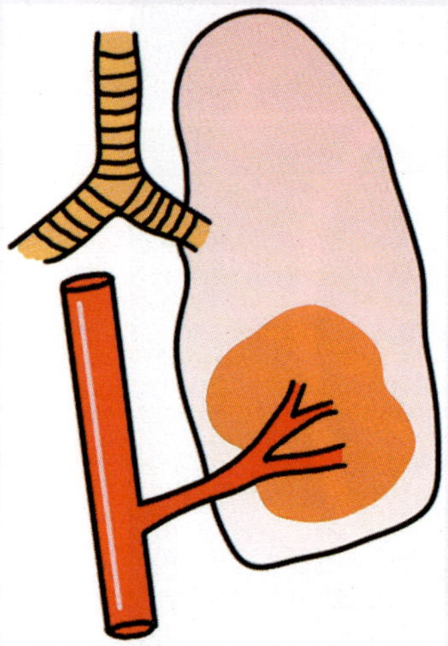	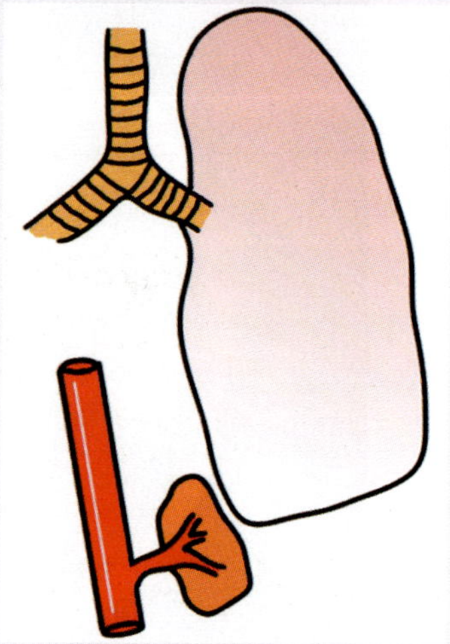
More common (75%)	Less common (25%)
Presents in older children and young adults	Presents in neonates
History of recurrent chest infections/pneumonia	Neonates present with dyspnoea, cyanosis and failure to thrive
Usually located in the left lower lobe	Usually left sided, situated between the lower lobe and left diaphragm
No separate pleural covering, aeration via pores of Kohn	Has a pleural covering but no aeration
Venous drainage supply is by the pulmonary veins	Venous drainage supply is by the systemic veins
Associated anomalies are uncommon	Associated anomalies are common: Congenital lobar emphysema (CLE), CCAM and bronchogenic cysts

Note: Both have arterial supply by aorta (thoracic or abdominal aorta)

FURTHER READING

OSCE 1

Bushberg, et al. *The essentials of physics and medical imaging.* Williams & Wilkins Publisher.
Bushong, S. C. (2008). *Radiologic science for technologists: Physics, biology, and protection* (9th ed.). Mosby Elsevier.
Christensen's physics of diagnostic radiology (4th ed.).
Farr's physics for medical imaging (2nd ed.).
Dr. Satyendra Raghuwanshi, et al. *Radiology without tears* (3rd ed., Vol. I).

OSCE 2

Bushberg, et al. *The essentials of physics and medical imaging.* Williams & Wilkins Publisher.
Christensen's physics of diagnostic radiology (4th ed.).
Farr's physics for medical imaging (2nd ed.).
Dr. Satyendra Raghuwanshi, et al. *Radiology without tears* (3rd ed., Vol. I).

OSCE 3

Bushberg, et al. *The essentials of physics and medical imaging.* Williams & Wilkins Publisher.
Christensen's physics of diagnostic radiology (4th ed.).
Farr's physics for medical imaging (2nd ed.).
Dr. Satyendra Raghuwanshi, et al. *Radiology without tears* (3rd ed., Vol. I).

OSCE 4

Bushberg, J. T., Seibert, J. A., Leidholdt, E. M., Jr., et al. *The essential physics of medical imaging.* LWW. ISBN:0781780578.
Sprawls, P. *Physical principles of medical imaging.* Aspen Publishing. ISBN:083420309X.

OSCE 5

Bushberg, J. T., Seibert, J. A., Leidholdt, E. M., Jr., et al. *The essential physics of medical imaging.* LWW. ISBN:0781780578.
Sprawls, P. *Physical principles of medical imaging.* Aspen Publishing. ISBN:083420309X.

OSCE 6

Bushberg, et al. *The essentials of physics and medical imaging.* Williams & Wilkins Publisher.
Bushong, S. C. (2008). *Radiologic science for technologists: Physics, biology, and protection* (9th ed.). Mosby Elsevier.
Christensen's physics of diagnostic radiology (4th ed.).
Farr's physics for medical imaging (2nd ed.).
Dr. Satyendra Raghuwanshi, et al. *Radiology without tears* (3rd ed., Vol. I).

OSCE 7

MAGNETOM Skyra Planning Guide. Siemens Medical Systems. (2013). *Contains a detailed fringe field map for this 3.0T scanner and lists other siting requirements.*
Turner, B. D. (2007, May). Shielding issues for medical products. *Conformity*, 48–53.

OSCE 8

Bushberg, J. T., Seibert, J.A., Leidholdt, E. M., Jr., et al. *The essential physics of medical imaging.* LWW. ISBN:0781780578.
Feldman, M. K., Katyal, S., & Blackwood, M. S. (2009). US artifacts. *RadioGraphics, 29*(4), 1179–1189. https://doi.org/10.1148/rg.294085199

OSCE 9

ACR Manual on Contrast Media. (2020).
GE Healthcare. *Drug information on Omnipaque.* Revised 12/2022.

OSCE 10

Fakhran, S., Alhilali, L., Kale, H., et al. (2015). Assessment of rates of acute adverse reactions to gadobenate dimeglumine: Review of more than 130,000 administrations in 7.5 years. *AJR American Journal of Roentgenology, 204*(4), 703–706.
Gadolinium contrast agents. *Questions and answers in MRI.* https://mriquestions.com/so-many-gd-agents.html
Guglielmo, F. F., Mitchell, D. G., & Gupta, S. (2014). Gadolinium contrast agent selection and optimal use for body MR imaging. *Radiologic Clinics of North America, 52*(4), 637–656.
Dr. Satyendra Raghuwanshi, et al., *Radiology without tears* (3rd ed., Vol. I).

OSCE 11

Chalazonitis, A., Tzovara, I., Laspas, F., et al. Hysterosalpingography: Technique and applications. *Current Problems in Diagnostic Radiology, 38*(5), 199–205.
Creasy, J. L., Clark, R. L., Cuttino, J. T., et al. (1985). Salpingitis isthmica nodosa: Radiologic and clinical correlates. *Radiology, 154*(3), 597–600.
Ott, D. J., Fayez, J. A., & Chen, M. Y. M. (1998). Techniques of hysterosalpingography. In D. J. Ott, J. A. Fayez, & R. J. Zagoria (Eds.). *Hysterosalpingography: A text and atlas* (2nd ed., pp. 11–27). Williams & Wilkins.
Tur-kaspa, I., Seidman, D. S., Soriano, D., et al. (1998). Hysterosalpingography with a balloon catheter versus a metal cannula: A prospective, randomized, blinded comparative study. *Human Reproduction, 13*(1), 75–77.

OSCE 12

Burke, C. T., & Mauro, M. A. (2004). Bronchial artery embolization. *Seminars in Interventional Radiology, 21*(1), 43–48.
Sopko, D. R., & Smith, T. P. (2011). Bronchial artery embolization for hemoptysis. *Seminars in Interventional Radiology, 28*(1), 48–62.
Dr. Satyendra Raghuwanshi, et al., *Radiology without tears* (3rd ed., Vol. I).
Yoon, W., Kim, J. K., Kim, Y. H., et al. (2002). Bronchial and nonbronchial systemic artery embolization for life-threatening hemoptysis: A comprehensive review. *RadioGraphics, 22*(6), 1395–1409. https://doi.org/10.1148/rg.226015180.

OSCE 13

Goel, A., Yu, Y., Havinga, D., et al. Goldman classification of urethral injuries. Reference article, Radiopaedia.org. https://doi.org/10.53347/rID-32017

Goldman, S. M., Sandler, C. M., Corriere, J. N., et al. (1997). Blunt urethral trauma: A unified, anatomical mechanical classification. *Journal of Urology*, *157*(1), 85–89.

Kawashima, A., Sandler, C. M., Wasserman, N. F., et al. (2004). Imaging of urethral disease: A pictorial review. *RadioGraphics*, *24*(Suppl 1), S195–S216.

Urethral injuries after pelvic trauma: Evaluation with urethrography1 – scientific figure on ResearchGate. https://www.researchgate.net/figure/Schematic-shows-the-normal-male-urethral-anatomy-in-the-sagittal-plane-During_fig1_23399613 [accessed 6 Apr, 2023]

OSCE 14

Buchberger, W., Strasser, K., Heim, K., Müller, E., & Schröcksnadel, H. (1991). Phylloides tumor: Findings on mammography, sonography, and aspiration cytology in 10 cases. *AJR American Journal of Roentgenology, 157*(4),715–719.

Farria, D., Gorczyca, D., Barsky, S., Sinha, S., & Bassett, L. (1996). Benign phyllodes tumor of the breast: MR imaging features. *AJR American Journal of Roentgenology, 167*(1), 187–189.

Gaillard, F., Niknejad, M., Knipe, H., et al. Phyllodes tumour. Reference article, Radiopaedia.org. https://doi.org/10.53347/rID-1872

Lifshitz, O., Whitman, G., Sahin, A., & Yang, W. (2003). Radiologic-pathologic conferences of the University of Texas M.D. Anderson Cancer Center. Phyllodes tumor of the breast. *AJR American Journal of Roentgenology, 180*(2), 332.

Weissleder, R. (2007). *Primer of diagnostic imaging*. Elsevier. https://www.amazon.co.uk/Primer-Diagnostic-Imaging-Mukesh-Harisinghani-dp-0323357741/dp/0323357741/ref=dp_ob_title_bk

Yabuuchi, H., Soeda, H., Matsuo, Y., et al. (2006). Phyllodes tumor of the breast: Correlation between MR findings and histologic grade. *Radiology, 241*(3), 702–709.

OSCE 15

ACR BI-RADS Atlas: Breast Imaging Reporting and Data System. American College of Radiology. https://www.acr.org/Clinical-Resources/Reporting-and-Data-Systems/Bi-Rads

Ben Kridis, W., Toumi, N., Daoud, E., et al. (2022). Breast cancer diagnosis and women cancer concerns: A single-center experience. *BMJ Supportive & Palliative Care*, bmjspcare-2021-003361. https://doi.org/10.1136/bmjspcare-2021-003361

OSCE 16

Baxi, L. V., & Walsh, C. A. (2010). Monoamniotic twins in contemporary practice: A single-center study of perinatal outcomes. *The Journal of Maternal-Fetal & Neonatal Medicine*, *23*(6), 506–510.

Cordero, L., Franco, A., & Joy, S. D. (2006). Monochorionic monoamniotic twins: Neonatal outcome. *Journal of Perinatology*, *26*(3), 170–175.

Dørum, A., & Nesheim, B. I. (1991). Monochorionic monoamniotic twins – the most precarious of twin pregnancies. *Acta Obstetrica et Gynecologica Scandinavica*, *70*(4–5), 381–383.

Wladimiroff, J. W., & Eik-Nes, S. (2009). *Ultrasound in obstetrics and gynaecology*. Elsevier Science Health Science div. ISBN:0444518290.

OSCE 17

Grant, L. A., & Griffin, N. (2018). *Grainger & Allison's diagnostic radiology essentials*. Churchill Livingstone.

Snyder, C. L., Miller, K. A., Sharp, R. J., Murphy, J. P., Andrews, W. H., Holcomb, G., Gittes, G. K., & Ashcraft, K. W. (2001). Management of intestinal atresia in patients with gastroschisis. *Journal of Pediatric Surgery*, *36*(10), 1542–1545. https://doi.org/10.1053/jpsu.2001.27040

Sun, E. X., Shi, J., & Mandell, J. C. (2021). *Core radiology: A visual approach to diagnostic imaging*. Cambridge University Press.

OSCE 18

Cafe Roentgen. (2019, March 22). *PCPNDT Simplified: A guide for radiology residents*. Cafe Roentgen. https://caferoentgen.com/2019/03/22/pcpndt-simplified-a-guide-for-radiology-residents/

Department of Family Welfare, Government of India. (2004). *Handbook on PNDT Act, 1994 and Amendments (revised edition).*

Onkar, P., Mitra, K. (2012). Important points in the PC-PNDT Act. *Indian Journal of Radiology and Imaging, 22*.

OSCE 19

ACR Committee on MR Safety. *ACR manual on MR safety, version 1.0*. American College of Radiology, 2020 ACR guidelines on MRI safety.

Sammet, S. (2016). Magnetic resonance safety. *Abdominal radiology (New York)*, *41*(3), 444–445.

Tsai, L. L., Grant, A. K., Mortele, K. J., Kung, J. W., & Smith, M. P. (2015). A practical guide to MR imaging safety: What radiologists need to know. *RadioGraphics*, *35*(6), 1722–1737.

OSCE 20

Gaillard, F., Machang'a, K., Knipe H, et al. Achalasia. Reference article, Radiopaedia.org (Accessed on 01 Dec 2023). https://doi.org/10.53347/rID-835

Woodfield, C. A., Levine, M. S., Rubesin, S. E., Langlotz, C. P., & Laufer, I. (2000). Diagnosis of primary versus secondary achalasia. *American Journal of Roentgenology, 175*(3), 727–731. doi:10.2214/ajr.175.3.1750727 (https://doi.org/10.2214/ajr.175.3.1750727)

OSCE 21

Grant, L. A., & Griffin, N. (2018). *Grainger & Allison's diagnostic radiology essentials*. Churchill Livingstone.

Pedrosa, I., Saíz, A., Arrazola, J., Ferreirós, J., & Pedrosa, C. S. (2000). Hydatid disease: Radiologic and pathologic features and complications. *RadioGraphics*, *20*(3), 795–817. doi:10.1148/radiographics.20.3.g00ma06795 (https://doi.org/10.1148/radiographics.20.3.g00ma06795)

OSCE 22

Grant, L. A., & Griffin, N. (2018). *Grainger & Allison's diagnostic radiology essentials*. Churchill Livingstone.

Saad, N. E. A., Saad, W. E. A., Davies, M. G., Waldman, D. L., Fultz, P. J., & Rubens, D. J. (2005). Pseudoaneurysms and the role of minimally invasive techniques in their management. *RadioGraphics*, *25*(suppl_1), S173–S189. doi:10.1148/rg.25si055503 (https://doi.org/10.1148/rg.25si055503)

OSCE 23

Grant, L. A., & Griffin, N. (2018). *Grainger & Allison's diagnostic radiology essentials*. Churchill Livingstone.

Outwater, E. K., Siegelman, E. S., & Hunt, J. L. (2001). Ovarian teratomas: Tumor types and imaging characteristics. *RadioGraphics*, *21*(2), 475–490. doi:10.1148/radiographics.21.2.g01mr09475 (https://doi.org/10.1148/radiographics.21.2.g01mr09475)

OSCE 24

Crocetti, M., Barone, M., & Oski, F. (2004). *Oski's essential pediatrics*. ISBN: 9780781737708.

Devos, A., & Blickman, J. (2007). *Radiological imaging of the digestive tract in infants and children*. ISBN: 9783540407331.

Norton, J., Barie, P., Bollinger, R., et al. (2008). *Surgery*. ISBN: 9780387308005.

OSCE 25

Ellis, C. N. (2008). Colonic adenomatous polyposis syndromes: Clinical management. *Clinics in Colon and Rectal Surgery*, *21*(4), 256–262. https://doi.org/10.1055/s-0028-1089940 – Free text at PubMed – PubMed citation.

Gaillard, F., & Kumar, S. Polyposis syndromes. Reference article, Radiopaedia.org (Accessed on 24 Sep 2022). https://doi.org/10.53347/rID-1907

Shussman, N., & Wexner, S. D. (2014). Colorectal polyps and polyposis syndromes. *Gastroenterology Report (Oxf)*, *2*(1), 1–15. https://doi.org/10.1093/gastro/got041 – Free text at PubMed – PubMed citation.

OSCE 26

Kawsar, H. I., Shahnewaz, J., Ricaurte, B., et al. (2012). Barium aspiration. *Case Reports, 2012*, bcr0220125891.

OSCE 27

Agarwal, S., Goel, S., Sankhwar, S., et al. (2018). Circumcaval ureter/retrocaval ureter. *Case Reports, 2018*, bcr-2018-225449.

Radswiki, T., & Niknejad, M. Circumcaval ureter. Reference article, Radiopaedia.org (Accessed on 01 Oct 2022). https://doi.org/10.53347/rID-12815

OSCE 28

Choi, S. H., Han, J. K., Kim, S. H., Lee, J. M., Lee, K. H., Kim, Y. J., ... Choi, B. I. (2004). Intussusception in adults: From stomach to rectum. *American Journal of Roentgenology*, *183*(3), 691–698. doi:10.2214/ajr.183.3.1830691 (https://doi.org/10.2214/ajr.183.3.1830691)

Khasawneh, R., El-Heis, M., Al-Omari, M., Al-Qaralleh, M. A., Al-Manasra, A. rahman, Alqudah, A. A., &Awad, S. (2021). The radiological characteristics of childhood intussusception including unusual features and rare pathological lead points. *Heliyon*, *7*(6), e07231. doi:10.1016/j.heliyon.2021.e07231 (https://doi.org/10.1016/j.heliyon.2021.e07231)

OSCE 29

Bonatti, M., Vezzali, N., Lombardo, F., Ferro, F., Zamboni, G., Tauber, M., & Bonatti, G. (2017). Gallbladder adenomyomatosis: Imaging findings, tricks and pitfalls. *Insights Into Imaging*, *8*(2), 243–253. https://doi.org/10.1007/s13244-017-0544-7

Boscak, A. R., Al-Hawary, M. M., & Ramsburgh, S. R. (2006). Adenomyomatosis of the gallbladder. *RadioGraphics*, *26*(3), 941–946. https://doi.org/10.1148/rg.263055180

Rumack, C. M., & Levine, D. (2023). *Diagnostic ultrasound, 2-volume set*. Elsevier.

Ryu, Y., Abdeldjalil, B., Molinari, A., et al. Adenomyomatosis of the gallbladder. Reference article, Radiopaedia.org. https://doi.org/10.53347/rID-7056

OSCE 30

Almeida, A., Melão, L., Viamonte, B., Cunha, R., & Pereira, J. M. (2009). Epiploic appendagitis: An entity frequently unknown to clinicians—diagnostic imaging, pitfalls, and look-alikes. *American Journal of Roentgenology*, *193*(5), 1243–1251. https://doi.org/10.2214/ajr.08.2071

Gaillard, F., Glick, Y., Rizk, M., et al. Epiploic appendagitis. Reference article, Radiopaedia.org. https://doi.org/10.53347/rID-1296

Singh, A. K., Gervais, D. A., Hahn, P. F., Sagar, P., Müeller, P. R., & Novelline, R. A. (2005). Acute epiploic appendagitis and its mimics. *RadioGraphics*, *25*(6), 1521–1534. https://doi.org/10.1148/rg.256055030

OSCE 31

Gaillard, F., Niknejad, M., Knipe, H., et al. Neuroblastoma vs Wilms tumor. Reference article, Radiopaedia.org (Accessed on 09 Nov 2023). https://doi.org/10.53347/rID-8154

Lowe, L. H., Isuani, B. H., Heller, R. M., Stein, S. M., Johnson, J. E., Navarro, O. M., & Hernanz-Schulman, M. (2000). Pediatric renal masses: Wilms tumor and beyond. *RadioGraphics*, *20*(6), 1585–1603. https://doi.org/10.1148/radiographics.20.6.g00nv051585

O'Brien, W. T. (2018). *Top 3 differentials in radiology: A case review*. Thieme Medical Publishers.

OSCE 32

Gaillard, F., Saber, M., Ibrahim, D., et al. Cortical nephrocalcinosis. Reference article, Radiopaedia.org. https://doi.org/10.53347/rID-9914

Gaillard, F., Shah, V., Baba, Y., et al. Medullary nephrocalcinosis. Reference article, Radiopaedia.org. https://doi.org/10.53347/rID-9913

Grant, L. A., & Griffin, N. (2018). *Grainger & Allison's diagnostic radiology essentials*. Churchill Livingstone.

Sun, E. X., Shi, J., & Mandell, J. C. (2021). *Core radiology: A visual approach to diagnostic imaging*. Cambridge University Press.

OSCE 33

Dahnert, W. F. (2017). *Radiology review manual*. Wolters Kluwer Health. ISBN: 9781496360694.

Gaillard, F., Anan, R., Silverstone, L., et al. Autosomal dominant polycystic kidney disease. Reference article, Radiopaedia.org. https://doi.org/10.53347/rID-10257

Grant, L. A., & Griffin, N. (2018). *Grainger & Allison's diagnostic radiology essentials*. Churchill Livingstone.

Sun, E. X., Shi, J., & Mandell, J. C. (2021). *Core radiology: A visual approach to diagnostic imaging*. Cambridge University Press.

OSCE 34

Amini B, Yap J, Kearns C, et al. Pyloric stenosis. Reference article, Radiopaedia.org. https://doi.org/10.53347/rID-1941

Dahnert, W. F. (2017). *Radiology review manual*. Wolters Kluwer Health. ISBN: 9781496360694.

Grant, L. A., & Griffin, N. (2018). *Grainger & Allison's diagnostic radiology essentials*. Churchill Livingstone.

Sun, E. X., Shi, J., & Mandell, J. C. (2021). *Core radiology: A visual approach to diagnostic imaging*. Cambridge University Press.

OSCE 35

Dahnert, W. F. (2017). *Radiology review manual*. Wolters Kluwer Health. ISBN: 9781496360694.

Grant, L. A., & Griffin, N. (2018). *Grainger & Allison's diagnostic radiology essentials*. Churchill Livingstone.

Sun, E. X., Shi, J., & Mandell, J. C. (2021). *Core radiology: A visual approach to diagnostic imaging*. Cambridge University Press.

OSCE 36

Horton, K. M., Lawler, L. P., & Fishman, E. K. (2003). CT findings in sclerosing mesenteritis (panniculitis): Spectrum of disease. *RadioGraphics*, *23*(6), 1561–1567. https://doi.org/10.1148/rg.1103035010

McLaughlin, P. D., Filippone, A., & Maher, M. M. (2013). The 'misty mesentery': Mesenteric panniculitis and its mimics. *American Journal of Roentgenology*, *200*(2), W116–W123. https://doi.org/10.2214/ajr.12.8493

Singh, G., Bell, D., Sharma, R., et al. Sclerosing mesenteritis. Reference article, Radiopaedia.org. https://doi.org/10.53347/rID-4975

OSCE 37

Chang, S. T., Jeffrey, R. B., & Olcott, E. W. (2014). Three-step sequential positioning algorithm during sonographic evaluation for appendicitis increases appendiceal visualization rate and reduces CT use. *American Journal of Roentgenology*, *203*(5), 1006–1012. https://doi.org/10.2214/ajr.13.12334

Grant, L. A., & Griffin, N. (2018). *Grainger & Allison's diagnostic radiology essentials*. Churchill Livingstone.

Jacob, D., Glick, Y., Silverstone, L., et al. Acute appendicitis. Reference article, Radiopaedia.org (Accessed on 31 Dec 2023). https://doi.org/10.53347/rID-922

Schaaf, K. A., Melnychuk, E., Ellison, R. D., & Snover, A. J. (2019). Two rare cases of appendicitis: Amyand's hernia and De Garengeot's hernia. *Case Reports in Emergency Medicine*, *2019*, 1–4. https://doi.org/10.1155/2019/6759206

OSCE 38

Brennan, G. B., Rosenberg, R. D., & Arora, S. (2004). Bouveret syndrome. *RadioGraphics*, *24*(4), 1171–1175. https://doi.org/10.1148/rg.244035222

Carnevale, A., Motta, L., Labaj, O., Cossu, A., Uccelli, L., & Giganti, M. (2020). Rolling in the deep: Imaging findings and diagnostic pearls in gallstone ileus. *Surgery Research and Practice*, *2020*, 1–10. https://doi.org/10.1155/2020/1421753

Gaillard, F., El-Feky, M., Rizk, M., et al. Gallstone ileus. Reference article, Radiopaedia.org. https://doi.org/10.53347/rID-1366

Lassandro, F., Romano, S., Ragozzino, A., Rossi, G., Valente, T., Ferrara, I., Romano, L., & Grassi, R. (2005). Role of helical CT in diagnosis of gallstone ileus and related conditions. *American Journal of Roentgenology*, *185*(5), 1159–1165. https://doi.org/10.2214/ajr.04.1371

OSCE 39

Kumar, N., Sundriyal, D., Wadhawan, P., & Charaniya, R. (2014). "Rice-grain" or "cigar-shaped" calcification: Radiological clue and minor criteria for neurocysticercosis. *Case Reports*, 2014 (Jun 27 1), bcr2014205363–bcr2014205363. doi:10.1136/bcr-2014-205363 (https://doi.org/10.1136/bcr-2014-205363)

OSCE 40

Grant, L. A., & Griffin, N. (2018). *Grainger & Allison's diagnostic radiology essentials*. Churchill Livingstone.

UnalErzurumlu, Z., Celenk, P., Bulut, E., &Barıs, Y. S. (2015). CT imaging of craniofacial fibrous dysplasia. *Case Reports in Dentistry*, *2015*, 1–4. doi:10.1155/2015/134123 (https://doi.org/10.1155/2015/134123)

OSCE 41

Ellatif, M., Sharif, B., Lindsay, D. et al. (2021). An update on the imaging of diaphyseal aclasis. *Skeletal Radiology*, 50, 1941–1962.

Grant, L. A., & Griffin, N. (2018). *Grainger & Allison's diagnostic radiology essentials*. Churchill Livingstone.

Wolfgang, F. D. (2017). *Radiology review manual*. Wolters Kluwer Health. ISBN: 9781496360694.

OSCE 42

Bickle, I., & Patel, M. Speech bubble sign. Reference article, Radiopaedia.org. (Accessed on 14 Aug 2022) https://doi.org/10.53347/rID-48471

Perdikakis, E., & Skiadas, V. (2013). MRI characteristics of cysts and "cyst-like" lesions in and around the knee: What the radiologist needs to know. *Insights into Imaging*, *4*(3), 257–272. doi:10.1007/s13244-013-0240-1 (https://doi.org/10.1007/s13244-013-0240-1)

OSCE 43

Liu, S.-Z., Zhou, X., Song, A., Wang, Y.-P., & Liu, Y. (2019). The corduroy appearance & the polka dot sign. *QJM: An International Journal of Medicine*. doi:10.1093/qjmed/hcz184 (https://doi.org/10.1093/qjmed/hcz184)

OSCE 44

Gómez Roselló, E., QuilesGranado, A. M., Artajona Garcia, M., et al. (2020). Facial fractures: Classification and highlights for a useful report. *Insights Imaging*, *11*, 49. https://doi.org/10.1186/s13244-020-00847-w

OSCE 45

Jang, J. H., Ward, M. M., Rucker, A. N., Reveille, J. D., Davis, J. C., Weisman, M. H., & Learch, T. J. (2011). Ankylosing spondylitis: Patterns of radiographic involvement—A re-examination of accepted principles in a cohort of 769 patients. *Radiology*, *258*(1), 192–198. https://doi.org/10.1148/radiol.10100426

Østergaard, M., & Lambert, R. G. (2012). Imaging in ankylosing spondylitis. *Therapeutic Advances in Musculoskeletal Disease*, *4*(4), 301–311. https://doi.org/10.1177/1759720x11436240

Prasad, C. B., Sankar, J., Dhir, V., & Jain, S. (2022). Trolley-track sign in ankylosing spondylitis. *QJM: An International Journal of Medicine*, *116*(3), 231–232. https://doi.org/10.1093/qjmed/hcac247

Wolfgang, F. D. (2017). *Radiology review manual*. Wolters Kluwer Health. ISBN: 9781496360694.

OSCE 46

Gandhi, M., Rac, M. W. F., & McKinney, J. (2019). Radial ray malformation. *American Journal of Obstetrics and Gynecology*, *221*(6), B16–B18. doi:10.1016/j.ajog.2019.09.024 (https://doi.org/10.1016/j.ajog.2019.09.024)

OSCE 47

Gonçalves, L., & Kroon, H. Chronic osteomyelitis. Case 7989. https://www.eurorad.org/case/7989: DOI:10.1594/EURORAD/CASE.7989

Kothari, N. A., Pelchovitz, D. J., & Meyer, J. S. (2001). Imaging of musculoskeletal infections. *Radiologic Clinics of North America*, *39*(4), 653–671. (PMID: 11549164).

Oudjhane, K., & Azouz, E. M. (2001). Imaging of osteomyelitis in children. *Radiologic Clinics of North America*, *39*(2), 251–266. (PMID: 11316358).

Pineda, C., Vargas, A., & Rodreguez, A. V. (2006). Imaging of osteomyelitis: Current concepts. *Infectious Disease Clinics of North America*, *20*(4), 789–825. (PMID: 17118291).

OSCE 48

Dangman, B. C., Hoffer, F. A., Rand, F. F., et al. (1992). Osteomyelitis in children: Gadolinium enhanced MR imaging. *Radiology*, *182*, 743. (PMID: 1535888).

Green, N. E., Beauchamp, R. D., & Griffin, P. P. (1981). Primary subacute epiphyseal osteomyelitis. *The Journal of Bone and Joint Surgery (Am)*, *63*, 107. (PMID: 7451513).

Grey, A. C., Davies, A. M., Mangham, D. C., et al. (1998). The 'penumbra' sign on T1-weighted MR imaging in subacute osteomyelitis: Frequency cause and significance. *Clinical Radiology*, *53*, 587–592. (PMID: 9744584).

Resnick. D., & Niwanyama, G. (2005). Osteomyelitis, septic arthritis and soft tissue infection: Mechanisms and situations. In D. Resnick (Ed.), *Diagnosis of bone and joint disorders* (3rd ed., p. 2338). W. B. Saunders Co.

Stephens, M. M., & MacAuley, P. (1988). Brodie's abscess. A long-term review. *Clinical Orthopaedics and Related Research*, *234*, 211. (PMID: 3409578).

OSCE 49

Turcotte, R. E. (2006). Giant cell tumour of bone. *Orthopedic Clinics of North America*, *37*, 35–51.

Werner, M. (2006). Giant cell tumour of the bone: Morphological, biological and histogenetical aspects. *International Orthopaedics*, *30*, 484–489. (PMID: 17013643).

OSCE 50

Killeen, K. L. (1998). The fallen fragment sign. *Radiology*, *207*(1), 261–262. doi:10.1148/radiology.207.1.9530325 (https://doi.org/10.1148/radiology.207.1.9530325)

Ramesh, N., et al. Simple (unicameral) bone cyst. *Eurorad*, 16 Nov 2022, www.eurorad.org/case/1749

OSCE 51

Dalbeth, N., & Doyle, A. J. (2012). Imaging of gout – An overview. *Best Practice & Research: Clinical Rheumatology*, *26*, 823–838. (PMID: 23273794).

Neogi, T., Jansen, T. L., Dalbeth, N., et al. (2015). 2015 Gout classification criteria: An American College of Rheumatology/European League Against Rheumatism collaborative initiative. *Arthritis & Rheumatology*, *67*, 2557–2568. (PMID: 26359487).

Richette, P., & Badin, T. (2010). Gout. *Lancet*, *9711*, 318–328. (PMID: 19692116).

OSCE 52

Kgoebane, K., Ally, M. M. T. M., Duim-Beytell, M. C., & Suleman, F. E. The role of imaging in rheumatoid arthritis. (2018, July 11). *South African Journal of Radiology*, *22*(1), 1316. https://doi.org/10.4102/sajr.v22i1.1316. PMID: 31754498; PMCID: PMC6837821.

Stanislavsky, A., Hacking, C., Guan, H., et al. Rheumatoid arthritis (musculoskeletal manifestations). Reference article, Radiopaedia.org. https://doi.org/10.53347/rID-12370

Vyas, S., Bhalla, A. S., Ranjan, P., Kumar, S., Kumar, U., & Gupta, A. K. (2016). Rheumatoid arthritis revisited – advanced imaging review. *Polish Journal of Radiology*, 81, 629–635. doi:10.12659/PJR.899317 (https://doi.org/10.12659/PJR.899317)

OSCE 53

Chew, F. S. (Ed.). (1997). Trauma in adults: Upper body. In *Skeletal radiology. The bare bones* (2nd ed., pp. 23–60). Williams & Wilkins.

Greenspan, A. (Ed.). (2000). Upper limb. Shoulder girdle and elbow. In *Orthopaedic radiology. A practical approach* (3rd ed., pp. 89–150). Lippincott.

Parlorio, E. Anterior dislocation of the glenohumeral joint associated with an unusually extensive fracture of the glenoid rim (bony Bankart lesion). https://www.eurorad.org/case/2418

Resnick, D., & Kang, H. S. (Eds.). (1997). *Internal derangements of joints. Emphasis on MR imaging* (pp. 163–333). WB Saunders Co.

OSCE 54

Roselló, E. G., Granado, A. M. Q., Garcia, M. A., et al. (2020). Facial fractures: Classification and highlights for a useful report. *Insights Imaging*, *11*, 49. https://doi.org/10.1186/s13244-020-00847-w

OSCE 55

Grant, L. A., & Griffin, N. (2018). *Grainger and Allison's diagnostic radiology essentials* (2nd ed.). Elsevier. ISBN: 9780702073113.

OSCE 56

Agha, M., Eid, A. F., &Sallam, M. (2013). Sickle cell anemia: Imaging from head to toe. *The Egyptian Journal of Radiology and Nuclear Medicine*, *44*(3), 547–561. doi:10.1016/j.ejrnm.2013.06.005 (https://doi.org/10.1016/j.ejrnm.2013.06.005)

Ejindu, V. C., Hine, A. L., Mashayekhi, M., Shorvon, P. J., & Misra, R. R. (2007). Musculoskeletal manifestations of sickle cell disease. *RadioGraphics*, *27*(4), 1005–1021. doi:10.1148/rg.274065142 (https://doi.org/10.1148/rg.274065142)

OSCE 57

Dahnert, W. F. (2017). *Radiology review manual*. Wolters Kluwer Health. ISBN: 9781496360694.

Kracoff, S. L. (2020). Radiographic characteristics of the hand in Apert syndrome. *The Journal of Hand Surgery (Asian-Pacific Volume)*, *25*(1), 82–86. doi:10.1142/S2424835520500113 (https://doi.org/10.1142/S2424835520500113)

OSCE 58

Mujtaba, B., Taher, A., Fiala, M. J., Nassar, S., Madewell, J. E., Hanafy, A. K., & Aslam, R. (2019, September 24). Heterotopic ossification: Radiological and pathological review. *Radiology and Oncology*, *53*(3), 275–284. https://doi.org/10.2478/raon-2019-0039. PMID: 31553710; PMCID: PMC6765162.

Weerakkody, Y., Yap, J., Niknejad, M., et al. Heterotopic ossification. Reference article, Radiopaedia.org. https://doi.org/10.53347/rID-19159

OSCE 59

Salam, H., Yap, J., Yu Jin, T., et al. Proximal femoral focal deficiency. Reference article, Radiopaedia.org. https://doi.org/10.53347/rID-8727

Uduma, F. U., Dim, E. M., & Njeze, N. R. (2020). Proximal femoral focal deficiency – a rare congenital entity: Two case reports and a review of the literature. *Journal of Medical Case Reports*, *14*(1). doi:10.1186/s13256-020-2350-y (https://doi.org/10.1186/s13256-020-2350-y)

OSCE 60

Gaillard, F., Lustosa, L., Knipe, H., et al. Slipped upper femoral epiphysis. Reference article, Radiopaedia.org. https://doi.org/10.53347/rID-2056

Hesper, T., Zilkens, C., Bittersohl, B., & Krauspe, R. (2017). Imaging modalities in patients with slipped capital femoral epiphysis. *Journal of Children's Orthopaedics*, *11*(2), 99–106. doi:10.1302/1863-2548-11-160276 (https://doi.org/10.1302/1863-2548-11-160276)

Rebich, E. J., Lee, S. S., & Schlechter, J. A. (2018). The S sign: A new radiographic tool to aid in the diagnosis of slipped capital femoral epiphysis. *The Journal of Emergency Medicine*, *54*(6), 835–843. doi:10.1016/j.jemermed.2018.01.023 (https://doi.org/10.1016/j.jemermed.2018.01.023)

OSCE 61

Adams, J. E. (2018). Radiology of rickets and osteomalacia. *Vitamin D*, 975–1006. doi:10.1016/B978-0-12-809965-0.00054-9 (https://doi.org/10.1016/B978-0-12-809965-0.00054-9)

Chang, C. Y., Rosenthal, D. I., Mitchell, D. M., Handa, A., Kattapuram, S. V., & Huang, A. J. (2016). Imaging findings of metabolic bone disease. *RadioGraphics*, *36*(6), 1871–1887. doi:10.1148/rg.2016160004 (https://doi.org/10.1148/rg.2016160004)

Niknejad, M., Roberts, D., Puwiwattanangkura, P., et al. Osteomalacia. Reference article, Radiopaedia.org (Accessed on 21 Feb 2023). https://doi.org/10.53347/rID-21389

OSCE 62

Niknejad, M., Sharma, R., Roberts, D., et al. Fluorosis. Reference article, Radiopaedia.org (Accessed on 21 Feb 2023). https://doi.org/10.53347/rID-21142

Wang, Y., Yin, Y., Gilula, L. A., & Wilson, A. J. (1994). Endemic fluorosis of the skeleton: Radiographic features in 127 patients. *American Journal of Roentgenology*, *162*(1), 93–98.

OSCE 63

Bennett, J., Suliburk, J. W., & Morón, F. E. (2020). Osseous manifestations of primary hyperparathyroidism: Imaging findings. *International Journal of Endocrinology*, *2020*, 1–10. doi:10.1155/2020/3146535 (https://doi.org/10.1155/2020/3146535)

Chang, C. Y., Rosenthal, D. I., Mitchell, D. M., Handa, A., Kattapuram, S. V., & Huang, A. J. (2016). Imaging findings of metabolic bone disease. *RadioGraphics*, *36*(6), 1871–1887. doi:10.1148/rg.2016160004 (https://doi.org/10.1148/rg.2016160004)

OSCE 64

Dixon, A., Hacking, C., Knipe, H., et al. Bone infarction. Reference article, Radiopaedia.org. https://doi.org/10.53347/rID-10017

Kosaraju, V., Harwani, A., Partovi, S., Bhojwani, N., Garg, V., Ayyappan, S., Kosmas, C., & Robbin, M. (2017). Imaging of musculoskeletal manifestations in sickle cell disease patients. *British Journal of Radiology*, *90*(1073), 20160130. https://doi.org/10.1259/bjr.20160130

Learning Radiology. *Learning Radiology – Bone Infarct, Medullary Bone Infarct, Osteonecrosis*. learningradiology.com/notes/bonenotes/boneinfarct.htm

OSCE 65

Sadiqi, J., Rasouly, N., Hamidi, H., & Siraj, S. (2017). Radiographic features of Ollier's disease – two case reports. *BMC Medical Imaging*, *17*(1). doi:10.1186/s12880-017-0230-8 (https://doi.org/10.1186/s12880-017-0230-8)

Zwenneke Flach, H., Ginai, A. Z., & Wolter Oosterhuis, J. (2001). Best Cases from the AFIP. *RadioGraphics*, *21*(5), 1311–1316. doi:10.1148/radiographics.21.5.g01se301311 (https://doi.org/10.1148/radiographics.21.5.g01se301311)

OSCE 66

Gaillard, F., Hacking, C., El-Feky, M., et al. Aneurysmal bone cyst. Reference article, Radiopaedia.org. https://doi.org/10.53347/rID-894

JMSR. *JMSR*. jmsronline.com/archive-article/Fluid-fluid-levels-in-bone-tumors-and-tumoral-lesions

Restrepo, R., Zahrah, D., Pelaez, L., Temple, H. T., & Murakami, J. W. (2022, August). Update on aneurysmal bone cyst: Pathophysiology, histology, imaging and treatment. *Pediatric Radiology*, *52*(9), 1601–1614. https://doi.org/10.1007/s00247-022-05396-6. Epub 2022 Aug 9. PMID: 35941207; PMCID: PMC9360065.

OSCE 67

Amini, B., Hacking, C., Knipe, H., et al. Giant cell tumor of bone. Reference article, Radiopaedia.org. https://doi.org/10.53347/rID-1385

Chakarun, C. J., Forrester, D. M., Gottsegen, C. J., Patel, D. B., White, E. A., & Matcuk, G. R. (2013). Giant cell tumor of bone: Review, mimics, and new developments in treatment. *RadioGraphics*, *33*(1), 197–211. doi:10.1148/rg.331125089 (https://doi.org/10.1148/rg.331125089)

Purohit, S., & Pardiwala, D. N. (2007, April). Imaging of giant cell tumor of bone. *Indian Journal of Orthopaedics*, *41*(2):91–96. https://doi.org/10.4103/0019-5413.32037. PMID: 21139758; PMCID: PMC2989147.

OSCE 68

Chai, J. W., Hong, S. H., Choi, J.-Y., Koh, Y. H., Lee, J. W., Choi, J.-A., & Kang, H. S. (2010). Radiologic diagnosis of osteoid osteoma: From simple to challenging findings. *RadioGraphics*, *30*(3), 737–749. doi:10.1148/rg.303095120 (https://doi.org/10.1148/rg.303095120)

Gaillard, F., Jones, J., Weerakkody, Y., et al. Double density sign (osteoid osteoma). Reference article, Radiopaedia.org (Accessed on 24 Feb 2023) https://doi.org/10.53347/rID-8428

Yuce, G., Aytekin, N., Eren, S., Genç, B., Ateş, Ö. F., & Canyiğit, M. (2020). Is radiofrequency ablation safe and effective in treating osteoid osteomas? A prospective single-center study with atypical cases. *Journal of Orthopaedic Surgery*, *28*(3), 230949902096055. doi:10.1177/2309499020960555 (https://doi.org/10.1177/2309499020960555)

OSCE 69

Aggarwal, S., Goulatia, R. K., Sood, A., Prasad, K., Ahuja, G. K., Mitchell, M. J., & Kumar, A. (1990). POEMS syndrome: A rare variety of plasma cell dyscrasia. *American Journal of Roentgenology*, *155*(2), 339–341. doi:10.2214/ajr.155.2.2115264 (https://doi.org/10.2214/ajr.155.2.2115264)

Healy, C. F., Murray, J. G., Eustace, S. J., Madewell, J., O'Gorman, P. J., & O'Sullivan, P. (2011). Multiple myeloma: A review of imaging features and radiological techniques. *Bone Marrow Research*, *2011*, 1–9. doi:10.1155/2011/583439 (https://doi.org/10.1155/2011/583439)

Mudgal, P., Weerakkody, Y., Murphy, A., et al. Skeletal survey. Reference article, Radiopaedia.org (Accessed on 24 Feb 2023). https://doi.org/10.53347/rID-28346

Ormond Filho, A. G., Carneiro, B. C., Pastore, D., Silva, I. P., Yamashita, S. R., Consolo, F. D., & Nico, M. A. C. (2019). Whole-body imaging of multiple myeloma: Diagnostic criteria. *RadioGraphics*, *39*(4), 1077–1097. doi:10.1148/rg.2019180096 (https://doi.org/10.1148/rg.2019180096)

OSCE 70

Radswiki, T., Bell, D., Weerakkody, Y., et al. Chondroectodermal dysplasia. Reference article, Radiopaedia.org. https://doi.org/10.53347/rID-15022

Singh, S., Arya, V., Daniel, M. J., Vasudevan, V. (2012, January). Ellis-van Creveld syndrome: A case report. *International Journal of Clinical Pediatric Dentistry*, *5*(1), 72–74. https://doi.org/10.5005/jp-journals-10005-1138. Epub 2012 Feb 24. PMID: 25206139; PMCID: PMC4093642.

OSCE 71

Jones, J., Raeesa, F., Veiga, M., et al. Acromegaly. Reference article, Radiopaedia.org. https://doi.org/10.53347/rID-5748

Woo, C. C. (1988, June). Radiological features and diagnosis of acromegaly. *Journal of Manipulative and Physiological Therapeutics*, *11*(3), 206–213. PMID: 3392475.

OSCE 72

Applied Radiology. *Common and uncommon imaging manifestations of hemophilia*. https://appliedradiology.com/articles/common-and-uncommon-imaging-manifestations-of-hemophilia.

Ray, A., Colville, J. G., Hartley, R., & Rowbotham, E. The musculoskeletal manifestations of haemophilia: A review of the imaging findings. (2022, October). *Clinical Radiology*, *77*(10), 730–737. https://doi.org/10.1016/j.crad.2022.06.022. Epub 2022 Aug 16. PMID: 35985846.

Dixon A, Murphy A, Kang O, et al. Arnold-Hilgartner classification of haemophilic arthropathy. Reference article, Radiopaedia.org. https://doi.org/10.53347/rID-9546

OSCE 73

Harisinghani, M. G., et al. (2018). Primer of *diagnostic imaging* (6th ed.). Elsevier. www.elsevier.com/books/primer-of-diagnostic-imaging/978-0-323-35774-6.

Radswiki, T., Knipe, H., Yap, J., et al. Thalassemia. Reference article, Radiopaedia.org. https://doi.org/10.53347/rID-15616

OSCE 74

AlArifi, M., Al Essa, A., Mashour, M., Mohamed Aly, A., Tayara, B., & Al Absi, E. (2019). Macrodystrophia lipomatosa of the finger: A case report. *Case Reports in Oncology*, *12*(1), 63–68. doi:10.1159/000496685 (https://doi.org/10.1159/000496685)

Murphey, M. D., Carroll, J. F., Flemming, D. J., Pope, T. L., Gannon, F. H., & Kransdorf, M. J. (2004). From the archives of the AFIP. *Radio-Graphics*, *24*(5), 1433–1466. doi:10.1148/rg.245045120 (https://doi.org/10.1148/rg.245045120)

OSCE 75

Gaillard, F., Iqbal, S., El-Feky, M., et al. Ficat and Arlet classification of avascular necrosis of femoral head. Reference article, Radiopaedia.org (Accessed on 25 Feb 2023). https://doi.org/10.53347/rID-951

Stoica, Z., Dumitrescu, D., Popescu, M., Gheonea, I., Gabor, M., & Bogdan, N. Imaging of avascular necrosis of femoral head: Familiar methods and newer trends. (2009, January). *Current Health Sciences Journal*, *35*(1), 23–28. Epub 2009 Mar 21. PMID: 24778812; PMCID: PMC3945237.

OSCE 76

Radswiki, T., Knipe, H., Lustosa, L., et al. Bipartite patella. Reference article, Radiopaedia.org. https://doi.org/10.53347/rID-12216

Theodorou, S. J., et al. *The painful bipartite patella: Imaging evaluation*. www.eurorad.org, 9 May 2014,CASE 11735. https://www.eurorad.org/case/11735. DOI:10.1594/EURORAD/CASE.11735

OSCE 77

Jha, P., Feger, J., Knipe, H., et al. Patellofemoral instability. Reference article, Radiopaedia.org. https://doi.org/10.53347/rID-16281

Radsource. (2010, August 2). Patella alta and baja – Radsource. radsource.us/patella-alta-and-baja

Yılmaz, B., Ozdemir, G., Sirin, E., Cicek, E. D., Anıl, B. S., & Bulbun, G. (2017, April–June). Evaluation of patella alta using MRI measurements in adolescents. *Indian Journal of Radiology and Imaging*, *27*(2), 181–186. https://doi.org/10.4103/ijri.IJRI_222_16. PMID: 28744079; PMCID: PMC5510316.

OSCE 78

Caldwell, R., Shorten, P., & Morrell, N. T. (2019). Common upper extremity fracture eponyms: A look into what they really mean. *The Journal of Hand Surgery*, *44*(4), 331–334. https://doi.org/10.1016/j.jhsa.2018.07.012

Jones, J., Worsley, C., Catchpoole, S., et al. Eponymous fractures. Reference article, Radiopaedia.org. https://doi.org/10.53347/rID-8948

The Radiology Assistant. (2008, January 12). *Fractures*. https://radiologyassistant.nl/musculoskeletal/wrist/fractures

Wong, P. K., Hanna, T. N., Shuaib, W., Sanders, S. M., & Khosa, F. (2015). What's in a name? Upper extremity fracture eponyms (Part 1). *International Journal of Emergency Medicine*, *8*(1). https://doi.org/10.1186/s12245-015-0075-2 Raghuwanshi PART F-3

OSCE 79

Fink, J. R. (2010). Imaging of cerebellopontine angle masses: Self-assessment module. *American Journal of Roentgenology*, *195* (3_supplement), S15–S21. doi:10.2214/AJR.09.7191 (https://doi.org/10.2214/AJR.09.7191)

Grant, L. A., & Griffin, N. (2018). *Grainger & Allison's diagnostic radiology essentials*. Churchill Livingstone.

OSCE 80

Grant, L. A., & Griffin, N. (2018). *Grainger & Allison's diagnostic radiology essentials*. Churchill Livingstone.

Upadhyaya, V., & Upadhyaya, D. N. (2020). An interesting case of MISME syndrome. *Journal of Peripheral Nerve Surgery*, *2020*(3), 41–43. https://doi.org/10.1055/s-0040-1703998

OSCE 81

Mehta, T. S., & Levine, D. (2007). Ultrasound and MR imaging of fetal neural tube defects. *Ultrasound Clinics*, *2*(2), 187–201. https://doi.org/10.1016/j.cult.2007.07.005

Singh, J. K., et al. (2015). Ultrasound evaluation of anencephaly in antenatal scan. *Eurorad*. CASE 12643. https://doi.org/10.1594/eurorad/case.12643. ISSN:1563-4086.

OSCE 82

Kunimatsu, A., Kunimatsu, N., Kamiya, K., Katsura, M., Mori, H., & Ohtomo, K. (2016). Variants of meningiomas: A review of imaging findings and clinical features. *Japanese Journal of Radiology*, *34*(7), 459–469. doi:10.1007/s11604-016-0550-6 (https://doi.org/10.1007/s11604-016-0550-6)

Nadgir, R. (2016, May 15). *Neuroradiology: The requisites* (4th ed.). https://shop.elsevier.com/books/neuroradiology-the-requisites/nadgir/978-1-4557-7568-2

Smithuis, R., & Montanera, W. (2008, July 2). *The radiology assistant: Systematic approach to brain tumors*. https://radiologyassistant.nl/neuroradiology/brain-tumor/systematic-approach#tumor-spread-intra-versus-extraaxial

OSCE 83

Kimura-Hayama, E. T., Higuera, J. A., Corona-Cedillo, R., Chávez-Macías, L., Perochena, A., Quiroz-Rojas, L. Y., ... Criales, J. L. (2010). Neurocysticercosis: Radiologic-pathologic correlation. *RadioGraphics*, *30*(6), 1705–1719. doi:10.1148/rg.306105522 (https://doi.org/10.1148/rg.306105522)

Nadgir, R. (2016, 15 May). *Neuroradiology: The requisites* (4th ed.). https://shop.elsevier.com/books/neuroradiology-the-requisites/nadgir/978-1-4557-7568-2

Osborn, A. G., Hedlund, G. L., & Salzman, K. L. (2018). *Osborn's brain, imaging, pathology, and anatomy* (2nd ed.). Elsevier.

OSCE 84

Chiapparini, L., Saletti, V., Solero, C. L., Bruzzone, M. G., & Valentini, L. G. (2011). Neuroradiological diagnosis of Chiari malformations. *Neurological Sciences, 32*(S3), 283–286. doi:10.1007/s10072-011-0695-0 (https://doi.org/10.1007/s10072-011-0695-0)

Grant, L. A., & Griffin, N. (2018). *Grainger & Allison's diagnostic radiology essentials*. Churchill Livingstone.

Jones J, Sharma R, Gaillard F, et al. Chiari malformations. Reference article, Radiopaedia.org (Accessed on 02 Oct 2023). https://doi.org/10.53347/rID-5781

Osborn, A. G., Hedlund, G. L., & Salzman, K. L. (2018). *Osborn's brain, imaging, pathology, and anatomy* (2nd ed.). Elsevier.

OSCE 85

Awal, S. S. (2023). Arachnoid cysts | Radiology case. In *Radiology vibes*. Retrieved from https://radiologyvibes.com/case-details/1103

Osborn, A. G., & Preece, M. T. (2006). Intracranial cysts: Radiologic-pathologic correlation and imaging approach. *Radiology, 239*(3), 650–664. doi:10.1148/radiol.2393050823 (https://doi.org/10.1148/radiol.2393050823)

OSCE 86

Yuh, E. L., Barkovich, A. J., & Gupta, N. (2009). Imaging of ependymomas: MRI and CT. *Child's Nervous System, 25*(10), 1203–1213. doi:10.1007/s00381-009-0878-7 (https://doi.org/10.1007/s00381-009-0878-7)

OSCE 87

Dahnert, W. F. (2017). *Radiology review manual*. Wolters Kluwer Health. ISBN: 9781496360694.

Grant, L. A., & Griffin, N. (2018). *Grainger & Allison's diagnostic radiology essentials*. Churchill Livingstone.

Suroyo, I., & Budianto, T. (2020). The role of diagnostic and interventional radiology in juvenile nasopharyngeal angiofibroma: A case report and literature review. *Radiology Case Reports, 15*(7), 812–815.

OSCE 88

Awal, S. S. (2023). Fahr disease. *Radiology vibes | Online learning platform for radiologists*. Retrieved from https://radiologyvibes.com/case-details/1090

Govindarajan, A. (2013, November 27). Imaging in Fahr's disease: How CT and MRI differ? *BMJ Case Reports, 2013*(1), bcr2013201523-bcr2013201523. doi:10.1136/bcr-2013-201523 (https://doi.org/10.1136/bcr-2013-201523)

OSCE 89

Chapman & Nakielny's aids to radiological differential diagnosis – 9780702075391 | Elsevier Health. (n.d.). Elsevier UK. https://www.uk.elsevierhealth.com/chapman-nakielnys-aids-to-radiological-differential-diagnosis-9780702075391.html

Hansford, B. G., Albert, D., & Yang, E. (2013). Classic neuroimaging findings of nonketotic hyperglycemia on computed tomography and magnetic resonance imaging with absence of typical movement disorder symptoms (hemichorea-hemiballism). *Journal of Radiology Case Reports, 7*(8). doi:10.3941/jrcr.v7i8.1470 (https://doi.org/10.3941/jrcr.v7i8.1470)

OSCE 90

Grant, L. A., & Griffin, N. (2018). *Grainger & Allison's diagnostic radiology essentials*. Churchill Livingstone.

Osborn, A. G., Hedlund, G. L., & Salzman, K. L. (2017). *Osborn's brain*. Elsevier.

OSCE 91

Hallinan, J. T. P. D., Pillay, P., Koh, L. H. L., Goh, K. Y., & Yu, W.-Y. (2016). Eye globe abnormalities on MR and CT in adults: An anatomical approach. *Korean Journal of Radiology, 17*(5), 664. doi:10.3348/kjr.2016.17.5.664 (https://doi.org/10.3348/kjr.2016.17.5.664)

Lane, J. I., Watson, R. E., Witte, R. J., & McCannel, C. A. (2003). Retinal detachment: Imaging of surgical treatments and complications. *RadioGraphics, 23*(4), 983–994. https://doi.org/10.1148/rg.234025163

OSCE 92

Badve, C. A., Mallikarjunappa, M. K., Iyer, R. S., Ishak, G. E., & Khanna, P. C. (2013, June). Craniosynostosis: Imaging review and primer on computed tomography. *Pediatric Radiology, 43*(6),728–742; quiz 725-7. https://doi.org/10.1007/s00247-013-2673-6. Epub 2013 May 2. (PMID: 23636536).

Kim, H. J., Roh, H. G., & Lee, I. W. (2016, May). Craniosynostosis: Updates in radiologic diagnosis. *Journal of Korean Neurosurgical Society, 59*(3), 219–226. https://doi.org/10.3340/jkns.2016.59.3.219. Epub 2016 May 10. PMCID: PMC4877543. (PMID: 27226852)

OSCE 93

Matlung, S. E., Bilo, R. A. C., Kubat, B., & van Rijn, R. R. (2011). Multicystic encephalomalacia as an end-stage finding in abusive head trauma. *Forensic Science, Medicine and Pathology, 7*, 355–363. https://doi.org/10.1007/s12024-011-9236-7

Naidich, T. P., & Chakera, T. M. (1984, August). Multicystic encephalomalacia: CT appearance and pathological correlation. *Journal of Computer Assisted Tomography, 8*(4), 631–636. PMID: 6736360.

OSCE 94

Michel, S. J. (2004). The Mount Fuji sign. *Radiology, 232*(2), 449–450. doi:10.1148/radiol.2322021556 (https://doi.org/10.1148/radiol.2322021556)

Pillai, P., Sharma, R., MacKenzie, L., Reilly, E. F., Beery, P. R., 2nd, Papadimos, T. J., & Stawicki, S. P. (2017, January–March). Traumatic tension pneumocephalus – two cases and comprehensive review of literature. *International Journal of Critical Illness and Injury Science, 7*(1), 58–64. https://doi.org/10.4103/IJCIIS.IJCIIS_8_17. PMID: 28382259; PMCID: PMC5364769.

OSCE 95

Grant, L. A., & Griffin, N. (2018). *Grainger & Allison's diagnostic radiology essentials*. Churchill Livingstone.

Zaleska-Dorobisz, U., Bladowska, J., Biel, A., Pałka, L. W., & Hołownia, D. (2010, April). MRI diagnosis of diastematomyelia in a 78-year-old woman: Case report and literature review. *Polish Journal of Radiology, 75*(2), 82–87. PMID: 22802781; PMCID: PMC3389875.

OSCE 96

Hacein-Bey, L., & Provenzale, J. M. (2011). Current imaging assessment and treatment of intracranial aneurysms. *American Journal of Roentgenology*, (1), 32–44. doi:10.2214/AJR.10.5329 (https://doi.org/10.2214/AJR.10.5329)

Stafa, A., & Leonardi, M. (2008). Role of neuroradiology in evaluating cerebral aneurysms. *Interventional Neuroradiology*, *14*(1_suppl), 23–37. doi:10.1177/15910199080140S106 (https://doi.org/10.1177/15910199080140S106)

Tomandl, B. F., Köstner, N. C., Schempershofe, M., Huk, W. J., Strauss, C., Anker, L., & Hastreiter, P. (2004). CT angiography of intracranial aneurysms: A focus on postprocessing. *RadioGraphics*, *24*(3), 637–655. doi:10.1148/rg.243035126 (https://doi.org/10.1148/rg.243035126)

OSCE 97

Gaillard, F., Ranchod, A., Picker, B., et al. Subarachnoid haemorrhage. Reference article, Radiopaedia.org (Accessed on 16 Sep 2023). https://doi.org/10.53347/rID-2119

Khatri, G. D., Sarikaya, B., Cross, N. M., & Medverd, J. R. (2021). The role of imaging in the management of non-traumatic subarachnoid hemorrhage: A practical review. *Emergency Radiology*, *28*(4), 797–808. doi:10.1007/s10140-021-01900-x (https://doi.org/10.1007/s10140-021-01900-x)

Marcolini, E., & Hine, J. (2019). Approach to the diagnosis and management of subarachnoid hemorrhage. *Western Journal of Emergency Medicine*, *20*(2), 203–211. doi:10.5811/westjem.2019.1.37352 (https://doi.org/10.5811/westjem.2019.1.37352)

OSCE 98

Kanekar, S. G., Zacharia, T., & Roller, R. (2012). Imaging of stroke: Part 2, Pathophysiology at the molecular and cellular levels and corresponding imaging changes. *American Journal of Roentgenology*, *198*(1), 63–74. doi:10.2214/AJR.10.7312 (https://doi.org/10.2214/AJR.10.7312)

Murphy, A., Baba, Y., Kube, J., et al. Windowing (CT). Reference article, Radiopaedia.org (Accessed on 19 Oct 2023). https://doi.org/10.53347/rID-52108

Osborn, A. G., Hedlund, G. L., & Salzman, K. L. (2018). *Osborn's brain, imaging, pathology, and anatomy* (2nd ed.). Elsevier.

Petitti, N. (1998). The hyperdense middle cerebral artery sign. *Radiology*, *208*, 687–688.

OSCE 99

Jeng, Y., Chen, D. Y.-T., Hsu, H.-L., Huang, Y.-L., Chen, C.-J., & Tseng, Y.-C. (2015). Spinal dural arteriovenous fistula: Imaging features and its mimics. *Korean Journal of Radiology*, *16*(5), 1119. doi:10.3348/kjr.2015.16.5.1119 (https://doi.org/10.3348/kjr.2015.16.5.1119)

OSCE 100

Nadgir, R. (2016, May 15). *Neuroradiology: The requisites* (4th ed.). Elsevier. https://shop.elsevier.com/books/neuroradiology-the-requisites/nadgir/978-1-4557-7568-2

Osborn, A. G., Hedlund, G. L., Salzman, K. L. (2018). *Osborn's brain, imaging, pathology, and anatomy* (2nd ed.). Elsevier.

Payne, W. N. (2023, May 22). *Contrecoup brain injury*. StatPearls – NCBI Bookshelf. https://www.ncbi.nlm.nih.gov/books/NBK536965/

OSCE 101

Awal, S. S. (2022). Thyroglossal duct cyst | Radiology case. *Radiology vibes*. Retrieved from https://radiologyvibes.com/case-details/84

Grant, L. A., & Griffin, N. (2018). *Grainger & Allison's diagnostic radiology essentials*. Churchill Livingstone.

OSCE 102

Nadgir, R. (2016, May 15). *Neuroradiology: The requisites* (4th ed.). Elsevier. https://shop.elsevier.com/books/neuroradiology-the-requisites/nadgir/978-1-4557-7568-2

Osborn, A. G., Hedlund, G. L., & Salzman, K. L. (2018) *Osborn's brain, imaging, pathology, and anatomy* (2nd ed.). Elsevier.

Shirley, M. D., Tang, H., Gallione, C. J., Baugher, J. D., Frelin, L. P., Cohen, B. A., North, P. E., Marchuk, D. A., Comi, A. M., & Pevsner, J. (2013). Sturge–Weber syndrome and port-wine stains caused by somatic mutation in GNAQ. *The New England Journal of Medicine*, *368*(21), 1971–1979. https://doi.org/10.1056/nejmoa1213507

OSCE 103

Manoukian, S. B., & Kowal, D. J. (2015). Comprehensive imaging manifestations of tuberous sclerosis. *American Journal of Roentgenology*, *204*(5), 933–943. https://doi.org/10.2214/ajr.13.12235

Marcinowski F, Atkinson H, Rasuli B, et al. Tuberous sclerosis. Reference article, Radiopaedia.org (Accessed on 30 Oct 2023). https://doi.org/10.53347/rID-2224

Wang, M. X., Segaran, N., Bhalla, S., Pickhardt, P. J., Lubner, M. G., Katabathina, V. S., & Ganeshan, D. (2021). Tuberous sclerosis: Current update. *RadioGraphics*, *41*(7), 1992–2010. https://doi.org/10.1148/rg.2021210103

OSCE 104

Jones, J., El-Feky, M., Bickle, I., et al. Hydranencephaly. Reference article, Radiopaedia.org (Accessed on 30 Oct 2023). https://doi.org/10.53347/rID-8187

Nadgir, R. (2016, May 15). *Neuroradiology: The requisites* (4th ed.). Elsevier. https://shop.elsevier.com/books/neuroradiology-the-requisites/nadgir/978-1-4557-7568-2

Osborn, A. G., Hedlund, G. L., & Salzman, K. L. (2018). *Osborn's brain, imaging, pathology, and anatomy* (2nd ed.). Elsevier.

OSCE 105

The Radiology Assistant: Neonatal Brain US. (2006, April 1). https://radiologyassistant.nl/pediatrics/spine/neonatal-brain-us

Dahnert, W. F. (2017). *Radiology review manual*. Wolters Kluwer Health. ISBN: 9781496360694.

OSCE 106

Araujo-Castro, M., Cancela, A. A., Vior, C., Pascual-Corrales, E., & Berrocal, V. R. (2022). Radiological KNOSP, Revised-KNOSP, and Hardy–Wilson Classifications for the prediction of surgical outcomes in the endoscopic endonasal surgery of pituitary adenomas: study of 228 cases. *Frontiers in Oncology, 11*. https://doi.org/10.3389/fonc.2021.807040

Osborn, A. G., Hedlund, G. L., & Salzman, K. L. (2018). *Osborn's brain, imaging, pathology, and anatomy* (2nd ed.). Elsevier.

Shih, R., Schroeder, J. W., & Koeller, K. K. (2021). Primary tumors of the pituitary gland: Radiologic-pathologic correlation. *RadioGraphics*, *41*(7), 2029–2046. https://doi.org/10.1148/rg.2021200203

Weerakkody Y, Knipe H, Yap J, et al. Pituitary macroadenoma. Reference article, Radiopaedia.org. https://doi.org/10.53347/rID-9801

OSCE 107

Dahnert, W. F. (2017). *Radiology review manual*. Wolters Kluwer Health. ISBN: 9781496360694.

Grant, L. A., & Griffin, N. (2018). *Grainger & Allison's diagnostic radiology essentials*. Churchill Livingstone.

Rumack, C. M., & Levine, D. (2023). *Diagnostic ultrasound, 2-volume set*. Elsevier.

Sun, E. X., Shi, J., & Mandell, J. (2021). *Core radiology: A visual approach to diagnostic imaging*. https://www.amazon.co.uk/Core-Radiology-Approach-Diagnostic-Imaging/dp/1108965911

OSCE 108

Kiverniti, E. (2008, March 1). Küttner's tumour: An unusual cause of salivary gland enlargement. *PubMed Central (PMC)*. https://www.ncbi.nlm.nih.gov/pmc/articles/PMC2532958/

Weerakkody, Y., Hartung, M., Lee, S., et al. Sialadenitis. Reference article, Radiopaedia.org (Accessed on 31 Oct 2023). https://doi.org/10.53347/rID-19998

OSCE 109

Chung, J. H., Cox, C. W., Montner, S. M., Adegunsoye, A., Oldham, J. M., Husain, A. N., Vij, R., Noth, I., Lynch, D. A., & Strek, M. E. (2018). CT features of the usual interstitial pneumonia pattern: Differentiating connective tissue disease-associated interstitial lung disease from idiopathic pulmonary fibrosis. *American Journal of Roentgenology, 210*(2), 307–313. https://doi.org/10.2214/ajr.17.18384

Mueller-Mang, C., Grosse, C., Schmid, K., Stiebellehner, L., & Bankier, A. A. (2007). What every radiologist should know about idiopathic interstitial pneumonias. *RadioGraphics, 27*(3), 595–615. https://doi.org/10.1148/rg.273065130

OSCE 110

Franquet, T., Müller, N. L., Giménez, A., Guembe, P., de la Torre, J., & Bagué, S. (2001). Spectrum of pulmonary aspergillosis: Histologic, clinical, and radiologic findings. *RadioGraphics, 21*(4), 825–837. doi:10.1148/radiographics.21.4.g01jl03825 (https://doi.org/10.1148/radiographics.21.4.g01jl03825)

Grant, L. A., & Griffin, N. (2018). *Grainger & Allison's diagnostic radiology essentials e-book*. Elsevier Health Sciences.

Panse, P. M., Smith, M. L., Cummings, K. W., Jensen, E. A., Gotway, M. B., & Jokerst, C. (2016). The many faces of pulmonary aspergillosis: Imaging findings with pathologic correlation. *Radiology of Infectious Diseases, 3*(4), 192–200. https://doi.org/10.1016/j.jrid.2016.10.002

OSCE 111

Bruzzi, J. F., Komaki, R., Walsh, G. L., Truong, M. T., Gladish, G. W., Munden, R. F., & Erasmus, J. J. (2008). Imaging of non–small cell lung cancer of the superior sulcus. *RadioGraphics, 28*(2), 551–560. doi:10.1148/rg.282075709 (https://doi.org/10.1148/rg.282075709)

Gaillard, F., Sharma, R., Bickle, I., et al. Pancoast tumour. Reference article, Radiopaedia.org (Accessed on 15 Aug 2023). https://doi.org/10.53347/rID-1829

Marulli, G., Battistella, L., Mammana, M., Calabrese, F., & Rea, F. (2016, June). Superior sulcus tumors (Pancoast tumors). *Annals of Translational Medicine, 4*(12), 239. https://doi.org/10.21037/atm.2016.06.16. PMID: 27429965; PMCID: PMC4930518.

OSCE 112

Grant, L. A., & Griffin, N. (2018). *Grainger & Allison's diagnostic radiology essentials e-book*. Elsevier Health Sciences.

Hassan, M., Asciak, R., Rizk, R., Shaarawy, H., Gleeson, F. V., & Rahman, N. M. (2018). Lung abscess or empyema? Taking a closer look. *Thorax, 73*(9), 887–889. doi:10.1136/thoraxjnl-2018-211604 (https://doi.org/10.1136/thoraxjnl-2018-211604)

Stark, D. D., Federle, M., Goodman, P. C., Podrasky, A. E., & Webb, W. R. (1983). Differentiating lung abscess and empyema: Radiography and computed tomography. *American Journal of Roentgenology, 141*(1), 163–167. https://doi.org/10.2214/ajr.141.1.163

OSCE 113

Jeong, Y. J., & Lee, K. S. (2008). Pulmonary tuberculosis: Up-to-date imaging and management. *American Journal of Roentgenology, 191*(3), 834–844. https://doi.org/10.2214/ajr.07.3896

Nachiappan, A. C., Rahbar, K., Shi, X., Guy, E., Barbosa, E. J. M., Shroff, G. S., Ocazionez, D., Schlesinger, A. E., Katz, S. I., & Hammer, M. M. (2017). Pulmonary tuberculosis: Role of radiology in diagnosis and management. *RadioGraphics*, 37(1), 52–72. https://doi.org/10.1148/rg.2017160032

Vohra, S. (2023, April 15). *Miliary tuberculosis*. StatPearls – NCBI Bookshelf. https://www.ncbi.nlm.nih.gov/books/NBK562300/

OSCE 114

Da Silva Gomes, M. R., Alves, M., Correia, J. B., & Santos, L. (2013). Empyema necessitans: Very late complication of pulmonary tuberculosis. *Case Reports*. https://doi.org/10.1136/bcr-2013-202072

Grant, L. A., & Griffin, N. (2018). *Grainger & Allison's diagnostic radiology essentials e-book*. Elsevier Health Sciences.

Kraus, G. J. (2007). The split pleura sign. *Radiology, 243*(1), 297–298. https://doi.org/10.1148/radiol.2431041658

Stark, D. D., Federle, M., Goodman, P. C., Podrasky, A. E., & Webb, W. R. (1983). Differentiating lung abscess and empyema: Radiography and computed tomography. *American Journal of Roentgenology, 141*(1), 163–167. https://doi.org/10.2214/ajr.141.1.163

Weerakkody Y, El-Feky M, Anan R, et al. Pleural empyema. Reference article, Radiopaedia.org (Accessed on 17 Aug 2023). https://doi.org/10.53347/rID-7336

OSCE 115

Cantin, L., Bankier, A. A., & Eisenberg, R. L. (2009). Bronchiectasis. *American Journal of Roentgenology, 193*(3), W158–W171. https://doi.org/10.2214/ajr.09.3053

Grant, L. A., & Griffin, N. (2018). *Grainger & Allison's diagnostic radiology essentials e-book*. Elsevier Health Sciences.

Milliron, B., Henry, T. S., Veeraraghavan, S., & Little, B. P. (2015). Bronchiectasis: Mechanisms and imaging clues of associated common and uncommon diseases. *RadioGraphics, 35*(4), 1011–1030. https://doi.org/10.1148/rg.2015140214

OSCE 116

Grant, L. A., & Griffin, N. (2018). *Grainger & Allison's diagnostic radiology essentials e-book*. Elsevier Health Sciences.

Harisinghani, M. G., Chen, J. W., & Weissleder, R. (2018). *Primer of diagnostic imaging*. Elsevier Health Sciences.

OSCE 117

Gaillard, F., El-Feky, M., Rasuli, B., et al. Pulmonary metastases. Reference article, Radiopaedia.org (Accessed on 05 Sep 2023). https://doi.org/10.53347/rID-8854

Tanay Patel, M. (2023, January 30). Lung metastases imaging. Practice essentials, Radiography, Computed tomography. https://emedicine.medscape.com/article/358090-overview

Webb, W. R., & Higgins, C. B. (2017). *Thoracic imaging: Pulmonary and cardiovascular radiology*. Lippincott Williams & Wilkins.

OSCE 118

Grant, L. A., & Griffin, N. (2018). *Grainger & Allison's diagnostic radiology essentials*. Churchill Livingstone.

Weerakkody, Y., Baba, Y., Bell, D., et al. Ebstein anomaly. Reference article, Radiopaedia.org. https://doi.org/10.53347/rID-7365

Weerakkody, Y., Mellam, Y., Yap, J., et al. Tetralogy of Fallot. Reference article, Radiopaedia.org. https://doi.org/10.53347/rID-7356
Weissleder, R. (2011). *Primer of diagnostic imaging*. Mosby.

OSCE 119

Frazier, A. A., Franks, T. J., Cooke, E. O., Mohammed, T. H., Pugatch, R. D., & Galvin, J. R. (2008). Pulmonary alveolar proteinosis. *RadioGraphics*, *28*(3), 883–899. https://doi.org/10.1148/rg.283075219
Rossi, S. E., Erasmus, J. J., Volpacchio, M., Franquet, T., Castiglioni, T., & McAdams, H. P. (2003). "Crazy-paving" pattern at thin-section CT of the lungs: Radiologic-pathologic overview. *RadioGraphics*, *23*(6), 1509–1519. https://doi.org/10.1148/rg.236035101

OSCE 120

Grant, L. A., & Griffin, N. (2018). *Grainger & Allison's diagnostic radiology essentials*. Churchill Livingstone.
Webb, W. R., & Higgins, C. B. (2017). *Thoracic imaging: Pulmonary and cardiovascular radiology*. Lippincott Williams & Wilkins.

OSCE 121

Aslam, A., De Luis Cardenas, J., Morrison, R., Lagisetty, K. H., Litmanovich, D., Sella, E., Lee, E. M., & Agarwal, P. P. (2022). Tracheobronchomalacia and excessive dynamic airway collapse: current concepts and future directions. *RadioGraphics*, *42*(4), 1012–1027. https://doi.org/10.1148/rg.210155
Maller, V., Saber, M., Plessis, V., et al. Tracheomalacia (differential). Reference article, Radiopaedia.org. https://doi.org/10.53347/rID-4999

OSCE 122

Bonde, A., Singh, R., Prasad, S. R., Kamireddy, D., Aggarwal, A., Ramani, N. S., Saboo, S. S., Shanbhogue, K., Dasyam, A. K., & Katabathina, V. S. (2023). Mesotheliomas and benign mesothelial tumors: Update on pathologic and imaging findings. *RadioGraphics*, *43*(3). https://doi.org/10.1148/rg.220128
Wang, Z. J., Reddy, G. P., Gotway, M. B., Higgins, C. B., Jablons, D. M., Ramaswamy, M., Hawkins, R. A., & Webb, W. R. (2004). Malignant pleural mesothelioma: Evaluation with CT, MR imaging, and PET. *RadioGraphics*, *24*(1), 105–119. https://doi.org/10.1148/rg.241035058
Webb, W. R., & Higgins, C. B. (2017). *Thoracic imaging: Pulmonary and cardiovascular radiology*. Lippincott Williams & Wilkins.

OSCE 123

Gaillard, F., Weerakkody, Y., El-Feky, M., et al. Eggshell calcification (lymph nodes). Reference article, Radiopaedia.org. https://doi.org/10.53347/rID-1262
Grant, L. A., & Griffin, N. (2018). *Grainger & Allison's diagnostic radiology essentials*. Churchill Livingstone.
Lanzafame, M., & Vento, S. (2021). Mini-review: Silico-tuberculosis. *Journal of Clinical Tuberculosis and Other Mycobacterial Diseases*, *23*, 100218. https://doi.org/10.1016/j.jctube.2021.100218
Sarı, G., Gokcek, A., Koyuncu, A., & Şimşek, C. (2022). Computed tomography findings in progressive massive fibrosis: Analyses of 90 cases. *PubMed*, *113*(1), e2022002. https://doi.org/10.23749/mdl.v113i1.12303

OSCE 124

Croake, A., & Croake, M. F. (2019). Subcutaneous emphysema. In *Springer eBooks* (pp. 147–149). https://doi.org/10.1007/978-3-030-26044-6_41
Grant, L. A., & Griffin, N. (2018). *Grainger & Allison's diagnostic radiology essentials*. Churchill Livingstone.
Kukuruza, K. (2023, July 17). *Subcutaneous emphysema*. StatPearls - NCBI Bookshelf. https://www.ncbi.nlm.nih.gov/books/NBK542192/
Yamaguchi, S., Takeda, M., Takahashi, T., Yamahata, H., Mitsuhara, T., Niiro, T., Hanakita, J., Hida, K., Arita, K., & Kurisu, K. (2015). Ginkgo leaf sign: A highly predictive imaging feature of spinal meningioma. *Journal of Neurosurgery*, *23*(5), 642–646. https://doi.org/10.3171/2015.3.spine1598

OSCE 125

Ali, S., Kaplan, S. L., Kaufman, T., Fenerty, S., Kozin, S. H., & Zlotolow, D. A. (2015). Madelung deformity and Madelung-type deformities: A review of the clinical and radiological characteristics. *Pediatric Radiology*, *45*(12), 1856–1863. https://doi.org/10.1007/s00247-015-3390-0
Di Muzio, B., Baba, Y., Botros, S., et al. Madelung disease. Reference article, Radiopaedia.org. https://doi.org/10.53347/rID-12161
Finsterer, J., & Scorza, F. A. (2021). Mediastinal and pleural lipomatosis as a manifestation of myotonic dystrophy type 1. *Lung India*. https://doi.org/10.4103/lungindia.lungindia_25_21
Quynguyên, K., Hoeffel, C., Lê, L. H., & Phan, H. T. (1998). Mediastinal lipomatosis. *Southern Medical Journal*, *91*(12), 1169–1172. https://doi.org/10.1097/00007611-199812000-00016

OSCE 126

Grant, L. A., & Griffin, N. (2018). *Grainger & Allison's diagnostic radiology essentials*. Churchill Livingstone.
Mullins, M. E., Stein, J. A., Saini, S. S., & Mueller, P. R. (2001). Prevalence of incidental Bochdalek's hernia in a large adult population. *American Journal of Roentgenology*, *177*(2), 363–366. https://doi.org/10.2214/ajr.177.2.1770363

OSCE 127

Brauner, E., Lapidot, M., Kremer, R., Best, L., & Kluger, Y. (2011) Aberrant right subclavian artery - suggested mechanism for esophageal foreign body impaction: Case report. *World Journal of Emergency Surgery*, *6*(1), 12. https://doi.org/10.1186/1749-7922-6-12
Evens, A., et al. (2019, July–August). Pediatric vascular rings and slings *Applied Radiology*, *48*(4), 26+. *Gale Academic OneFile*. https://appliedradiology.com/articles/pediatric-vascular-rings-and-slings. Accessed 31 Oct. 2023.
Hanneman, K., Newman, B., & Chan, F. P. (2017). Congenital variants and anomalies of the aortic arch. *RadioGraphics*, *37*(1), 32–51. https://doi.org/10.1148/rg.2017160033
Robb, C. L., Bhalla, S., & Raptis, C. A. (2022). Subclavian artery: Anatomic review and imaging evaluation of abnormalities. *RadioGraphics*, *42*(7), 2149–2165. https://doi.org/10.1148/rg.220064

OSCE 128

Castañer, E., Gallardo, X., Ballesteros, E., Andreu, M., Pallardó, Y., Mata, J. M., & Riera, L. (2009). CT diagnosis of chronic pulmonary thromboembolism. *RadioGraphics*, *29*(1), 31–50. doi:10.1148/rg.291085061 (https://doi.org/10.1148/rg.291085061)
D'Souza, D., Hacking, C., Weerakkody, Y., et al. Pulmonary embolism. Reference article, Radiopaedia.org. https://doi.org/10.53347/rID-1937
Grant, L. A., & Griffin, N. (2018). *Grainger & Allison's diagnostic radiology essentials e-book*. Elsevier Health Sciences.
Lin, E. (2008). *Practical differential diagnosis for CT and MRI*. Thieme.

OSCE 129

Gaillard, F., Weerakkody, Y., Baba, Y., et al. Bronchiectasis. Reference article, Radiopaedia.org. https://doi.org/10.53347/rID-1021

Kennedy, M. P., Noone, P. G., Leigh, M. W., Zariwala, M. A., Minnix, S. L., Knowles, M. R., & Molina, P. L. (2007). High-resolution CT of patients with primary ciliary dyskinesia. *American Journal of Roentgenology, 188*(5), 1232–1238. https://doi.org/10.2214/ajr.06.0965

Wahba, M., Baba, Y., Bickle, I., et al. Kartagener syndrome. Reference article, Radiopaedia.org. https://doi.org/10.53347/rID-6892

OSCE 130

Agrawal, R. et al. Pulmonary sequestration. Reference article, Radiopaedia.org. https://radiopaedia.org/articles/pulmonary-sequestration?lang=gb

Felker, R. E., & Tonkin, I. L. (1990). Imaging of pulmonary sequestration. *American Journal of Roentgenology, 154*(2), 241–249. https://doi.org/10.2214/ajr.154.2.2105007

Grant, L. A., & Griffin, N. (2018). *Grainger & Allison's diagnostic radiology essentials e-book*. Elsevier Health Sciences.

Webb, W. R., & Higgins, C. B. (2017). *Thoracic imaging: Pulmonary and cardiovascular radiology*. Lippincott Williams & Wilkins.

OSCE INDEX

INDEX